Exploring the Role of Social Media in Health Promotion

Exploring the Role of Social Media in Health Promotion

Special Issue Editors

Michael Stellefson
J. Don Chaney
Beth H. Chaney
Samantha R. Paige

MDPI • Basel • Beijing • Wuhan • Barcelona • Belgrade • Manchester • Tokyo • Cluj • Tianjin

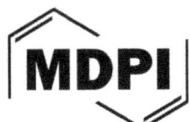

Special Issue Editors

Michael Stellefson
East Carolina University
USA

J. Don Chaney
East Carolina University
USA

Beth H. Chaney
East Carolina University
USA

Samantha R. Paige
University of Florida
USA

Editorial Office
MDPI
St. Alban-Anlage 66
4052 Basel, Switzerland

This is a reprint of articles from the Special Issue published online in the open access journal *International Journal of Environmental Research and Public Health* (ISSN 1660-4601) (available at: https://www.mdpi.com/journal/ijerph/special_issues/media_health).

For citation purposes, cite each article independently as indicated on the article page online and as indicated below:

LastName, A.A.; LastName, B.B.; LastName, C.C. Article Title. *Journal Name* **Year**, *Article Number*, Page Range.

ISBN 978-3-03936-328-5 (Pbk)
ISBN 978-3-03936-329-2 (PDF)

© 2020 by the authors. Articles in this book are Open Access and distributed under the Creative Commons Attribution (CC BY) license, which allows users to download, copy and build upon published articles, as long as the author and publisher are properly credited, which ensures maximum dissemination and a wider impact of our publications.

The book as a whole is distributed by MDPI under the terms and conditions of the Creative Commons license CC BY-NC-ND.

Contents

About the Special Issue Editors vii

Michael Stellefson, Samantha R. Paige, Beth H. Chaney and J. Don Chaney
Social Media and Health Promotion
Reprinted from: *Int. J. Environ. Res. Public Health* **2020**, *17*, 3323, doi:10.3390/ijerph17093323 . . . 1

Dongxiao Gu, Jingjing Guo, Changyong Liang, Wenxing Lu, Shuping Zhao, Bing Liu and Tianyue Long
Social Media-Based Health Management Systems and Sustained Health Engagement: TPB Perspective
Reprinted from: *Int. J. Environ. Res. Public Health* **2019**, *16*, 1495, doi:10.3390/ijerph16091495 . . . 7

Trevor Bopp, Joshua D. Vadeboncoeur, Michael Stellefson and Melissa Weinsz
Moving Beyond the Gym: A Content Analysis of YouTube as an Information Resource for Physical Literacy
Reprinted from: *Int. J. Environ. Res. Public Health* **2019**, *16*, 3335, doi:10.3390/ijerph16183335 . . . 23

Ming-Yan Wang, Peng-Zhu Zhang, Cheng-Yang Zhou and Neng-Ye Lai
Effect of Emotion, Expectation, and Privacy on Purchase Intention in WeChat Health Product Consumption: The Mediating Role of Trust
Reprinted from: *Int. J. Environ. Res. Public Health* **2019**, *16*, 3861, doi:10.3390/ijerph16203861 . . 41

Yuehua Zhao, Jin Zhang and Min Wu
Finding Users' Voice on Social Media: An Investigation of Online Support Groups for Autism-Affected Users on Facebook
Reprinted from: *Int. J. Environ. Res. Public Health* **2019**, *16*, 4804, doi:10.3390/ijerph16234804 . . 61

Avery Apperson, Michael Stellefson, Samantha R. Paige, Beth H. Chaney, J. Don Chaney, Min Qi Wang and Arjun Mohan
Facebook Groups on Chronic Obstructive Pulmonary Disease: Social Media Content Analysis
Reprinted from: *Int. J. Environ. Res. Public Health* **2019**, *16*, 3789, doi:10.3390/ijerph16203789 . . . 75

Chengyan Zhu, Xiaolin Xu, Wei Zhang, Jianmin Chen and Richard Evans
How Health Communication via Tik Tok Makes a Difference: A Content Analysis of Tik Tok Accounts Run by Chinese Provincial Health Committees
Reprinted from: *Int. J. Environ. Res. Public Health* **2020**, *17*, 192, doi:10.3390/ijerph17010192 . . . 93

Samantha R. Paige, Rachel E. Damiani, Elizabeth Flood-Grady, Janice L. Krieger and Michael Stellefson
The Perceived Availability of Online Social Support: Exploring the Contributions of Illness and Rural Identities in Adults with Chronic Respiratory Illness
Reprinted from: *Int. J. Environ. Res. Public Health* **2020**, *17*, 242, doi:10.3390/ijerph17010242 . . . 107

Salvatore Giorgi, David B. Yaden, Johannes C. Eichstaedt, Robert D. Ashford, Anneke E.K. Buffone, H. Andrew Schwartz, Lyle H. Ungar and Brenda Curtis
Cultural Differences in Tweeting about Drinking Across the US
Reprinted from: *Int. J. Environ. Res. Public Health* **2020**, *17*, 1125, doi:10.3390/ijerph17041125 . . 123

Trevor Bopp and Michael Stellefson
Practical and Ethical Considerations for Schools Using Social Media to Promote Physical Literacy in Youth
Reprinted from: *Int. J. Environ. Res. Public Health* **2020**, *17*, 1225, doi:10.3390/ijerph17041225 . . . 137

Nikol Kvardova, Hana Machackova and David Smahel
The Direct and Indirect Effects of Online Social Support, Neuroticism, and Web Content Internalization on the Drive for Thinness among Women Visiting Health-Oriented Websites
Reprinted from: *Int. J. Environ. Res. Public Health* **2020**, *17*, 2416, doi:10.3390/ijerph17072416 . . . **147**

Michael Stellefson, Samantha R. Paige, Beth H. Chaney and J. Don Chaney
Evolving Role of Social Media in Health Promotion: Updated Responsibilities for Health Education Specialists
Reprinted from: *Int. J. Environ. Res. Public Health* **2020**, *17*, 1153, doi:10.3390/ijerph17041153 . . . **161**

About the Special Issue Editors

Michael Stellefson (Associate Professor, Department of Health Education and Promotion, East Carolina University). Dr. Stellefson's research aims to: (1) evaluate web-based educational tools for chronic disease self-management and (2) measure and promote eHealth literacy about chronic diseases and their self-management by patients and their caregivers.

J. Don Chaney is Professor and Chair in the Department of Health Education and Promotion at East Carolina University. Dr. Chaney's research interests primarily include technology applications in health education and promotion, with specific expertise in the area of distance education course delivery.

Beth H. Chaney is an Associate Professor in Health Education and Promotion at East Carolina University. Dr. Chaney's research includes instrument development and evaluation in health education and promotion, and she has worked in the areas of quality assessment of distance education technology, eHealth literacy with chronic disease, and alcohol use/misuse among specific populations.

Samantha R. Paige is a Postdoctoral Research Fellow in the STEM Translational Communication Center at the University of Florida. Dr. Paige's research has a strong focus on the intersection of technology and healthcare communication in decision making among rural, medically underserved populations at risk of and living with chronic illnesses.

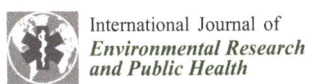 International Journal of *Environmental Research and Public Health*

Editorial

Social Media and Health Promotion

Michael Stellefson [1,*], Samantha R. Paige [2], Beth H. Chaney [1] and J. Don Chaney [1]

[1] Department of Health Education and Promotion, East Carolina University, Greenville, NC 27858, USA; chaneye@ecu.edu (B.H.C.); chaneyd@ecu.edu (J.D.C.)
[2] STEM Translational Communication Center, University of Florida, Gainesville, FL 32611, USA; paigesr190@ufl.edu
* Correspondence: stellefsonm17@ecu.edu

Received: 30 April 2020; Accepted: 7 May 2020; Published: 11 May 2020

With over 3 billion users worldwide, social media has become a staple of daily life for people across the globe. Social media allows virtual network members to quickly cultivate and exchange information and ideas in the form of video, image, text, and multimedia. The success of social media is grounded in its ability to adapt to the dynamic social contexts of its users and evolve with the sophistication of technology. In the health promotion profession, we have recognized the power and success of social media in achieving goals and objectives of public health, including behavioral, organizational, and policy change [1]. However, as health promotion researchers and practitioners, we simply cannot ignore the fact that these powerful tools also present a number of challenges (e.g., managing misinformation) and complications (e.g., ensuring compliance with privacy protections) that may eventually hinder our efforts and become a detriment to public health [2]. Our Special Issue includes a collection of innovative studies to help us better understand these challenges and complications and what they mean for the future of health promotion.

Unique to other special issues related to this topic is our focus on supplementing traditional approaches of health promotion with principles of translational health communication. We present 11 papers that employ theories of both behavior change and social influence to understand how social media is used by diverse audience segments in various health contexts. Strong attention is placed on the social, physical, and geographic factors that facilitate and hinder its use as an effective behavior change and decision-making tool. Perhaps most notable within the issue is its collective focus on using social media as a dissemination tool and ensuring that current and emerging collaborative technologies are appropriate for the audience(s) and message(s). In our opinion, this Special Issue generates a breadth of new knowledge about social media in health promotion, but, most importantly, it harnesses core principles of two interrelated fields (i.e., health promotion and translational health communication) to demonstrate the depth of the challenges and complications we seek to understand and overcome. In the following paragraphs, we provide a brief synopsis of each article, highlighting its contribution to the aims of our Special Issue.

Kvardova, Machackova, and Smahel [3] used the Tripartite Influence Model, a theoretical framework that explains eating disturbances with socio-cultural factors, to expand knowledge about the role of health-related websites in the development of eating disorders. Among young adult women, the drive for thinness was positively correlated with online social support, web content internalization, as well as neuroticism. These findings confirmed what is hypothesized in the Tripartite Influence Model: body image concerns and eating disorders are directly affected by socio-cultural factors (e.g., media pressures, peer criticism) and indirectly through the internalization of the medialized body ideals. The authors acknowledge the potential impact of health-oriented websites on young women and their drive for thinness, especially in the context of the internalization of body appearance standards; likewise, it is suggested that future research consider how social media influencers can be especially protective or detrimental to women's perception of body ideals.

Giorgi and colleagues [4] examined geo-located language in public tweets mentioning the term "drunk" and correlated this language with the prevalence of self-reported excessive alcohol consumption as reported in the United States (U.S.) Behavioral Risk Factor Surveillance System. Linguistic markers associated with excessive drinking were subsequently identified in different regions and cultural communities as identified by the American Community Project. The frequency with which people tweeted the word "drunk" (as a percentage of all tweets) was moderately correlated with excess drinking at both the county and state level. Of particular note, communities differed both in terms of how much they tweet about drinking and how they tweet about drinking. Results showed that tweets about being drunk were predictive of different "styles" of excessive drinking behavior across many types of communities derived from demographic and socio-economic indicators. The particular words, phrases, and linguistic themes associated with alcohol abuse within particular regions and communities can provide insight into sociocultural alcohol use and may help to shape targeted public health messages that recognize the cultural determinants of alcohol use and abuse.

Recognizing that Provincial Health Committees (PHCs) in China have started to adopt the microvideo sharing platform, Tik Tok, to engage with local residents and communicate health-related information, Zhu and colleagues [5] examined 31 verified PHC Tik Tok accounts. Findings suggested that in provinces with greater economic prosperity, local health departments delivered better quality health education to provinces with citizens more likely to have a higher level of health literacy than to provinces with low economic prosperity. The top 100 most liked health communication microvideos were mainly from six PHCs. With the growing number of Tik Tok users, especially among young individuals, the authors suggest that PHCs should continue to refine use of Tik Tok to grow engagement levels with all citizens. Most notably, the authors recommend that use of Tik Tok become part of each PHC's social media ecosystem that functions to communicate health information to citizens on a more personal level.

Through Natural Language Processing methods, Zhao, Zhang, and Wu [6] investigated five Facebook-based autism support groups. An interactive visualization method (i.e., pyLDAvis) was employed to visualize intertopic distance maps that explored how group members shared information and interacted with one another. In doing so, topics that autism-affected users were most concerned with emerged, along with how these issues were addressed on Facebook. By studying these support groups using text mining and data visualization, researchers were able to gather data on issues that individuals living with autism were concerned about (e.g., parenting, education, and behavior traits). Healthcare professionals can reference this social media data to enhance communication with their patients and informal caregivers. Findings from this study showed that latent Dirichlet allocation is feasible to use when attempting to determine important support topics posted on Facebook autism support groups.

Using the theories of reasoned action and expectancy confirmation, Wang, Zhang, Zhou, and Lai [7] analyzed the effects of cognitive factors on WeChat users' health product purchase intentions. In this study, social media services had a higher penetration rate among younger user groups. Trust experienced by customers fully mediated the relationship between emotional price and purchase intention among WeChat users. However, there was no evidence that trust played a mediating role between emotional products and purchase intention. Results indicated that social media has gradually formed an important environment conducive to health communication. However, in order for the public to benefit from such an environment, health service providers must seek to resolve issues related to public mistrust and misinformation on social media.

Trust in online resources also contributes to an individual's willingness to participate in online support groups found on social media. Through social media content analysis, Apperson and colleagues [8] examined Chronic Obstructive Pulmonary Disease (COPD) self-management information shared within Facebook groups dedicated to the condition. Findings suggested that the purpose of most COPD Facebook groups was to provide support (19/26, 73.1%), while the remaining groups (7/26, 26.9%) built awareness or shared health information. The findings from this study show that members of these Facebook groups shared various experiences managing COPD. Medications, for example, were the most addressed self-management topic on the COPD Facebook groups, while engagement, in the form of "likes", were highest for posts that demonstrated some form of social support. Overall, the study showed that COPD Facebook group members search for information regarding specific self-management topics and also share their disease-related experiences on the platform. Therefore, use of the social media platform has potential for providing emotional and informational support to users living with COPD.

Furthering this work, Paige and colleagues [9] drew from social identity theory to examine how communal COPD illness and rural identities influence the degree that a person feels they have online health-related support available to them, should they need it. A survey of social media and clinic-based cohorts demonstrated that socio-demographics, specifically low income and high education, were associated with communal COPD illness identity; however, illness-related experiences (i.e., receiving a physician diagnosis of COPD, identifying as a current/recent smoker) and reporting more severe respiratory symptoms explained the greatest amount of variance in shaping this identity. As expected, a COPD diagnosis and identifying with other patients who live with the condition was associated with a greater degree of available online social support. Interestingly, rural identity moderated the effect of COPD illness identity (and not a COPD diagnosis) on the perceived availability of online social support. This study demonstrates that determining whether social media is the right health promotion tool for a person extends beyond their diagnostic status; rather, there is a need to consider the role of social identities in determining whether social media is an acceptable health promotion and decision-making tool for behavior change.

With the rapid increase of mobile internet and the emerging popularity of social networks, Gu and colleagues [10] surveyed adults in East China about their use of social media-based health management systems (SocialHMS). These health management systems have been extensively used in patient decision making, chronic disease management, and health information inquiries. One of the great benefits of using SocialHMS is that it provides a convenient method for people to obtain health services. The study explored factors influencing sustained health engagement of SocialHMS while utilizing the theoretical underpinnings of the Theory of Planned Behavior, the big-five theory, and trust theory. Results provided a holistic understanding of the sustained use of SocialHMS both by users and researchers in the context of information systems and healthcare. The authors suggest that social media developers can improve SocialHMS based on individual openness to experience and by matching users to tailored health content based on their respective personality characteristics.

Bopp and colleagues [11] reported on the content, exposure, engagement, and information quality of uploaded physical literacy videos found on YouTube. Over half of the videos demonstrated the concept of physical literacy through unstructured play, otherwise known as "free play". However, less than half of the videos were deemed to be of high quality according to HONCode guidelines for trustworthy online health information. Videos focusing on physical activity and behaviors had higher overall quality ratings, followed closely by videos addressing affective domains, such as motivation, confidence, and self-esteem. Moreover, the authors assessed the content delivery method and quality. Content and content delivery method were the most significant factors impacting the quality evaluation. Videos that focused on physical activity behaviors had the strongest indication of high-quality ratings, followed by videos covering affective domains of physical literacy. Findings support that YouTube has the potential to enhance video resources; virtual networking opportunities; as well as the sharing, dissemination, accumulation, and enrichment of physical literacy information, especially for youth.

Given the increased use of social media in schools, Bopp and Stellefson [12] provide a critical commentary about challenges and opportunities for using social media to improve physical literacy among youth. Based on the positive relationship between increased physical activity and positive health outcomes, best practices of social media use in the healthcare industry are described for physical educators practicing in schools. Opportunities are discussed for using the ALL-ENGAGE model as a framework for facilitating youth engagement about physical literacy on social media. The authors describe how school administrators should engage with physical educators and the public to address physical activity and misconceptions or misinformation about physical literacy on social media. For example, educators and school systems are encouraged to locate and use social media tools to aid them in enhancing physical literacy among students. Extending upon this recommendation, our commentary, by Stellefson, Paige, Chaney, and Chaney [13], argues that professionals who deliver health education, such as those in public health and school systems, need to be wary of designing and sharing social media interventions or campaigns that are most suited to population segments that are text-, tech- and eHealth-literate. To provide explicit guidance based on our recommendations, we present communication and advocacy roles and responsibilities of health education specialists in the context of social media research and practice.

The global expansion of social media has resulted in various platforms transforming into promising avenues for the delivery of health promotion messages, self-management education, and interventions. This Special Issue highlights the versatility and flexibility of social media, in that it can be used effectively with a variety of health promotion topics and with many populations (i.e., adolescents, adults, and patients living with a chronic illness). In exploring the depth of challenges and complications related to using social media for health promotion, these studies demonstrate the value of theory- and model-driven approaches in understanding factors that have a fundamental effect on how social media can be used and optimized for health promotion. The factors explored in this Special Issue included socio-cultural identity, trust in online resources, and literacy levels, among others. Of particular note, is that the results of these studies draw our attention to considering a triad of factors associated with health promotion on social media, including what information is exchanged, how it is communicated, and by whom is it delivered and received. As we consider the potential fit of social media for a particular audience or disease context, we must weigh these factors in addition to the affordances of various online health promotion programs.

Furthermore, these eleven papers present new opportunities for the development of future social media interventions and analyses. While we believe that researchers and practitioners should tackle these new opportunities head on, it is important to recognize that significant headwinds are likely to come from individuals or entities using social media to promote alternative views on health-related issues or unhealthy behaviors that are not backed by scientific evidence. Therefore, to prevent the spread of health-related misinformation, health education specialists must be vigilant in monitoring and evaluating public health advocacy and communication occurring on social media. The authors in our Special Issue highlight innovative methodologies to efficiently and effectively tackle these endeavors. We firmly believe that results from these studies will expand and build upon traditional health education approaches and improve participative engagement in health promotion through systematic online community building that supports improvements in public health outcomes.

Author Contributions: M.S. outlined and wrote the first draft of the editorial; S.R.P. provided revisions to the first draft and contributed to its concept. B.H.C. provided revisions to the first draft. All authors have read, edited, and agreed to the published version of the manuscript. All authors have read and agreed to the published version of the manuscript.

Funding: This research received no external funding.

Acknowledgments: The authors wish to acknowledge the support of the *IJERPH* staff and the work of the anonymous reviewers.

Conflicts of Interest: The authors declare no conflict of interest.

References

1. Korda, H.; Itani, Z. Harnessing Social Media for Health Promotion and Behavior Change. *Health Promot. Pract.* **2013**, *14*, 15–23. [CrossRef] [PubMed]
2. Conrad, E.; Becker, M.; Powell, B. Improving Health Promotion Through the Integration of Technology, Crowdsourcing and Social Media. *Health Promot. Pract.* **2020**, *21*, 228–237. [CrossRef] [PubMed]

3. Kvardova, N.; Machackova, H.; Smahel, D. The Direct and Indirect Effects of Online Social Support, Neuroticism, and Web Content Internalization on the Drive for Thinness among Women Visiting Health-oriented Websites. *Int. J. Environ. Res. Public Health* **2020**, *17*, 2416. [CrossRef] [PubMed]
4. Giorgi, S.; Yaden, D.B.; Eichstaedt, J.C.; Ashford, R.D.; Buffone, A.E.; Schwartz, H.A.; Ungar, L.H.; Curtis, B. Cultural Differences in Tweeting about Drinking Across the US. *Int. J. Environ. Res. Public Health* **2020**, *17*, 1125. [CrossRef] [PubMed]
5. Paige, S.R.; Damiani, R.E.; Flood-Grady, E.; Krieger, J.L.; Stellefson, M. The Perceived Availability of Online Social Support: Exploring the Contributions of Illness and Rural Identities in Adults with Chronic Respiratory Illness. *Int. J. Environ. Res. Public Health* **2020**, *17*, 242. [CrossRef] [PubMed]
6. Zhu, C.; Xu, X.; Zhang, W.; Chen, J.; Evans, R. How Health Communication via Tik Tok Makes a Difference: A Content Analysis of Tik Tok Accounts Run by Chinese Provincial Health Committees. *Int. J. Environ. Res. Public Health* **2020**, *17*, 192. [CrossRef] [PubMed]
7. Zhao, Y.; Zhang, J.; Wu, M. Finding Users' Voice on Social Media: An Investigation of Online Support Groups for Autism-Affected Users on Facebook. *Int. J. Environ. Res. Public Health* **2019**, *16*, 4804. [CrossRef] [PubMed]
8. Wang, M.-Y.; Zhang, P.-Z.; Zhou, C.-Y.; Lai, N.-Y. Effect of Emotion, Expectation, and Privacy on Purchase Intention in WeChat Health Product Consumption: The Mediating Role of Trust. *Int. J. Environ. Res. Public Health* **2019**, *16*, 3861. [CrossRef] [PubMed]
9. Apperson, A.; Stellefson, M.; Paige, S.R.; Chaney, B.H.; Chaney, J.D.; Wang, M.Q.; Mohan, A. Facebook Groups on Chronic Obstructive Pulmonary Disease: Social Media Content Analysis. *Int. J. Environ. Res. Public Health* **2019**, *16*, 3789. [CrossRef] [PubMed]
10. Gu, D.; Guo, J.; Liang, C.; Lu, W.; Zhao, S.; Liu, B.; Long, T. Social Media-Based Health Management Systems and Sustained Health Engagement: TPB Perspective. *Int. J. Environ. Res. Public Health* **2019**, *16*, 1495. [CrossRef] [PubMed]
11. Bopp, T.; Vadeboncoeur, J.D.; Stellefson, M.; Weinsz, M. Moving Beyond the Gym: A Content Analysis of YouTube as an Information Resource for Physical Literacy. *Int. J. Environ. Res. Public Health* **2019**, *16*, 3335. [CrossRef] [PubMed]
12. Bopp, T.; Stellefson, M. Practical and Ethical Considerations for Schools Using Social Media to Promote Physical Literacy in Youth. *Int. J. Environ. Res. Public Health* **2020**, *17*, 1225. [CrossRef] [PubMed]
13. Stellefson, M.; Paige, S.R.; Chaney, B.H.; Chaney, J.D. Evolving Role of Social Media in Health Promotion: Updated Responsibilities for Health Education Specialists. *Int. J. Environ. Res. Public Health* **2020**, *17*, 1153. [CrossRef] [PubMed]

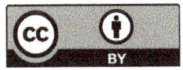

© 2020 by the authors. Licensee MDPI, Basel, Switzerland. This article is an open access article distributed under the terms and conditions of the Creative Commons Attribution (CC BY) license (http://creativecommons.org/licenses/by/4.0/).

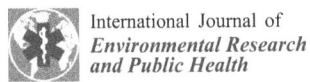

Article

Social Media-Based Health Management Systems and Sustained Health Engagement: TPB Perspective

Dongxiao Gu [1,2,*], Jingjing Guo [1], Changyong Liang [1], Wenxing Lu [1], Shuping Zhao [1], Bing Liu [3] and Tianyue Long [1]

1. The School of Management, Hefei University of Technology, Hefei 230009, China; 2017170627@mail.hfut.edu.cn (J.G.); cyliang@hfut.edu.cn (C.L.); luwenxing@163.com (W.L.); zhaoshuping1753@126.com (S.Z.); mikehfut0551@163.com (T.L.)
2. The School of Informatics, Computing and Engineering, Bloomington, IN 47405-3907, USA
3. China Academy of Social Management & School of Sociology, Beijing Normal University, Beijing 100000, China; liubing@bnu.edu.cn
* Correspondence: gudongxiao@hfut.edu.cn; Tel.: +86-181-2391-7616

Received: 18 March 2019; Accepted: 25 April 2019; Published: 27 April 2019

Abstract: *Background:* With the popularity of mobile Internet and social networks, an increasing number of social media-based health management systems (SocialHMS) have emerged in recent years. These social media-based systems have been widely used in registration, payment, decision-making, chronic diseases management, health information and medical expenses inquiry, etc., and they greatly facilitate the convenience for people to obtain health services. *Objective:* This study aimed to investigate the factors influencing sustained health engagement of SocialHMS by combining the theory of planned behavior (TPB) with the big-five theory and the trust theory. *Method:* We completed an empirical analysis based on the 494 pieces of data collected from Anhui Medical University first affiliated hospital (AMU) in East China through structural equation modeling and SmartPLS (statistical analysis software). *Results:* Openness to new experience has a significantly positive influence on attitude (path coefficient = 0.671, t = 24.0571, R^2 = 0.451), perceived behavioral control (path coefficient = 0.752, t = 32.2893, R^2 = 0.565), and perceived risk (path coefficient = 0.651, t = 18.5940, R^2 = 0.424), respectively. Attitude, perceived behavioral control, subjective norms, and trust have a significantly positive influence on sustained health engagement (path coefficients = 0.206, 0.305, 0.197, 0.183 respectively, t = 3.6684, 4.9158, 4.3414, and 3.3715, respectively). The explained variance of the above factors to the sustained health engagement of SocialHMS is 60.7% (R^2 = 0.607). Perceived risk has a significantly negative influence on trust (path coefficient = 0.825, t = 46.9598, R^2 = 0.681). *Conclusions:* Attitude, perceived behavioral control, subjective norm, and trust are the determinants that affect sustained health engagement. The users' personality trait of openness to new experience and perceived risk were also found to be important factors for sustained health engagement. For hospital managers, there is the possibility to take appropriate measures based on users' personality to further enhance the implementation and utilization of SocialHMS. As for system suppliers, they can provide the optimal design for SocialHMS so as to meet users' needs.

Keywords: social media-based health management systems; theory of planned behavior; openness to new experience; sustained health engagement

1. Introduction

With the rapidly increasing development of mobile Internet and the popularity of social networks, an increasing number of social media-based health management systems (SocialHMS) have emerged in recent years [1]. These social media-based systems have been widely used in registration [2], payment, decision making, chronic diseases management, health information and medical expenses inquiry [3], etc., and they greatly facilitate the convenience for people to obtain health services [4,5]. WeChat is one of the most popular social media platforms in China. In the medical field, the application of WeChat can provide patients with functions such as inquiry, appointment, number taking, payment, etc. As long as they pay attention to the public account of the hospital, they can realize more convenient services in WeChat. For example, in terms of Anhui Provincial Hospital, patients can pay attention to the WeChat public number of the hospital, so that they can not only view the relevant information of doctors and experts in the department but also select an appropriate doctor to make an appointment according to their own symptoms and conditions. What is more, they can make use of other advantages of the public number, such as checking the hospital address and ride information, visiting the waiting team information, checking test results, paying online, and checking medical expenses. By using WeChat as a social media platform to develop a health management system, it is possible for patients to shorten the waiting time, appointment arrangement, registration, and examination in the treatment process, so that they can reasonably arrange the waiting and treatment time. When patients know their waiting time for medical treatment, they can arrange their daily affairs flexibly. With the continuous improvement of social media, the application development of social media-based health management system is constantly changing. In addition, the functions of such systems are getting closer and closer to becoming perfect, and the process is more convenient, and meanwhile, the service is more and more optimized. First, a social media-based health management system can realize the connection between patient information and hospital system data, so that data analysis can provide better personalized medical services for patients. For example, the patient can pay attention to the WeChat public number of the hospital and seek medical treatment through the public number before they come to the hospital. Second, information such as charges is transparent, and patients can obtain more information, which is conducive to reducing information asymmetry and improving the relationship between doctors and patients. Third, through a social media-based health management system, patients can actively participate in the system, increasing sustained health engagement [6]. Fourth, after collecting data through a social media-based health management system, analysis can be performed to rationally allocate medical resources and change the state of imbalance of existing medical resources. In short, the benefits of the application of social media-based health management systems are numerous, such as that: (1) They bring convenience to patients' medical services; (2) they accelerates the transformation of the medical industry; and (3) they make medical services develop in the direction of intelligence, personalization, and autonomy. For instance, Le Zhang et al. proposed the implementation process and significance of developing a medical information service system based on the WeChat public platform. The system is mainly composed of micro-sites and micro-medical networks, which can provide static and dynamic information inquiry services, as well as appointment registration and consulting services. Through this system, patients can receive medical services on the mobile phone in real time, hence simplifying medical procedures and improving patient satisfaction [7]. Further, Haolin studied the performance of social media-based conversation agents in the quit smoking program. The results showed that the presence of social media-based health management systems significantly increased participants' engagement and smoking cessation effectiveness [8]. What is more, Velasco et al. found that the social media-based mobile Internet health information exchange is regarded as an opportunity to improve public health supervision. On the basis of the traditional systems in which doctors and laboratories report infectious diseases to government agencies, infectious disease cases can be identified more quickly with the help of social media innovation. Social media-based health management systems could allow surveillance epidemiologists to identify potential public health threats, such as rare new diseases and early warning of epidemics [9]. Medical cyber-physical systems (MCPS), which present a new level of integrated intelligence that is characterized by interaction and coordination of computing processes with physical processes, can provide pregnant women with advanced medical care to achieve eugenics [10]. However, one problem of concern is that some patients lose interest in using it and cease using it. Several studies have indicated that users of hospital information systems (HIS) stop using a system after the system has been implemented and adopted by the healthcare organization [11].

Discontinuance wastes a large amount of quality improvement money spent on implementing the system [12]. More importantly, regarding social media-based health management systems (SocialHMS) as a continuous application is important because continuity is the prerequisite for the success of SocialHMS implementations. The significance of behavior continuity in achieving goals has been recognized for a long time in different contexts, including quality improvement [13] and organization success [14]. Thus, it becomes necessary to study factors influencing sustained health engagement and to understand how to use them to enhance the system use and benefits [15].

At present, most of the exiting studies in the area of SocialHMS are focused on the acceptance, development, and application of these systems [16]. In addition, most of the studies about information system (IS) continuance are focused on business-oriented IS such as corporate IS [17–19] and e-commerce [20]. Generalizing the outcomes of these studies to the HIS domain is not possible, given the dependence of factors influencing continuance on the context of IS use [21]. Under these circumstances, researchers have called for the study of continuance in the HIS context [22].

Theory of planned behavior (TPB) has been widely accepted as an effective model, which can explain the behavior intention. Further, it is the expansion of theory of reasoned action (TRA), which holds the opinion that any factor could indirectly influence use behavior through attitude and subjective norms [23]. However, the results of many studies show that user's behavior intention does not always lead to actual behavior. Thus, TPB extends TRA by adding a new component, "perceived behavioral control" to cover nonvolitional behaviors for predicting behavioral intention and actual behavior [24]. According to TPB, individual behaviors can be explained by the behavioral intention which is influenced by attitude, subjective norms, and perceived behavioral control. Attitude towards behavior can reflect likes and dislikes, as well as affective feedbacks, such as whether an experience is pleasant or not [25]. Subjective norm refers to an individual's perception of social pressure when taking some actions [26]. Perceived behavioral control could be further subdivided into external and internal control factors. Internal control factors refer to an individual's ability, skill, emotion, the impulse of certain behaviors, etc. External control factors refer to the intervening degree of that environment and facilities for some certain behavior occurring [27]. However, TPB has been criticized for focusing on cognitive factors but ignoring the affect and identity [28].

In the area of social personality psychology, the big five personality types, which are also known as the five-factor model (FFM), have received wide interest and approval [29,30]. This model possesses a high degree of stability in examining cross-cultural phenomena like language benefited from its unique dimensions and levels. Two core issues have been settled in FFM: (1) Distinguishing individual difference and describing order; and (2) structure existing in the individual difference construct [31]. Five relatively stable factors of FFM have been discovered after evaluating and analyzing the experimental results and factors. They are: (1) Extrovert (voluble, confident, and energetic); (2) easy-going (kind, good-natured, cooperative); (3) reliable (cautious, responsible, organized); (4) emotionally stability (calm, non-jittery, good-tempered); and (5) elegant (wise, educated, independent-thinking). All these five factors are highly regarded as the big five, in which the latter has been confirmed by other social-personality psychologists in their strict inspections and studies [32]. From the factors of FFM, openness to experience may be associated with an individual's behavior intention. The greater the openness of a user, the more willing and confident they are to try new things [33], which reflects an individual's way of receiving information and processing tendencies.

Perceived risk originates from psychology and has been introduced to the marketing field [34]. It refers to an individual's perceptions and cognition concerning various objective risks in one's environment and emphasizes an individual's experience obtained from intuitive judgment and subjective feeling, as these affect cognitions. Research has found that in certain scenarios, as a result of decision-making variables, behavior intention is related to the level of risk perception of decision makers [35,36].

To sum up, this study is to investigate the factors influencing continuous use of SocialHMS via the integrated research model which combines TPB with openness experience and perceived risk.

The research model is presented in Figure 1. By taking account of numerous literature and actual conditions, we propose eight research hypotheses broken into three categories: (1) Openness to new experience; (2) theory of planned behavior; and (3) perceived risk and trust.

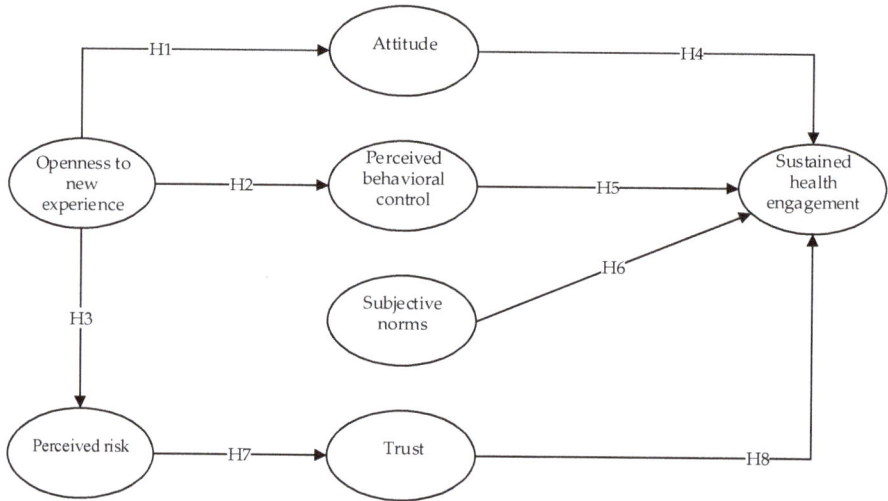

Figure 1. Research model.

1.1. Openness to Experience

Openness to experience, which is from the NEO Personality Inventory (NEO-PI-R) scale defining FFM, is correlated with curiosity, broad-ranging interests, and open-mindedness [37]. Among the factors of FFM, openness to experience may be associated with an individual's behavior intention because it is a reflection of the characteristics of those individuals who are more open to new ideas and experiences, and more willing and confident to try new things, which reflects an individual's way of receiving information and processing tendencies. Further, it is a very important variable that can influence the individual's behavior. Firstly, Lim and Lee found that openness of medical staff and active communication are important for nursing students in order to have a positive attitude toward complementary and alternative therapies [38]. Secondly, Bandura proposed his ternary interaction model that human motivation is generated by one's behavior, cognitive style, and environment [39]. An individual will not only respond to the external environment, but also adopt some strategies to change the environment they are in. Hascher and Hagenauer examined that openness to experience can positively predict a teacher's self-efficacy [40]. Hull and Booker's model also consistently identified openness to experience as a significant contributor to teacher self-efficacy [41]. This research employs the self-efficacy model to evaluate patient performance and feedback on their effectiveness of the SocialHMS. In addition, some research found that the perceived behavioral control based on personal experience and expected blocks will also affect behavior [42]. Thirdly, in the process of using SocialHMS, the user may be confronted with various risks, some of which could be sensed while some could not; some could be exaggerated while some could be diminished. Existing research has shown that perceived risks of consumers from different groups have different impacts on purchase intention [43]. Based on the openness to experience, it is certain that a user with a high degree of openness is good at absorbing new experiences, being brave to take the challenge, and effectively using various strategies to cope with the changes when facing unknowns. Meanwhile, the user of this kind would actively search for innovation when tackling problems, and therefore, can adjust to new changes quickly. In this study, SocialHMS can be viewed as a kind of new experience. These social media-based systems are used in registration, payment, decision-making, chronic diseases management, health information and medical expenses inquiry, etc. A user with a high degree of openness is more willing and confident to accept and use SocialHMS, and they can adjust to the new changes quickly.

Thus, the following are three hypotheses related to openness to experience:

Hypothesis 1 (H1): *Openness to new experience has a significant positive relationship with attitudes towards using the SocialHMS system.*

Hypothesis 2 (H2): *Openness to new experience has a significant positive relationship with perceived behavioral control over use of the SocialHMS system.*

Hypothesis 3 (H3): *Openness to new experience has a significant positive relationship with perceived risk of using the SocialHMS system.*

1.2. Theory of Planned Behavior

Perceived behavioral control has been defined as the perceived difficulty of performing a behavior and points out that an individual's behavior is restricted by his or her own ability to perform the behavior along with influences from the external environment. This reflects one's cognition about the factors that can either promote or impede the action, thus affecting the possibility to conduct this action. Ajzen cited numerous studies supporting the correlation between the behavior intention and perceived behavior control [42]. He believed that a stronger perceived behavior control led to a stronger behavior intention. Lots of studies showed that perceived behavior control could predict the behavior intention, such as predicting the user's intention of using the new software [44]. Perceived behavior control could coordinate the relationship between behavior intention and using behavior, thus exerting a direct influence on the behavior intention. Users' confidence concerning the difficulty of using SocialHMS could influence the capability of controlling the information system, hence affecting their intention to use SocialHMS.

Attitude refers to an individual's evaluation of personal behaviors. Attitude towards behavior is determined by the product function sum of belief and outcome evaluation. The attitude examined in this research is about the patients' adaptation to SocialHMS and whether they gained pleasure from it. Healthcare researchers consider attitude as an important factor in determining the user behavior in adopting guidelines or in SocialHMS use. This is evident in influential models created to explain the user's adoption of guidelines [45] and in attitude being the main predictor and guideline the use in healthcare studies [46,47]. Subjective norm refers to the individual's perception of what he or she believed about others' likelihood to sustain use of the SocialHMS [48]. Subjective norms could come from both internal and external avenues. Internal influence mainly refers to an influence that comes from friends, family, colleagues, leadership, etc., while external influence refers to mass media reports, the opinions of the experts but not individual information [49]. Venkatesh and Davis believed that when a social role wants an individual to perform a behavior, and when the social role can provide a corresponding reward or punishment, individuals tend to follow the social impact [50]. Research concerning this influence of social norms comes from examining users who are participating in virtual communities [51]. Bock and Zmud found that organizational climate forms subjective norms and strongly influences knowledge-sharing intentions among workers [52]. Further, the influence of this factor can be used to study the continuous use of IT systems. The use of SocialHMS can be regarded as a kind of social activity, and the users' behavior toward using SocialHMS can be observed by a range of the group. What is more, behavior toward using SocialHMS may affect the public's perception and evaluation of users. When both of the two points were perceived by users, it is likely that sustained health engagement will be affected.

Therefore, we proposed the following hypotheses:

Hypothesis 4 (H4): *Attitude has a significant positive relationship with sustained health engagement.*

Hypothesis 5 (H5): *Subjective norms have a significant positive relationship with sustained health engagement.*

Hypothesis 6 (H6): *Perceived behavioral control has a significant positive relationship with sustained health engagement.*

1.3. Perceived Risk and Trust

Perceived risk theory believes that as long as the output and outcome are uncertain, risk will be generated [53]. There are two uncertainties of every consequence in the decision to use SocialHMS. One is an uncertainty about the results (whether the results will satisfy their purpose), and the other is uncertainty about the failure of using the system. These uncertainties, when perceived by users, may create situations of risk. For example, some studies have shown that users will give up using the system if they perceive it as a threat to their professionalism [54]. Further, sense of privacy is the aspect of the form of perceived risk on the Internet environment, representing the worries and concerns over one's exposure of privacy [55]. According to the special use environment of SocialHMS, the patient's personal privacy information is sometimes recorded. Thus, the protection of privacy information will greatly affect patients' perceived risk level of SocialHMS. This may then affect patients' continuous use of the system.

Trust in our study refers to patients' trust that SocialHMS could provide the service they needed. McKnight had shown that trust has an impact on the intention for continuous use [56]. Based on the earlier research results, trust has the following characteristic, risk. That is to say, trust itself represents the intention to take risks; therefore, our study sought to explore the indirect impact of trust on sustained health engagement through perceived risk.

Thus, we proposed the following hypotheses:

Hypothesis 7 (H7): *Perceived risk has a significant negative relationship with the user trust in SocialHMS.*

Hypothesis 8 (H8): *The user trust in SocialHMS has a significant positive relationship with sustained health engagement.*

2. Methodology

2.1. Toolkits

The structural equation model (SEM) matured in the 1980s and is a better method in social science research, remedying the shortcomings of traditional statistical methods [57]. Several advantages of SEM are listed as follows: (1) It can process multiple dependent variables at the same time; (2) it allows independent variables and dependent variables to contain measurement errors; (3) it simultaneously estimates factor structure and factor relationship. The measurement of the structural equation model mainly includes two major evaluations. The first is the evaluation of the measurement model, including the relationship between the observed variables and the latent variables (data reliability and validity analysis). The strength of the model's interpretation of the latent variable is the R_2 value. The second is the evaluation of the structural model. That is, the relationship between latent variables supports whether the model hypothesis is supported. The structural equation model is established by partial least squares (PLS), and the measurement quality (measurement model) and mutual relationship (structural model) are evaluated. Though the ordinary least squares method as the estimation technique, PLS performs an iterative factor analysis set and applies a bootstrap method to estimate the significance of the path (*t* value). It is a powerful method for analyzing complex models using smaller samples. SmartPLS is developed in Java and can run on any platform. It provides three choices of internal weight modes: Centroid weight, factor weight, and path weight. It can set the number of iterations, iteration precision, and missing value processing. Thus, in this study, we used SmartPLS to evaluate the measurement properties and tested the hypotheses. Note that SmartPLS is a statistical analysis software designed by the development team of Ring, Wende, and Will of the University of Hamburg, Germany in 2005.

The rationality and reliability of the questionnaire are reflected in the form of the scale. The rationality of the scale determines the reliability and availability of data collection. Therefore, before statistical analysis of the results of the questionnaire, the credibility of the data should be analyzed to ensure the availability of the data and the credibility of the interpretation of the model. Only when the credibility of the data is within the acceptable range are the data collection results of the questionnaire reasonable and reliable, and the value of further analysis and statistics available. Cronbach's alpha reliability coefficient is used to measure the reliability analysis of the data. The higher the value, the higher the reliability of the table. It is generally accepted that a reliability coefficient above 0.7 is acceptable, and less than 0.7 indicates that the item of the scale needs to be adjusted [58]. Therefore, the threshold used herein is that the Cronbach's alpha coefficient be greater than 0.7.

Validity analysis, also known as effectiveness analysis, is mainly to detect whether each measurement question accurately expresses the meaning of each research variable [59]. Accurate expression means high degree of agreement, and high degree of data validity. Regarding the analysis of data validity, this study conducted two aspects of analysis, one being the analysis of convergence validity and the other the analysis of differential validity. For convergence validity, this paper measured two aspects: (1) Composite reliability (CR); and (2) average variance extracted (AVE). In general, composite reliability is greater than 0.6, indicating that the inherent consistency of all measurement questions is higher. Average variance extracted (AVE) is greater than 0.5, indicating that the measurement questions can better reflect the characteristics of each research variable in the model [60]. For differential validity, the analysis can be performed by the square root of the AVE value. The data for the diagonal position are the square root of the mean variance extraction rate (AVE value) for each study variable. When the square root of the mean variance extraction rate (AVE value) of each measurement question is greater than the correlation coefficient between the variables [61], it indicates that there is a strong discriminant coefficient between the variables, that is, the difference between each measurement variable is better. In general, the larger the R^2 value, the stronger the model's interpretation of each latent variable.

2.2. Sample and Data Collection

Considering the large number of existing studies that have adopted online survey research methods to collect data, we followed a similar data collection method by designing a survey questionnaire to collect data. Measures for the seven variables in our research model were adapted from previous studies. We referred to the relevant research and looked at the variables as well as the relationships among them. Then, by consulting the item of each variable in literature and combining the characteristic of this study, we increased and modified the related question appropriately. Finally, we designed the questionnaire of this study. Our questionnaire adopts a Likert 7-grade scale ranging from 1 (Highly Disagree) to 7 (Highly Agree).

The data collection of this study was carried out in Anhui Medical University first affiliated hospital (AMU), which is a 3A hospital in East China. 3A represents the highest level of hospital in China. The hospital has implemented SocialHMS for 3 years and already has many users. All respondents had 2–3 years of experience using SocialHMS. Firstly, in order to ensure the structural integrity of the questionnaire [62], the English reference scale in the questionnaire was translated into Chinese by a professional translator. After the preliminary design of the questionnaire, in order to ensure the validity and reliability of the questionnaire, we implemented a pilot survey and collected 100 questionnaires in AMU Hospital in June 2014. According to the collected data from the preliminary survey and the advice of the respondents, we adjusted the questions that were difficult to understand. Then, we analyzed the reliability and validity of the data using SmartPLS2.0 and confirmed the good reliability and validity of the questionnaire. The effort to determine reliability is described further along in the data analysis section. Finally, we conducted a survey in the hospital from October 2014 to March 2015. In order to achieve a reasonable response rate, we granted small gifts such as pre-paid phone cards, brush pots, and a creative small fan to each respondent. Each item was valued at about ¥30, about $5. A total of 550 questionnaires were handed out, and we received 532 questionnaires, of which 494 were valid. The return rate was 96.7%, and the valid response rate was 92.9%.

3. Results

3.1. Analysis of Measurement Model

The acceptability of the measurement model was assessed by the reliability of individual items, internal consistency between items, the model's convergent, and discriminant validity. Table 1 provides the descriptive statistics generated from the initial data, including the mean, standard deviation, and factor loading for each variable. Table 2 shows the Cronbach's alpha, composite reliability, average variance extracted (AVE), and square root of the AVE, as well as the correlations between the constructs. It is generally accepted that a reliability coefficient above 0.7 is acceptable. Therefore, the threshold used here is that Cronbach's alpha coefficient be greater than 0.7 [59]. As shown in Table 2, Cronbach's alpha of the seven constructs are all above the recommended criterion of 0.70, ranging from 0.7188 (Subjective norm) to 0.8571 (trust), which shows that the measures are reliable and internally consistent. Further, convergent validity and discriminant validity tests can be conducted by using SmartPLS2.0.

Convergent validity is generally assessed by the loadings of all the items; composite reliability (CR), average extracted variance (AVE), and discriminant validity should be evaluated by examining whether AVEs are higher than the interconstruct correlations. As shown in Table 1, the loadings of all the items are above the threshold of 0.75, indicating that the observed variables have high convergent validity. Furthermore, there is a high correlation between the observed variables and their belonging structure variables. Composite reliability that achieved 0.70 or above means the scale has good reliability. In general, composite reliability is greater than 0.6 and average variance extracted (AVE) is greater than 0.5, indicating that the reliability of this model is good [60]. Table 2 shows composite reliability is above 0.70 for all the variables in this study. Moreover, Table 2 shows AVE in this study is above 0.50 throughout, which denotes that the latent variables have a convergence ability that is quite ideal. When the square root of the mean variance extraction rate (AVE value) of each measurement question is greater than the correlation coefficient between the variables, it indicates that the difference between each measurement variable is better [58]. Further, the square root of the latent variables AVE value is greater than the absolute value of the correlation coefficient among latent variables. Thus, the discriminant validity of latent variables has been readjusted to meet standard.

Table 1. Reliability analysis of variables.

Construct	Item Statistics			
	Construct Items	Mean	Std. Deviation	Loading
Openness to New Experience	OtE1 *	5.44	1.35	0.856783
	OtE2 *	5.64	1.28	0.905741
	OtE3 *	5.26	1.44	0.837521
Attitude	Attitude1	6.07	1.1	0.826909
	Attitude2	6.02	1.1	0.827472
	Attitude3	6.02	1.05	0.848277
	Attitude4	5.93	1.16	0.822302
Perceived Behavioral Control	PBC1 *	5.77	1.2	0.829332
	PBC2 *	5.86	1.19	0.862304
	PBC3 *	5.65	1.28	0.820957
Subjective Norms	SN1	4.96	1.71	0.756089
	SN2	5.62	1.35	0.819427
	SN3	5.55	1.31	0.822804
Perceived Risk	PR1	5.75	1.26	0.891781
	PR2	5.63	1.24	0.917101
Trust	Trust1	5.6	1.23	0.804032
	Trust2	5.44	1.24	0.824332
	Trust3	5.61	1.23	0.847866
	Trust4	5.78	1.19	0.869369
Sustained Health Engagement	SU1	5.69	1.2	0.888886
	SU2	5.62	1.29	0.889958

* The construct items are used to explain the construct. For example, OtE1, OtE2, and OtE3 are scales of the openness to new experience. PBC1, PBC2, and PBC3 are scales of the perceived vehavioral control.

Therefore, the reliability of this study is good.

3.2. Analysis of Structural Model

Model fitting results are shown in Figure 2 and Table 3: The hypothesis of the impact of openness to experience personality trait on the attitude of use toward the SocialHMS (H1) is verified. In general, the *t* value is greater than 1.64, indicating that the hypothesis is supported [61]. Its path coefficient was 0.671 (*t* = 24.0571). Obviously, it reaches the significant level of 0.01, and the explained variance is 45.1%. The results show that the independence of the user's personality has a positive, significant influence on perceived usefulness. The path coefficient of openness to experience to perceived behavioral control is 0.752 (*t* = 32.2893), and this also reaches the significant level of 0.01, with an explained variance of 56.5%. Therefore, openness to experience has a positive significant influence on perceived behavioral control, and (H2) is verified. The path coefficient of openness to experience to perceived risk is 0.651 (*t* = 18.5940), and this also reaches the significant level of 0.01. Because the path coefficient is negative, the negative correlation of openness to experience to perceived risk can be verified. Thus, hypothesis H3 was supported. H7, the hypothesis of perceived risk to trust has been verified, too. Its path coefficient is 0.825 (*t* = 46.9598), reaching the significant level of 0.01, and the explained variance is 68.1%. The path coefficient of attitude (H4), perceived behavioral control (H5), subjective norms (H6), and trust (H8) in the intention of sustained use of the SocialHMS were 0.206 (*t* = 3.6684), 0.305 (*t* = 4.9158), 0.197 (*t* = 4.3414) and 0.183 (*t* = 3.3715), respectively. Therefore, H4, H5, H6, and H8 are verified. H4, H5, H6, and H8 reach the significant level of 0.01. Hence, we drew a conclusion that the perceived risk has a significant influence on the sustained intention to use SocialHMS. The explained variance of the above factors to the sustained health engagement of SocialHMS is 60.7%.

Table 2. Validity analysis of variables.

Construct Items	AVE [1]	Composite Reliability	Cronbach's Alpha	Attitude	SU	OtE	PBC	PR	SN	Trust
Attitude	0.6911	0.8995	0.851	0.8313 *						
SU	0.792	0.8839	0.7374	0.6929	0.89 *					
OtE	0.752	0.9008	0.835	0.6714	0.655	0.8672 *				
PBC	0.7018	0.8759	0.788	0.7796	0.7148	0.7515	0.8377 *			
PR	0.8182	0.9	0.7786	0.6281	0.6234	0.651	0.654	0.9045 *		
SN	0.64	0.8419	0.7188	0.6269	0.6351	0.6408	0.6208	0.6024	0.8 *	
Trust	0.7002	0.9032	0.8571	0.6897	0.6661	0.713	0.6961	0.8255	0.6562	0.8368 *

[1] AVE stands for average variance extract. * The bold number is the square root of AVE. The bold numbers listed diagonally are the square root of the variance shared between the constructs and their measures. The off-diagonal elements are the correlations among the constructs. For discriminate validity, the diagonal elements should be larger than the off-diagonal elements.

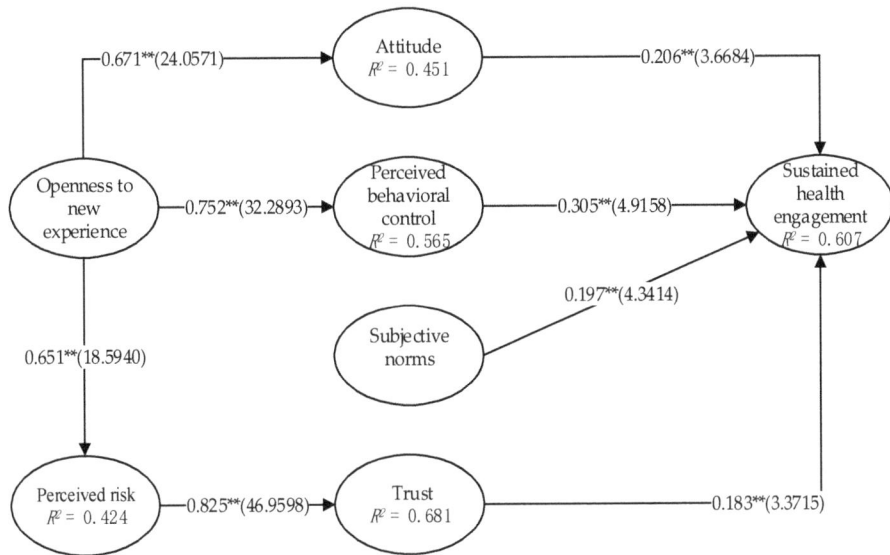

Figure 2. Model results. ** represents $p < 0.01$.

Table 3. Hypothesis testing results of the model.

Hypothesized Path.	Standardized Path Coefficients	t-Value	Results
H1: OtE -> Attitude	0.671	24.0571	Yes
H2: OtE -> PBC	0.752	32.2893	Yes
H3: OtE -> PR	0.651	18.594	Yes
H4: Attitude -> SU	0.206	3.6684	Yes
H5: PBC -> SU	0.305	4.9158	Yes
H6: SN -> SU	0.197	4.3414	Yes
H7: PR -> Trust	0.825	46.9598	Yes
H8: Trust -> SU	0.183	3.3715	Yes

4. Discussion

This paper studied the continuous use behavior of SocialHMS. As the experimental analysis results have shown, the 8 hypotheses proposed in the model have all been supported.

The analysis of H1, H2, and H3 showed that the openness to new experience personality trait has a significant positive impact on the attitude, perceived behavioral control, and perceived risk, thus improving sustained health engagement. The verified H4 and H5 show that the attitude and perceived behavioral control have a direct effect on sustained health engagement. The personality trait of openness to experience was a case in point. The greater the openness of a user, the more willing and confident they are to accept and use SocialHMS. Developers can improve SocialHMS based on the openness to experience and match the users through big data and cloud computing with each respective personality characteristic. System designers can improve the operation and function of SocialHMS. Then, system designers can design more humanized and more acceptable SocialHMS to enhance the user's sustained health engagement. Over time, web designers should seek to improve user attitudes towards, and perceived behavioral control by the use of the SocialHMS, which is likely to increase user engagement.

The empirical results of H6 indicated that subjective norms have a positive effect on the user's sustained health engagement. By enhancing the user's subjective norms, through official promotion, advertising, word of mouth, and system promoters can improve patients' positive cognition of the system [63], as well as effectively enhance the doctors' sustained health engagement.

The supported H7 indicated that perceived risk has a significant negative relationship with user trust in SocialHMS. The supported H8 shows that user trust in SocialHMS has a significant positive relationship with sustained health engagement. The support for these two hypotheses indicates that the lower the risk in the SocialHMS users perceive, the more trust they place in the system, and the more sustained health engagement will result. From this perspective, hospitals could improve patients' trust and strengthen their sustained health engagement through improving the SocialHMS safety features and strengthening patients' privacy safeguards [64].

5. Conclusions

Three theories including TPB, the big-five trait theory, and risk and trust theory were introduced in this study so as to, on the one hand, examine the relationship between openness experience and sustained health engagement and, on the other hand, examine how perceived risk affects sustained health engagement in the context of social media-based health management systems (SocialHMS). Our results revealed that attitude, perceived behavioral control, subjective norm, and trust are the determinants that affect sustained health engagement. The users' personality trait of openness to new experience and perceived risk were also found to be important factors for sustained health engagement. The results of this study integrate two research streams, IS and healthcare, to provide a holistic understanding of the sustained use of SocialHMS both by users and researchers. The research model is quite novel and combines the classic TPB model with both the big-five theory and risk and trust theory. This can be seen as an endeavor to extend the TPB model. In essence, the paper has provided a new perspective to the study of sustained health engagement, demonstrating the effect of personality (openness to new experience) on use of hospital systems [65]. It can also provide designers with a reference for system optimization [66], as well as for decision-making support for medical institutions [67], thus further improving the implementation of various intelligent technologies in hospitals. Designers can improve SocialHMS based on this personality perspective, and they can design more humanized and more acceptable hospital information systems to enhance the user's sustained health engagement. Through official promotion, advertising, and word of mouth, hospitals can improve patients' positive cognition of the system and effectively enhance doctors' sustained health engagement by enhancing the user's subjective norms. Hospitals could also improve patients' trust and strengthen their sustained health engagement through improving the SocialHMS safety features and strengthening patients' privacy safeguards.

Author Contributions: D.G. conceived the research; J.G. wrote the draft; S.Z., T.L., and B.L. collected the data and conducted data analysis; C.L. and W.L. provided some guiding suggestions and revised the paper.

Funding: This research is partially supported in the collection, analysis, and interpretation of data by the National Natural Science Foundation of China under Grant No. 71331002, 71771075, 71771077, 71573071, and 71601061.

Conflicts of Interest: The authors declare no conflict of interest.

References

1. De Brún, A.; McAuliffe, E. Social Network Analysis as a Methodological Approach to Explore Health Systems: A Case Study Exploring Support among Senior Managers/Executives in a Hospital Network. *Int. J. Environ. Res. Public Health* **2018**, *15*, 511. [CrossRef] [PubMed]
2. Khajeheian, D.; Colabi, A.M.; Shah, N.B.A.K.; Wan Mohamed Radzi, C.W.J.B.; Jenatabadi, H.S. Effect of Social Media on Child Obesity: Application of Structural Equation Modeling with the Taguchi Method. *Int. J. Environ. Res. Public Health* **2018**, *15*, 1343. [CrossRef] [PubMed]
3. Marqués-Sánchez, P.; Muñoz-Doyague, M.F.; Martínez, Y.V.; Everett, M.; Serrano-Fuentes, N.; Van Bogaert, P.; Vassilev, I.; Reeves, D. The Importance of External Contacts in Job Performance: A Study in Healthcare Organizations Using Social Network Analysis. *Int. J. Environ. Res. Public Health* **2018**, *15*, 1345. [CrossRef]

4. Mikkelsen, B.E.; Bloch, P.; Reinbach, H.C.; Buch-Andersen, T.; Winkle, L.L.; Toft, U.; Glumer, C.; Jensen, B.B.; Aagaaed-Hansen, J. Project SoL—A Community-Based, Multi-Component Health Promotion Intervention to Improve Healthy Eating and Physical Activity Practices among Danish Families with Young Children Part 2: Evaluation. *Int. J. Environ. Res. Public Health* **2018**, *15*, 1513. [CrossRef] [PubMed]
5. Wu, H.; Wu, S.; Wu, H.; Xia, Q.; Li, N. Living Arrangements and Health-Related Quality of Life in Chinese Adolescents Who Migrate from Rural to Urban Schools: Mediating Effect of Social Support. *Int. J. Environ. Res. Public Health* **2017**, *14*, 1249. [CrossRef] [PubMed]
6. Thomsen, M.S.; Nørrevang, O. A model for managing patient booking in a radiotherapy department with differentiated waiting times. *Acta Oncol.* **2009**, *48*, 251–258. [CrossRef] [PubMed]
7. Zhang, L.; Liu, Z.; Wu, S.; Wang, L.; Yang, G. Study on the medical information service system based on the WeChat platform. *Chin. Med. Devices* **2015**, *30*, 82–84.
8. Wang, H.; Zhang, Q.; Ip, M.; Lau, J.T.F. Social media-based conversational agents for health management and interventions. *Computer* **2018**, *51*, 26–33. [CrossRef]
9. Velasco, E.; Agheneza, T.; Denecke, K.; Kirchner, G.; Eckmanns, T. Social media and internet-based data in global systems for public health surveillance: A systematic review. *Milbank Q.* **2014**, *92*, 7–33. [CrossRef] [PubMed]
10. Li, G.-C.; Chen, C.-L.; Chen, H.-C.; Lin, F.; Gu, C. Design of a secure and effective medical cyber-physical system for ubiquitous telemonitoring pregnancy. *Concurr. Comput.* **2018**, *30*, e4236. [CrossRef]
11. Archer, N.; Cocosila, M. A Comparison of Physician Pre-Adoption and Adoption Views on Electronic Health Records in Canadian Medical Practices. *J. Med. Internet Res.* **2011**, *13*, e57. [CrossRef] [PubMed]
12. Baker, A. Crossing the Quality Chasm: A New Health System for the 21st Century. *BMJ* **2011**, *323*, 1192. [CrossRef]
13. Shortell, S.M.; O'Brien, J.L.; Carman, J.M.; Foster, R.W.; Hughes, E.F.; Boerstler, H.; O'Connor, E.J. Assessing the impact of continuous quality improvement/total quality management: Concept versus implementation. *Health Serv. Res.* **1995**, *30*, 377–401. [PubMed]
14. March, J.G. Continuity and change in theories of organizational action. *Adm. Sci. Q.* **1996**, *41*, 278–287. [CrossRef]
15. Otte, E.; Rousseau, R. Social network analysis: A powerful strategy, also for the information sciences. *J. Inf. Sci.* **2002**, *28*, 441–453. [CrossRef]
16. Fareedi, A.A.; Hassan, S. The impact of social media networks on healthcare process knowledge management (using of semantic web platforms). In Proceedings of the 2014 14th International Conference on Control, Automation and Systems, Seoul, South Korea, 22–25 October 2014; IEEE: Piscatvi, NJ, USA, 2014. [CrossRef]
17. Bhattacherjee, A. Understanding information systems continuance: An expectation-confirmation model. *MIS Q.* **2001**, *25*, 351–370. [CrossRef]
18. Bhattacherjee, A.; Premkumar, G. Understanding Changes in Belief and Attitude toward Information Technology Usage: A Theoretical Model and Longitudinal Test. *MIS Q.* **2004**, *28*, 229–254. [CrossRef]
19. Venkatesh, V.; Goyal, S. Expectation disconfirmation and technology adoption: Polynomial modeling and response surface analysis. *MIS Q.* **2010**, *34*, 281–303. [CrossRef]
20. Pavlou, P.; Fygenson, M. Understanding and predicting electronic commerce adoption: An extension of the theory of planned behavior. *MIS Q.* **2006**, *30*, 115–143. [CrossRef]
21. Venkatesh, V.; Thong, J.Y.L.; Chan, F.K.Y.; Hu, P.J.-H.; Brown, S.A. Extending the two-stage information systems continuance model: Incorporating UTAUT predictors and the role of context. *Inf. Syst. J.* **2011**, *21*, 527–555. [CrossRef]
22. Sun, Y.; Jeyaraj, A. Information technology adoption and continuance: A longitudinal study of individuals' behavioral intentions. *Inf. Manag.* **2013**, *50*, 457–465. [CrossRef]
23. Fishbein, M. A theory of reasoned action: Some applications and implications. *Nebr. Symp. Motiv.* **1980**, *27*, 65.
24. Ajzen, I. The theory of planned behavior, organizational behavior and human decision processes. *J. Leis. Res.* **1991**, *50*, 176–211.
25. Ajzen, I.; Fishbein, M. Attitudes and the Attitude-Behavior Relation: Reasoned and Automatic Processes. *Eur. Rev. Soc. Psychol.* **2000**, *11*, 1–33. [CrossRef]
26. Fishbein, M.; Ajzen, I. Belief, Attitude, Intention and Behaviour: An introduction to theory and research. *Philos. Rhetor.* **1977**, *41*, 842–844.

27. Ajzen, I. *Attitudes, Personality, and Behavior*; McGraw-Hill Education: New York, NY, USA, 2005.
28. Maio, G.R.; Haddock, G. *The Psychology of Attitudes and Attitude Change*; Sage: London, UK, 2019.
29. Saroglou, V.; Jaspard, J.-M. Personality and religion: From eysenck's taxonomy to the five-factor model. *Arch. Psychol. Relig.* **2000**, *23*, 41–70. [CrossRef]
30. Schmitt, D.P.; Allik, J.; Mccrae, R.R.; Benetmartínez, V. The Geographic Distribution of Big Five Personality Traits: Patterns and Profiles of Human Self-Description across 56 Nations. *J. Cross Cult. Psychol.* **2007**, *38*, 173–212. [CrossRef]
31. Larsen, R.J.; Buss, D.M. *Personality Psychology: Domains of Knowledge about Human Nature*; McGraw Hill Education: New York, NY, USA, 2017.
32. Kapogiannis, D.; Sutin, A.; Davatzikos, C.; Costa, P., Jr.; Resnick, S. The five factors of personality and regional cortical variability in the Baltimore longitudinal study of aging. *Hum. Brain Mapp.* **2013**, *34*, 2829–2840. [CrossRef]
33. Davis, D.D.; Bjornberg, N.H. Flourishing in the Workplace through Meditation and Mindfulness. *Ind. Organ. Psychol.* **2015**, *8*, 667–674. [CrossRef]
34. Bauer, R.A. Consumer Behavior as Risk Taking. In Proceedings of the 43rd National Conference of the American Marketing Assocation, Chicago, IL, USA, 15–17 June 1960; American Marketing Association: Chicago, IL, USA, 1960.
35. van der Weerd, W.; Timmermans, D.R.; Beaujean, D.J.; Oudhoff, J.; van Steenbergen, J.E. Monitoring the level of government trust, risk perception and intention of the general public to adopt protective measures during the influenza A (H1N1) pandemic in the Netherlands. *BMC Public Health* **2011**, *11*, 575. [CrossRef] [PubMed]
36. Liao, C.; Lin, H.-N.; Liu, Y.-P. Predicting the use of pirated software: A contingency model integrating perceived risk with the theory of planned behavior. *J. Bus. Ethics* **2010**, *91*, 237–252. [CrossRef]
37. McCrae, R.R.; Terracciano, A. Universal features of personality traits from the observer's perspective: Data from 50 cultures. *J. Pers. Soc. Psychol.* **2005**, *88*, 547. [CrossRef] [PubMed]
38. Lim, S.H.; Lee, J.Y. Nursing Students' Perception, Experience and Attitude on Complementary and Alternative Therapies. *J. East West Nurs. Res.* **2015**, *21*, 110–118.
39. Bandura, A. *Social Foundations of Thought and Action: A Social Cognitive Theory*; Prentice-Hall, Inc.: Englewood Cliffs, NJ, USA, 1986.
40. Hascher, T.; Hagenauer, G. Openness to theory and its importance for pre-service teachers' self-efficacy, emotions, and classroom behaviour in the teaching practicum. *Int. J. Educ. Res.* **2016**, *77*, 15–25. [CrossRef]
41. Hull, D.M.; Booker, D.D.; Näslund-Hadley, E.I. Teachers' self-efficacy in Belize and experimentation with teacher-led math inquiry. *Teach. Teach. Educ.* **2016**, *56*, 14–24. [CrossRef]
42. Manstead, A.S.R.; van Eekelen, S.A.M. Distinguishing between perceived behavioral control and self-efficacy in the domain of academic achievement intentions and behaviors. *J. Appl. Soc. Psychol.* **1998**, *28*, 1375–1392. [CrossRef]
43. Xie, C. The Influence of Perceived Risk on Purchase Intention—A Case study of Taobao Online Shopping of Fresh Fruit. *Asian Agric. Res.* **2017**, *9*, 30–35.
44. Miyazaki, A.D.; Fernandez, A. Consumer perceptions of privacy and security risks for online shopping. *J. Consum. Aff.* **2001**, *35*, 27–44. [CrossRef]
45. Pathman, D.E.; Konrad, T.R.; Freed, G.L.; Freeman, V.A.; Koch, G.G. The awareness-to-adherence model of the steps to clinical guideline compliance: The case of pediatric vaccine recommendations. *Med. Care* **1996**, *34*, 873–889. [CrossRef]
46. Howes, O.D.; Vergunst, F.; Gee, S.; Mcguire, P.; Kapur, S.; Taylor, D. Adherence to treatment guidelines in clinical practice: Study of antipsychotic treatment prior to clozapine initiation. *Br. J. Psychiatry* **2012**, *201*, 481–485. [CrossRef] [PubMed]
47. Solà, I.; Carrasco, J.M.; del Campo, P.D.; Gracia, J.; Orrego, C.; Martínez, F.; de Gaminde, I. Attitudes and perceptions about clinical guidelines: A qualitative study with Spanish physicians. *PLoS ONE* **2014**, *9*, e86065. [CrossRef] [PubMed]
48. Ajzen, I.; Madden, T.J. Prediction of goal-directed behavior: Attitudes, intentions, and perceived behavioral control. *J. Exp. Soc. Psychol.* **1986**, *22*, 453–474. [CrossRef]
49. Bhattacherjee, A. Acceptance of e-commerce services: The case of electronic brokerages. *IEEE Trans. Syst. Man. Cybern. A. Syst. Hum.* **2000**, *30*, 411–420. [CrossRef]

50. Venkatesh, V.; Davis, F.D. A theoretical extension of the technology acceptance model: Four longitudinal field studies. *Manag. Sci.* **2000**, *46*, 186–204. [CrossRef]
51. Bagozzi, R.P.; Dholakia, U.M. Intentional social action in virtual communities. *J. Interact. Mark.* **2002**, *16*, 2–21. [CrossRef]
52. Bock, G.-W.; Zmud, R.W.; Kim, Y.-G.; Lee, J.-N. Behavioral intention formation in knowledge sharing: Examining the roles of extrinsic motivators, social-psychological forces, and organizational climate. *MIS Q.* **2005**, *29*, 87–111. [CrossRef]
53. Fraedrich, J.P.; Ferrell, O. The impact of perceived risk and moral philosophy type on ethical decision making in business organizations. *J. Bus. Res.* **1992**, *24*, 283–295. [CrossRef]
54. Doolin, B. Power and resistance in the implementation of a medical management information system. *Inf. Syst. J.* **2004**, *14*, 343–362. [CrossRef]
55. Kesharwani, A.; Bisht, S.S. The impact of trust and perceived risk on internet banking adoption in India: An extension of technology acceptance model. *Int. J. Bank Mark.* **2012**, *30*, 303–322. [CrossRef]
56. McKnight, D.H.; Chervany, N.L. What trust means in e-commerce customer relationships: An interdisciplinary conceptual typology. *Int. J. Electron. Comer.* **2001**, *6*, 35–59. [CrossRef]
57. Weir, J.P. Quantifying test-retest reliability using the intraclass correlation coefficient and the sem. *J. Strength Cond. Res.* **2005**, *19*, 231–240. [PubMed]
58. Hair, J.F.; Black, W.C.; Babin, B.J.; Anderson, R.E.; Tatham, R.L. Multivariate Data Analysis. *Technometrics* **2013**, *49*, 103–104.
59. Carrasco, J.-L.; Jover, L. Assessing individual bioequivalence using the structural equation model. *Stat. Med.* **2003**, *22*, 901–912. [CrossRef] [PubMed]
60. Srinivasan, R.; Lilien, G.L.; Rangaswamy, A. Technological opportunism and radical technology adoption: An application to e-business. *J. Mark.* **2002**, *66*, 47–60. [CrossRef]
61. Multivariate Data Analysis: Pearson New International Education. Available online: https://is.muni.cz/el/1423/podzim2017/PSY028/um/_Hair_-_Multivariate_data_analysis_7th_revised.pdf (accessed on 18 March 2019).
62. Brislin, R.W. Cross-cultural research methods. *Environ. Cult.* **1980**, *4*, 47–82.
63. Sykes, T.A.; Venkatesh, V.; Gosain, S. Model of acceptance with peer support: A social network perspective to understand employees' system use. *MIS Q.* **2009**, *33*, 371–393. [CrossRef]
64. Vozniuk, A.; Holzer, A.C.; Govaerts, S.; Mazuze, J.; Gillet, D. Graspeo: A Social Media Platform for Knowledge Management in NGOs. In Proceedings of the International Conference on Information & Communication Technologies and Development, Singapore, 15–18 May 2015; EPFL Scientific Publications: Lausanne, Switzerland, 2015.
65. Cameron, D.; Smith, G.A.; Daniulaityte, R.; Sheth, A.P.; Dave, D.; Chen, L.; Anand, G.; Carlson, R.; Watkins, K.Z.; Falck, R. PREDOSE: A semantic web platform for drug abuse epidemiology using social media. *J. Biomed. Inform.* **2013**, *46*, 985–997. [CrossRef] [PubMed]
66. Razmerita, L.; Phillips-Wren, G.; Jain, L.C. *Innovations in Knowledge Management—The Impact of Social Media, Semantic Web and Cloud Computing*; Springer: Berlin, Germany, 2016.
67. Tyagi, A.; Tyagi, R. Social media: Opportunities and challenges for human resource management. *IJKBO* **2012**, *2*. [CrossRef]

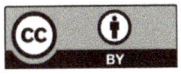

© 2019 by the authors. Licensee MDPI, Basel, Switzerland. This article is an open access article distributed under the terms and conditions of the Creative Commons Attribution (CC BY) license (http://creativecommons.org/licenses/by/4.0/).

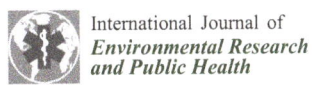

Article

Moving Beyond the Gym: A Content Analysis of YouTube as an Information Resource for Physical Literacy

Trevor Bopp [1,*], Joshua D. Vadeboncoeur [1], Michael Stellefson [2] and Melissa Weinsz [1]

1. Department of Sport Management, University of Florida, Gainesville, FL 32611, USA
2. Department of Health Education and Promotion, East Carolina University, Greenville, NC 27858, USA
* Correspondence: tbopp@ufl.edu; Tel.: +1-352-294-1663

Received: 5 July 2019; Accepted: 2 September 2019; Published: 10 September 2019

Abstract: The Internet, and particularly YouTube, has been found to be and continues to develop as a resourceful educational space for health-related information. Understanding physical literacy as a lifelong health-related outcome and facilitator of an active lifestyle, we sought to assess the content, exposure, engagement, and information quality of uploaded physical literacy videos on YouTube. Two researchers collected 300 YouTube videos on physical literacy and independently coded each video's: title, media source of upload, content topics related to physical literacy, content delivery style, and adherence to adapted Health on the Net Foundation Code of Conduct (HONcode) principles of information quality. Physical literacy videos that focused on physical activity and behaviors were the strongest predictor of high quality ratings, followed closely by videos covering affective domains (motivation, confidence, and self-esteem) of physical literacy. The content delivery method was also important, with videos utilizing presentations and testimonials containing high quality information about physical activity. Thus, providers of physical literacy and health-related online video content should be aware of and adhere to the expected quality standards. As health information expectations and ethical standards increase, the Internet, and specifically YouTube, has the potential to enhance video resources, virtual networking opportunities, as well as the sharing, dissemination, accumulation, and enrichment of physical literacy information for all.

Keywords: physical literacy; activity; social media; online resource; Internet; HONcode; YouTube

1. Introduction

Regular physical activity is a critical component of healthy living, particularly as it pertains to weight management, preventing chronic disease, and promoting psychological well-being [1,2]. It is especially important for youth to become physically active so as to mitigate health risk factors that can accumulate and negatively impact health outcomes over life course trajectories [3,4]. For example, obesity affects nearly 1 in 5 American children and adolescents [5]. Struggles with obesity and weight status present youth with challenges to performing basic movement skills [6], which subsequently impacts their self-confidence, and in turn, deters their participation in activities that are likely to develop fine motor skills necessary for physical activity [4]. Physical literacy is a foundational and enduring concept regarding one's "motivation, confidence, physical competence, knowledge, and understanding to value and take responsibility for engagement in physical activities for life [7]". Given its conceptualization as the basis for a life course trajectory of healthy living, physical literacy has evolved into a relevant lifelong learning outcome for all individuals, of all ages and ability levels.

According to Whitehead [8], the affective domain of physical literacy refers to the relationship among an individual's confidence, motivation, and self-esteem in relation to their level(s) of physical activity. Additionally, physical literacy is contingent upon the cognitive accrual and maintenance of, "knowledge and understanding to value and take responsibility" for engaging in physical activity across the life course [7]. Knowing how to live an active lifestyle establishes the cognitive foundation for an individual to become aware of and attach value to participation in physical activity [9]. Thus, physical literacy should influence attitudes toward physical activity, wherein "attention to understanding the importance of physical activity, health and wellbeing throughout the life course [10] (p. 120)" becomes of prime importance.

At present, scholarly conversations continue as to how to best implement, endorse, and teach physical literacy in educational settings and sport/physical activity programs [11,12]. For instance, the Society of Health and Physical Educators (SHAPE) provides resources and professional development opportunities to help youth develop into physically literate individuals, yet still faces challenges when attempting to "describe and demonstrate what physical literacy informed practice is and looks like without being overly perspective and restrictive [11] (p. 270)". A number of international organizations (e.g., Aspen, Canadian Sport for Life [CS4L], International Physical Literacy Association [IPLA]) also offer online platforms that provide informational resources, scholarly publications, strategies for promoting and implementing physical literacy curriculum and standards, and instructor training workshops on physical literacy. Despite the wealth of information made available online by these organizations physical educators, teachers, and those with a general interest in learning remain at a loss when searching for online physical literacy resources [13].

When considering physical literacy from a health perspective, both as an outcome and antecedent to an active and healthy lifestyle, it becomes a worthwhile endeavor to examine and understand how physical literacy information is shared and disseminated on the Internet, and in particular, among social media users. Social media has been found to be a popular and increasingly-accessible resource for health-related information [14]. YouTube is a public platform and people from wide ranging disciplines and contexts access it for information on broad range of topics and issues. As a continually developing online resource for health information, communication, and promotion, health education researchers have examined the use and effectiveness of specific popular social media sites such as YouTube [15–18], Pinterest [19,20], Instagram [21], and Facebook [22]. Given the popularity, reach, accessibility and unregulated governance of social media, it is critical that users seek and post/upload information from reputable, qualified and trusted health and medical sources. Therefore, the following section further details social media as a health-related information platform, with particular attention paid to YouTube.

Social Media and YouTube as Information Resources

As the Internet and social media allow for asynchronous and synchronous transmission and dissemination of information, it is critical for proponents of physical literacy (e.g., teachers, parents, students, etc.) to be aware of how physical literacy is portrayed online, especially through popular social media which is a common learning forum for youth health and wellness [23]. Given that youth have been found to place a relatively high value on the accessibility of information made available on social media [24], extent research has demonstrated that youth are not only pivoting to social media platforms for health-based information at increasing rates [14], but in doing so, are reporting benefits such as higher levels of socialization, knowledge procurement, and even socio-psychological support [25,26]. Likewise, it is in this vein that many individuals of adult-age may hold an unawareness of the potential opportunities that social media embodies as an emerging medium for health promotion amongst youth, much of which can be attributed to the complex nature behind how social media operates to influence youth [24]. For example, given the breadth of social media platforms (e.g., Facebook, Instagram, Snapchat, Twitter, YouTube), interactive applications and features made available to engage with said platforms, and "who" and "what" is accessing and/or creating content, each operates in conjunction to offer a contextually dynamic space that diverges from what is considered to be more traditional forms of public health pedagogies [27,28].

Nevertheless, as posited by Dudley et al. [29], "developing health literacy in young people is an important construct that should be considered in the context of engagement with social media," such that it can offer adolescents, "greater availability of information and with the potential for shared dialogue and positive normative beliefs that enhance healthy behaviors" (p. 157). Although in agreement with the aforementioned sentiments, Cale [30] cautioned that because health and physical education teachers and practitioners alike remain focused on instrumental outcomes rather than health benefits, the use of social media in physical education pedagogy may very well serve as yet another platform that replicates and reinforces the same static approaches already in practice. Furthermore, there is a lack of sourcing of health information from digital technologies on behalf of teachers and practitioners [31–33], thus prompting growing recommendations in the research literature for an intentional, "focus on adults' critical pedagogical response both to health and health-related social media," as means "to develop critically aware pedagogues who can support and develop critically aware youngsters" [30] (p. 216).

Moreover, as noted by Casey, Goodyear, and Armour [33], among the practitioners in their study, digital technologies were merely used to reinforce traditionally-held physical education pedagogical practices, the likes of which could be extrapolated to include the interrelationship(s) between social media technologies, health, and physical education [30]. It is no wonder that recent scholarship has placed an intentioned focus on the use of social media [34] and related emergent technologies [35] in the promotion of health-related and physical education information, as well as the bridging of physical education and digital technology through pedagogical (re)development [36,37]. For instance, and more narrowly, extant literature has deemed platforms such as Facebook, for example, to be an effective information resource in diverse contexts, such as through pedagogical design [38–40]) and more pointedly, for the purposes of sharing health information, both at the individual [41] and organizational [42] levels. As a result, understanding the dynamic functionality and interactivity of social media platforms, particularly concerning their influence on the health-related behavior(s) and knowledge of youth, becomes imperative. Thus, we are in alignment with Shaw, Mitchell, Welch, and Williamson's [43] assertion that all future inquiry on social media as a health intervention and information resource for youth must consider "the newness of using social media as a health intervention, the importance of the use of rigorous methodological processes when using social media as a health intervention, and the need to develop further knowledge on adolescents' use of social media (p. 8)".

While the aforementioned discussion demonstrates the recent (and yet, ongoing) investigation of social media platforms as health-related, information resources, little attention has been directed towards evaluating physical literacy videos on YouTube. For instance, although YouTube has been investigated as a source of information for a number of health-related topics [15–18,44,45], as well as a teaching aid in physical education [46], physical literacy has been absent from this line of inquiry. YouTube (www.youtube.com), with 1.8 billion registered users [47], is the largest and most utilized video-based social media platform globally [48]. The platform allows users to view, upload and rank video content as well as connect and communicate will fellow users. It is the second most popular search engine behind Google [48] and is used by 73% of U.S. adults, 94% of U.S. 18- to 24-year-olds, and 85% of U.S. teens ages 13–17 [49,50]. YouTube has been identified as a valuable learning resource that, when properly integrated into school settings, assists in the daily delivery of curriculum. Its broad reach and engagement capacity makes it the ideal technology for serving as a supplemental learning channel that extends the classroom environment beyond the school walls and into natural physical activity settings [51]. Furthermore, YouTube is one social media platform notably utilized for the sharing of patient education materials and healthcare information [15,16,18]. Thus, the purpose of this study was to assess the content, exposure, engagement, and information quality of uploaded YouTube videos on physical literacy. To this end, we address the following research questions regarding physical literacy videos posted on YouTube:

1. Is the information quality of YouTube videos on physical literacy associated with viewer attitudes?

2. Does the quality of physical literacy information in the YouTube videos vary based on media source?
3. Do the content properties in the physical literacy YouTube videos influence the (a) quality of information and (b) viewer attitudes?
4. Does the content delivery style of the physical literacy YouTube videos influence the (a) quality of information and (b) viewer attitudes?

2. Materials and Methods

According to Petrescu [52], on average, 71% of organic desktop searches in Google result in web users clicking on results from the first page, whereas a click-through rate of just under 6% exists for page two and three results. Moreover, on the first page alone, 68% of web users will click on results within the first five listings, as opposed to results 6 through 10, which account for only 4% of all clicks. As such, to account for user behavior and ensure that a screening method devoid of arbitrary page and/or video count limits was employed, we utilized the "playlist" feature on YouTube. This feature allows an account user to curate a playlist of up to a maximum of 150 selected videos. While no methodology can provide truly objective data collection, we believed the utilization of YouTube playlists to be an appropriate standard from which to conduct this study. Thus, on September 11, 2018, two members of the research team independently conducted an initial video search, whereby the keyword "physical literacy" was input into the YouTube search engine.

For each video, we wanted to know which properties of physical literacy were addressed and in which context, athletic or educational; as well as the media source that uploaded the YouTube videos and for which target audience they were intended. To address these questions, the following details were recorded for each retrieved video: title, media source of upload, date of upload (measured in number of days since initial posting), duration (measured in minutes, seconds), content topics related to physical literacy (e.g., affective, cognitive, physical), the style of content delivery (e.g., animation, presentation, demonstration), and adherence to adapted Health On the Net Foundation (HONcode) principles of video quality (measured in frequency of principles followed).

As it concerned the media source of upload, we assigned each video to one of seven total categories: (a) educational institution (e.g., university, research institute, primary/secondary school); (b) government agency/organization (e.g., local sport council, parks and recreation department, government-sponsored); (c) news media outlet; (d) non-profit organization; (e) physical education-based/development program (e.g., for-profit organization offering physical education-based services); (f) professional organization (e.g., teachers association, professional development/learning); and (g) user-generated content (UGC).

We were also interested in the quality of physical literacy information in the YouTube videos. Efforts to best determine and measure the quality of information via ethical guidelines for internet-derived health information, such as self-regulatory codes of ethics, rating tools, third-party reviewers, and both accreditation and certification systems, have been numerous and diverse in their approaches [53,54]. Yet, one of the more popular and industry accepted tools, HONcode, was selected for this study. HONcode is a code of ethics for web site managers to follow as it concerns the presentation of objective and verifiable medical and health-related information. Extant research reveals that the HONcode has been well accepted by health-related web sites on account of its comprehensive set of principles that assess the ethics, quality, transparency, and trustworthiness of online-derived health information [55,56]. Additionally, due to the relative lack of assessment tools for the evaluation of online platforms such as YouTube [57], Stellefson et al. [18] demonstrated the utility of the HONcode as such a tool, using an adaptation of the instrument to measure information quality of Chronic Obstructive Pulmonary Disease (COPD) patient education videos posted to YouTube.

In accordance with each of the eight HONcode principles and subsequent adaptations [18], we used six adapted principles to evaluate the quality of selected YouTube videos. Although HONcode was developed as a code of ethics for web site content, we followed the similar efforts of Stellefson et al. in adjusting the principles in a manner that would render applicability to video content, which included thematic alignment with physical literacy and the collapsing of certain principles deemed to be unsuitable for this particular study. For each video, the coder indicated on a binary scale (0 = No; 1 = Yes) whether or not each of the six principles was followed, at which point a summated score was computed to measure total adherence to the adapted HONcode principles. Again, given the respective aims of this study, one of which is to assess the relative quality of information in videos shared on YouTube, we believe the merits of the HONcode principles and our subsequent adaptation to be best suited to carry out our data collection.

Additional metrics collected included total video view counts, viewer engagement (e.g., the number of "likes" and "dislikes"), and number of posted viewer comments. As per YouTube's "Creator Academy" platform, a total of 18 example categories (e.g., education, entertainment, people & blogs, sports) are listed for content creators to organize and optimize the viewer reach of their videos. Thus, coders screened the listed category for each video (according to YouTube guidelines, only one category can be selected per video) and evaluated the relevance of the selected category per the video's content topic.

As it concerns the categorical organization of both content topics and the delivery of said content, the authors collaborated to devise a definitive list for each set of categories. In drawing upon Edwards et al. [10] systematic review of the physical literacy construct, we developed a set of adapted content subthemes and core categories (noted in parentheses), which included: affective (confidence, motivation, self-esteem); cognitive (knowledge and understanding, value and responsibility); physical capabilities (FMS/capacity to move, competence); target audience(s) (youth, adults, none); behavioral characteristics (health behaviors, physical activity); psychological, social, and attitudinal (academic performance, enjoyment, support); contextual (structural or unstructured sport, physical education); and additionally, the subthemes of pathway, environment, holistic/ontological, and pedagogical. Several categories were first utilized when assessing the style of content delivery, however, after discussing the perceived intentions and outcomes of each delivery style category, we collapsed them into four primary classifications: animation (e.g., picture, script); presentation (i.e., academic, in classroom, conference); demonstration (i.e., visual observation, instructional); and testimonial (e.g., organizational, individual).

In order to satisfy the inclusion criteria of this study, video content had to be audible in the English language and pertinent to physical literacy content topic. Both coders were informed of the respective criteria for locating and henceforth evaluating each video. For each video that satisfied our inclusion criteria, both coders saved the video to a YouTube playlist. As previously indicated, a maximum of 150 videos can be saved on a single playlist, which allowed the coders to save a total of 300 videos. Of those selected, all videos with content that did not relate to the aims and scope of this study ($n = 22$), were not in English ($n = 37$), and duplicate videos ($n = 91$) were subsequently excluded. Whenever disagreement arose between both coders as to whether a particular saved video did not meet the inclusion criteria, resolution was met by either common consensus through discussion or by way of a third member of the research team. In all, a total of 150 unique videos were saved and utilized for data analysis.

2.1. Data Reliability

Interrater reliability of codes was established to confirm an appropriate level of consensus between the two coders. To determine interrater reliability via Cohen's Kappa (k), or coefficient of agreement, 40 videos were randomly selected and coded by two independent researchers. A subsample size of 40 was deemed appropriate for conducting reliability analyses [58] and the k coefficient cutoff was set at the moderately acceptable value of 0.60 [59]. Using IBM SPSS software version 25 [60], coefficients of agreement were computed for coding the properties of physical literacy ($k = 0.82$), target audiences ($k = 0.90$), contexts ($k = 0.77$), and delivery style ($k = 0.83$). For a further breakdown of the reliability analyses see Table 1. Additionally, reliability of the adapted physical literacy HONCode principles was established using Lin's concordance correlation coefficient [61] and was determined to be almost perfect, $\rho_c = 0.90$. This metric was selected as it can serve as a robust measure between two coders when observing continuous variables [18,62].

Table 1. Interrater reliability scores for coding content and other focus areas in sample ($n = 40$) of physical literacy videos on YouTube.

Content & Focus Areas	Cohen's k
Properties of Physical Literacy	0.82
Affective	0.86
Confidence	0.94
Motivation	0.74
Self-Esteem	0.80
Cognitive	0.62
Knowledge/Understanding	0.71
Value/Responsibility	0.46
Physical	0.82
Fundamental Movement Skills	0.73
Competence	0.85
Behavioral	0.86
Health	0.80
Physical Activity	0.92
Psychosocial and Attitudinal	0.85
Academic Performance	0.91
Enjoyment	0.82
Support	0.74
Target Audiences	0.90
Youth	0.84
Adults	0.84
None	N/A
Contexts	0.77
Physical Education	0.75
Structured Sport	0.80
Unstructured Sport	0.71
Style of Content Delivery	0.83
Animation	0.88
Demonstration	0.85
Presentation	0.86
Testimonial	0.65

2.2. Data Analysis

IBM SPSS software version 25 [60] was utilized to run basic frequency and descriptive statistics to understand more about the affective, cognitive, behavioral, physical, psychological, social and attitudinal properties of physical literacy covered in the YouTube videos. Likewise, the target audiences, athletic/educational contexts, and media source of the YouTube videos were also examined via frequency and descriptive statistics. The quality of each video was determined by the adding together the number of adapted HONcode principles that each of the physical literacy YouTube videos met; adherence to 0–3 principles indicated low quality, while 4–6 principles suggested high quality [18]. Due to the non-normal distribution of data, the Mann-Whitney U test was conducted to determine associations between video quality of information and viewers' attitudes, via "likes" (Research Question 1). Similarly, Fisher's exact test was conducted to determine associations between media source of the YouTube videos and adherence to the adapted HONCode principles (Research Question 2). Binary logistic regression analyses were run to examine the influence of physical literacy YouTube video content properties on the quality of information (Research Question 3a) and viewer attitudes (Research Question 3b). Likewise, binary logistic regression analyses were run to determine the potential influence of the content delivery style of the physical literacy YouTube videos on the quality of information (Research Question 4a) and viewer attitudes (Research Question 4b).

2.3. Results

Demographic data and frequencies can be found in Table 2. However, prior to sharing the results of the research questions, we wanted to highlight several of the more critical aspects of the YouTube videos on physical literacy. The most prominent physical literacy properties covered in the YouTube videos were those centered on physical constructs (n = 122; 81.3%), followed closely by psychosocial and attitudinal concepts (n = 117; 78.0%), and behavioral aspects (n = 111; 74.0%). Affective components of physical literacy were present in the majority of the YouTube videos (n = 91; 60.7%), while the cognitive constructs were discussed in less than half of the videos (n = 67; 44.7%). Over half of the videos addressed these physical literacy domains in the context of unstructured play and physical activity (n = 84; 56.0%) with only 28 (18.7%) considering physical literacy in the context of structured sport and physical activity. The physical education space was the predominant context for 43.3% (n = 65) of the videos. Of the remaining 85 YouTube videos in which the information was presented outside the context of physical education, 38 (44.7%) were solely within the space of unstructured play, while one (1.2%) video focused only on structured sport. Thirty (35.3%) of these videos did not communicate information within the context of structured or unstructured play, while 16 (18.8%) videos considered both contexts.

Table 2. Frequencies of physical literacy content, topics, focus, and intent observed in sample of reviewed YouTube videos (n = 150).

Content & Focus Areas	n	Percentage
Properties of Physical Literacy		
Affective	91	60.7%
Confidence	87	58.0%
Motivation	68	45.3%
Self-Esteem	17	11.3%
Cognitive	67	44.7%
Knowledge/Understanding	64	42.7%
Value/Responsibility	37	24.7%
Physical	122	81.3%
Fundamental Movement Skills	112	74.7%
Competence	74	49.3%
Behavioral	111	74.0%
Health	57	38.0%
Physical Activity	109	72.7%
Psychosocial & Attitudinal	117	78.0%
Academic Performance	27	18.0%
Enjoyment	95	63.3%
Support	78	52.0%
Target Audiences		
Youth	133	88.7%
Adults	96	64.0%
None	5	3.3%
Contexts		
Physical Education	65	43.3%
Structured Sport	28	18.7%
Unstructured Sport	84	56.0%
Style of Content Delivery		
Animation	12	8.0%
Demonstration	74	49.3%
Presentation	56	37.3%
Testimonial	97	64.7%

The summation of content areas might add up to more than the number of videos in each properties because videos could contain more than one topic.

The media sources uploading these physical literacy videos to YouTube were diverse. The two largest media sources of content comprised almost two-thirds of the videos: user-generated (n = 47; 31.3%) and non-profit organizations (n = 46; 30.7%). Nearly one-third of the YouTube videos were uploaded by a government agency/organization (n = 18; 12.0%), while educational institutions posted only eight videos (5.3%). Regarding the audiences of the YouTube videos, over half (n = 84; 56%) portrayed physical literacy as a lifelong journey and were inclusive of both youth and adults. Forty nine (32.7%) videos specifically addressed physical literacy in youth, while only 12 (8%) were directed solely towards an adult population. Only five (3.3%) of the YouTube videos were judged to not have an intended audience.

2.3.1. Research Question 1: Is the Information Quality of YouTube Videos on Physical Literacy Associated with Viewer Attitudes?

Less than half of the YouTube videos were rated as being of high quality (n = 64; 42.7%), leaving the remaining 86 videos (57.3%) to be rated low quality. Principle #2, which requires videos to be clear in their mission to supplement and not replace information from certified/qualified educators and sources, was achieved by the most videos (n = 106; 70.7%). Principle #3, requiring videos to provide information and instruction in line with the most commonly accepted and understood conceptualizations of physical literacy, was the second most achieved (n = 91; 60.7%), while Principles #1 and #4, which required source information (n = 80; 53.3%) and credentials (n = 74; 49.3%), were each followed by nearly half of the videos. For further detail on the HONCode principles see Table A1. Results from the Mann-Whitney U test revealed a significant difference in the number of viewer likes given to low versus high quality YouTube videos, U = 3,377.50, z = 2.424, p = 0.015, r = 0.20, such that high quality videos, or those adhering to 4 or more adapted HONCode principles (Md = 3.00, n = 64), received more "likes" than low quality videos (Md = 1.00, n = 86).

2.3.2. Research Question 2: Does the Quality of Physical Literacy Information in the YouTube Videos Vary Based on Media Source?

Due to 4 of the 14 cells (28.6%) containing less than the expected count of 5, Fisher's exact test was conducted. The analysis revealed a statistically significant difference in adherence to the adapted HONCode principles based on the media source, Fisher's exact test = 39.36, p < 0.001. The greatest number of high quality videos, per adapted HONCode principles, were posted by non-profit organizations with 26 (56.5%). While this was just above half of the videos posted by such social media accounts, the largest proportion of high-quality videos were posted by professional associations (n = 12; 85.7%;). The vast majority of user-generated YouTube videos on physical literacy were of low-quality (n = 41; 87.2%).

2.3.3. Research Question 3a: Do the Content Properties in the YouTube Videos on Physical Literacy Influence the Quality of Information?

Binary logistic regression revealed that the physical literacy properties of the YouTube videos had a significant association with the quality of the videos, x^2 (5, N = 150) = 49.73, p < 0.001. The full model explained between 28.2% (Cox & Snell R square) and 37.9% (Nagelkerke R square) of the variance in quality, per the HONcode principles, correctly classified 72.7% of the videos. Table A2 shows that videos focused on physical activity behaviors were the strongest predictor of high quality ratings (Wald = 4.75, df = 1, 95% CI: 1.17–18.29, p = 0.029), with an odds ratio (OR) of 4.62. Videos containing affective content were also found to be a significant predictor (OR = 3.6) of a video being rated as high quality (Wald = 4.90, df = 1, 95% CI: 1.16–11.18, p = 0.027).

2.3.4. Research Question 3b: Do the Content Properties in the YouTube Videos on Physical Literacy Influence Viewer Attitudes?

Binary logistic regression revealed no significant findings regarding the influence of the physical literacy content properties and viewer attitudes.

2.3.5. Research Question 4a: Does the Content Delivery Style of the Physical Literacy YouTube Videos Influence the Quality of Information?

Binary logistic regression revealed that the delivery style on the YouTube videos' content had a significant impact on the quality of the videos, x^2 (4, N = 150) = 42.56, $p < 0.001$. The full model explained between 24.7% (Cox & Snell R square) and 33.2% (Nagelkerke R square) of the variance in quality, per the HONcode principles, correctly classifying 73.3% of the videos. Table A2 shows that videos delivering content using a presentation style were the strongest predictor (OR = 13.7) of a video achieving high quality status (Wald = 27.30, df = 1, 95% CI: 5.13–36.5, $p < 0.001$). Delivering content via testimonial style was also a significant predictor of a high quality video (Wald = 10.01, df = 1, 95% CI: 1.77–11.22, $p = 0.002$), with an OR of 4.5.

2.3.6. Research Question 4b: Does the Content Delivery Style of the Physical Literacy YouTube Videos Influence Viewer Attitudes?

The full model did not significantly explain any influence of the content delivery style of the physical literacy YouTube videos on viewer attitudes. However, videos delivering content through demonstration were found to be the strongest predictor, with an OR of 2.5, of viewers attitudes to "like" a video (Wald = 4.44, df = 1, 95% CI: 1.07–5.87, $p = 0.035$).

3. Discussion

The purpose of this study was to assess the content, exposure, engagement, and information quality of videos uploaded to YouTube, one of the most popular social media websites on the Internet [48]. More specifically, we sought to determine the qualities of videos as they relate to introducing, educating and serving the public as a shared resource(s) on physical literacy. What follows is a discussion of the results and implications of the data analysis.

3.1. Content and Delivery

When considering the value of physical literacy videos uploaded to YouTube, it is important to consider the content of said videos as well as the audience to whom the videos are directed. An overwhelming number of videos, 133, addressed physical literacy with consideration to youth while 96 targeted adults. This was an encouraging finding given that enhancing physical literacy should be a lifelong learning opportunity [63,64] that positively contributes to an enduring lifestyle of physical activity [56,65]. While physical literacy education and training seem inherently entangled in a pedagogical focus among physical educators [11,12], self-examination of one's movements and interaction with the environment and developing into a physically literate individual can take place in a variety of spaces, as evidenced by the diverse contexts in which the videos were recorded. Therefore, it is important for health and activity educators and practitioners, as well as individuals, to consider, communicate, and embrace physical literacy in the context of fluctuating environments during and well beyond youth.

Over half of the videos demonstrated the concept of physical literacy through unstructured play or free play. Unstructured play and/or activities typically occur as time permits, during which participants determine the rules, (dis)organization, as well as goals and intentions of their activities, play, and movement without the restrictions of developmental plans that may inhibit their expression and enjoyment [66]. The value of free or unstructured play is critical in the development of athletic skills, movement, health and physical activity [67,68] and can positively impact one's, particularly youth, progression toward becoming physically literate. Unfortunately, as evidenced by nearly one-third of the videos, physical literacy is often considered in the context of structured sport and physical activities or physical education sites. However, given that more videos placed physical literacy in the context of unstructured environments advocates for physical literacy as an individual lifelong journey. Thus, physical literacy instruction should reflect this journey by addressing physical pursuits and activities throughout the lifecourse, from early stages of physicality to adulthood [9]. As witnessed prior, the physical literacy videos posted on YouTube demonstrate this life course perspective of physical literacy, appropriately articulating and disseminating information to viewers as lifelong learners.

Given the breadth of one's lifelong progression towards physical literacy, a number of topics were presented in the YouTube videos on physical literacy. Being a construct largely focused on movement and one's ability to engage with the physical environment through a variety of movement forms, competencies and patterns [11,69], it was not surprising that most videos sought to educate viewers on elements of movement in the development of physical literacy. However, far too many videos failed to account for the wide array of physical skills and abilities that youth sport participants must masters. For physical literacy to advance towards becoming a universal health consideration for youth, one's subjective understanding of physical capacity to move must be considered. It is of likewise importance for physical educators and organizations to consider the factors that may hinder youth from becoming physically active. Thus, it becomes critical that physical literacy is understood as an individualized journey across one's life course as dictated by not only embodied interactions and potential, but also, institutional and structural constraints [8,70], many of which are not addressed when promoting physical literacy to youth.

The least focused on elements of physical literacy, although still present in over half of the videos, were those of affect and cognition. While not as salient as psychosocial and health-related behaviors, it is critical that video content focus more on the development of one's confidence, motivation, and especially self-esteem, as a lack any or all of these constructs may hinder one's disposition towards lifelong physical activity [8]. Likewise, when videos promote the continuing accumulation (or lack thereof) of physical literacy's affective and behavioral components, they begin to cultivate a foundation from which youth, in particular, can value and take personal responsibility for the lifetime and long-term positive impacts on a healthy lifestyle [9]. However, this is not to underscore our prior points concerning the relative power of embodied potential and structural constraints to the subsequent maintenance of physical literacy. Rather, to cultivate this foundation whereby individuals, especially youth, are provided the agency to lead physically active lives and henceforth internalize the value of such a lifestyle, is to stay vigilant. Along these same lines, the positive social aspects of physical literacy were evidenced in the videos. Content reinforced the development and strengthening of social networks and support systems through interactions with others, particularly in the formative years of children and adolescents, which is of vital importance [10].

3.2. Quality

Intended as a code of ethics, the comprehensive set of principles put forth by the HONcode benefits both users and managers of online content regarding objective, verifiable, ethical, transparent and trustworthy medical and health-related information. However, not even half of the videos were deemed to be of high quality, as providers of information may not have shared their health and education qualifications for providing such information or share the source from which they collected their information. Yet, the intended mission of many videos was simply to educate viewers, and as such, it was made clear that physical literacy information was being communicated in accordance with commonly accepted definitions or understandings and as a supplement, not a replacement, to the advice of a qualified physical education or health source. Regardless, as a result of these findings, it is suggested that developers and uploaders of YouTube videos on physical literacy better source their information and be more transparent with their credentials via disclaimers espousing the adherence to the HONcode.

Regarding the quality of information, it was discovered that the greatest proportion (85%) of high-quality videos belonged to professional associations, despite the largest number of high quality videos being posted by non-profit organizations. Further, the lowest number of high-quality videos were of the user-generated variety, who conversely, were also responsible for the highest number and greatest proportion of low-quality videos. This suggests not only the value that viewers place on reputable sources of information, but also the preference and trust they may have towards reputable professional and non-profit organizations. Given the scarcity of high-quality and excess of low-quality videos posted by individual YouTube users, it was promising to see the potential apprehension viewers might have towards sources of information coming from individuals and non-credentialed groups or organizations. Thus, when users are being instructed or advised to use YouTube for additional information, it is recommended that they be directed to physical literacy videos from reputable sources that post high quality videos.

Surprisingly, educational institutions posted only eight (5.3%) videos. This is troubling given the knowledge and research capabilities of people and working groups within such spaces. Furthermore, as a legitimate health outcome and antecedent, physical literacy serves as a cross-disciplinary interest in a number of related areas of study. However, it is rebranded so as to better fit the purpose and understanding within each discipline [71], adding further confusion to understanding and application within and among multiple fields of study [72]. Additionally, there exists an extensive number of characteristics said to be associated with physical literacy [73], which may be too numerous for a single educational entity to assume definitive expertise. To this point, institutions in Canada have combined efforts of multiple institutions to arrive at a consensus definition and develop curriculum and programming accordingly [73]. Educational institutions may also feel hesitant to create and upload physical literacy videos to YouTube due to the lack of academic curriculum that can appropriately teach physical literacy, per educational standards and expectations, to students and knowledge seekers that range in age, abilities, interest and learning styles [74,75]. Yet, as knowledge purveyors, it is incumbent upon academicians within these types of programs to share their information to a more diverse population of races, genders, age, and socioeconomic status. These efforts will ensure a more inclusive, physically literate society. For instance, Pew Research data suggests that Black youth are not only more frequent users of Internet and social media platforms, but also more likely to use smartphones for Internet access as compared to White youth [76]. However, while social media usage provides some benefits to teenagers, such as opportunities for interpersonal and individualized learning, increased social awareness, and greater digital literacy, Black youth continue to be subject to lower levels of digital literacy and technological skill development [77]. Taken together, physical literacy educators and researchers should view this disparity between digital media use and digital fluency as an opportunity to engage with and educate diverse viewers of online content and youth.

As it concerns the availability of online teaching and learning opportunities, as well as the sharing of knowledge and resources, there are several findings that speak to best practices for content and delivery of physical literacy videos on YouTube. Regarding the quality of videos, providing content in either a formal or informal presentation has the greatest association with adherence to the HONcode principles. As such, health-related information disseminated in this format is judged to be the most trustworthy and in accord with, yet not disparately impacted by, common physical literacy knowledge and trends. Similarly, physical literacy videos with personal testimonies could reach viewers in a more open and honest way, such that they are more likely to be deemed high quality than other content delivery methods. However, YouTube viewers were more than twice as likely to "like" videos in which the information was delivered as a demonstration or instruction. This is understandable given the large focus (122 videos) on physical abilities and FMS in this study's sample; as it is likely easier to understand and learn movement skills through visualizations including role models.

Lastly, videos that focused on the affective and behavioral components of physical literacy were judged as having the highest quality. Perhaps this has to do with the expertise warranted to speak appropriately and applicably on these components. This is not meant as a value judgment on the remaining core themes [10], but rather, these findings speak to the importance of understanding one's confidence, motivation, and self-esteem in relation to their level(s) of and behavior towards physical activity. One's mental health and physical well-being are not to be taken lightly, and speaking on the subject(s) requires a level of professionalism, knowledge and (possibly) credentials. The Internet is seemingly aware of this as uploaders of such content made sure they and their content were of high quality (e.g., ethical, trustworthy, transparent), affording them opportunities to speak to the affective and behavioral components that develop and facilitate a healthy and active lifestyle.

3.3. Study Limitations

Having to utilize YouTube's integrated search engine, there is a chance that relevant videos on the website were not included in this study. Likewise, not being privy to the procedures by which engagement and evaluative metrics are determined and measured, we had to rely on YouTube's controlled information in our assessment of physical literacy videos. Additionally, the information shared by uploaders of the videos was not always readily available or indicative of intentions leading to the creation and sharing of the physical literacy videos. Some of this limitation can be mitigated by collecting data on more videos and for a longer period of time. Other user metrics could also be collected to provide a more holistic view of user perceptions and quality of the uploaded videos. A longitudinal study in which viewer metrics are analyzed over a period of time could provide researchers and practitioners with better understandings of how and why videos trend, are sustained, and/or not viewed. Further, while this study was not limited to YouTube videos uploaded or viewed by users in a particular country, the use of the English language as inclusion criteria likely served to keep relevant, non-English speaking videos from being accounted for and coded.

From a design standpoint, several of the content and delivery coding procedures could serve to limit the interpretation of results. First, the coding of the content delivery style was not mutually exclusive. For instance, developers of a video could utilize both animation and presentation styles to send their message. Similarly, when considering the context of the videos (athletic or education, structured vs unstructured), both styles of play could be present in the videos, which could also be set in both environments. Thus, it is important to delve further into the role of structured vs unstructured play in both athletic and education contexts. Additionally, simply coding data collected from uploaded YouTube videos provides a limited perspective on site as an information resource for physical literacy. Future studies would benefit from taking a behavioral approach and collect self-reported data from watchers of the uploaded videos and users of YouTube to gain a stronger sense of their perceptions of the video website as an information resource.

Although well accepted by many organizations, the instrument is not without its shortcomings. As a self-regulatory tool that relies on codes of ethics, the HONcode may be limited in the sense that "self-regulation does not deter the unscrupulous, those who mostly need to have their ethical standards raised [78] (p. 236)". Specifically, it has been noted that studies utilizing HONcode reported incorrect data as it concerned criteria adherence and assessment [79–81]. Nevertheless, we submit said limitations of the HONcode principles, for instance, to be less a reflection of the instrument as an unfit measure of ensuring high ethical standards and more so the result of either limited accountability or a lack thereof on the part of web sites engaged in distributing health-related content. While the purview of the present study is narrower in that it is centered on content distribution by way of video, we believe the merits of the HONcode principles, as opposed to similarly constructed instruments, to be in alignment with the purposes of this study.

4. Conclusions

As researchers and practitioners alike, we must continue to concern ourselves with the quality of health-related information available on the Internet, particularly YouTube, and other social media outlets. As it relates to online information resources and videos for physical literacy, it is critical to keep in mind who is watching these videos, how the information is being conveyed, in what context is it delivered, if is it influenced by a particular type of curricula (i.e., educational), and whether or not consideration was made towards certain socio-demographic factors and inclusivity. Lastly, what are the social determinants of physical literacy for youth? While the aforementioned list of considerations is by no means an exhaustive list, it challenges us to be mindful of the many intersecting factors that may not only be impacting one's ability to become physically literate, but also the content, delivery, and quality of the resources intended to foster physical literacy in the first place. This study revealed that the content and content delivery method were most important in quality evaluations. Physical literacy videos that focused on physical activity and behaviors were the strongest predictor of high quality ratings, followed closely by videos covering affective domains (motivation, confidence, and self-esteem) of physical, literacy. The content delivery method was also important, with videos utilizing presentations and testimonials containing high quality information about physical literacy. Thus, providers of physical literacy and health-related online video content should be aware of and adhere to the expected quality standards.

The Internet is a resourceful educational space for health-related information and content [82,83]. Understanding physical literacy as a lifelong health-related outcome and facilitator of an active lifestyle, we sought to assess the content, exposure, engagement, and information quality of uploaded physical literacy video discussions, presentations, demonstrations and tutorials made available through YouTube. Our findings were encouraging in that they suggest the online physical literacy community has a desire for quality physical literacy information and content. Likewise, our findings speak to the quality standards expected of providers of health-related online video content. As expectations and ethical standards increase, the Internet, and specifically YouTube, has the potential to enhance video resources, virtual networking opportunities, as well as the sharing, dissemination, accumulation, and enrichment of physical literacy information for all.

Author Contributions: Individual contributions were as follows: conceptualization, T.B., J.D.V., and M.W.; methodology, T.B., J.D.V., and M.S.; validation, T.B., J.D.V., M.S., and M.W.; formal analysis, T.B. and M.S.; data curation, T.B., J.D.V. and M.W.; writing—original draft preparation, T.B. and J.D.V.; writing—review and editing, T.B., J.D.V. and M.S.; project administration, T.B.

Funding: This research received no external funding.

Conflicts of Interest: The authors declare no conflict of interest.

Appendix A

Table A1. Adapted HONcode principles rating information quality in sample of reviewed YouTube videos (n = 150).

Number	Description of Criteria	Video Adherence	
		n	Percentage
1	The video provides physical education or health-related information and/or advice given by professionals or organizations whose qualifications/training are displayed. A disclaimer must be made whenever physical education or health-related information and/or advice is offered by a non-qualified source.	80	53.3%
2	The intended mission of the video is to provide information that supports the development and/or self-management of the physically literate individual. If/when applicable, a disclaimer must be made indicating that any information presented within the video is not meant to complement or replace the advice of a qualified physical education or health source.	106	70.7%
3	The notion of physical literacy must be found in accordance with commonly accepted definitions, as per qualified health and physical education professionals and organizations. For instance, SHAPE America accepts the following definition of physical literacy as "the ability to move with competence and confidence in a wide variety of physical activities in multiple environments that benefit the healthy development of the whole person."	91	60.7%
4	For information presented in the video, a HTML link or bibliographic reference to external source data is provided. Additionally, the video makes readily accessible external source data, contact information, and/or an external link to a web site for further inquiry.	74	49.3%

Table A1. Cont.

Number	Description of Criteria	Video Adherence	
		n	Percentage
5	Information provided in the video respects the privacy and confidentiality of all featured presenters, participants, and other individuals.	16	10.7%
6	For commercial or non-commercial organizations, as well as personal or private web sites, the source of either funds or materials presented in the video are clearly disclosed.	63	42.0%

Table A2. Associations between Video Quality, Likes, Style of Delivery, and Physical Literacy Properties ($N = 150$).

Style of Delivery & Content Properties	High Quality n (%)	Low Quality n (%)	OR (95% CI)	p Value	Liked n (%)	Not Liked n (%)	OR (95% CI)	p Value
Animation								
Yes	4 (2.7)	8 (5.3)	2.12 (0.47, 9.49)	0.327	8 (5.3)	4 (2.7)	1.52 (0.37, 6.32)	0.564
No	60 (40)	78 (52)			96 (64)	42 (28)		
Demonstration								
Yes	26 (17.3)	48 (32)	1.43 (0.60, 3.40)	0.424	57 (38)	17 (11.3)	2.5 (1.07, 5.87)	0.035 *
No	38 (25.3)	38 (25.3)			47 (31.3)	29 (19.3)		
Presentation								
Yes	40 (26.7)	16 (10.7)	13.68 (5.13, 36.5)	0.000 ***	41 (27.3)	15 (10)	1.78 (0.75, 4.26)	0.194
No	24 (16)	70 (46.7)			63 (42)	31 (20.7)		
Testimonial								
Yes	47 (31.3)	50 (33.3)	4.46 (1.77, 11.22)	0.002 **	62 (41.3)	35 (23.3)	0.59 (0.26, 1.35)	0.212
No	17 (11.3)	36 (24)			42 (28)	11 (7.3)		
Affective Properties								
Addressed	56 (37.3)	35 (23.3)	3.60 (1.16, 11.18)	0.027 *	65 (43.3)	26 (17.3)	0.48 (0.16, 1.46)	0.198
Not Addressed	8 (5.3)	51 (34)			39 (26)	20 (13.3)		
Cognitive Properties								
Addressed	43 (28.7)	24 (16)	1.42 (0.55, 3.66)	0.465	50 (33.3)	17 (11.3)	1.45 (0.55, 3.80)	0.454
Not Addressed	21 (14)	62 (41.3)			54 (36)	29 (19.3)		
Physical Properties								
Addressed	62 (41.3)	60 (40)	2.91 (0.54, 15.65)	0.213	90 (60)	32 (21.3)	2.43 (0.84, 7.08)	0.103
Not Addressed	2 (1.3)	26 (17.3)			14 (9.3)	14 (9.3)		
Behavioral Properties								
Addressed	61 (40.7)	50 (33.3)	4.62 (1.17, 18.29)	0.029 *	82 (54.7)	29 (19.3)	1.66 (0.60, 4.56)	0.328
Not Addressed	3 (2)	36 (24)			22 (14.7)	17 (11.3)		
Psychosocial & Attitudinal Properties								
Addressed	57 (38)	60 (40)	1.58 (0.53, 4.75)	0.415	84 (56)	33 (22)	1.51 (0.61, 3.73)	0.372
Not Addressed	7 (4.7)	26 (17.3)			20 (13.3)	13 (8.7)		

Notes: * $p < 0.05$, ** $p < 0.01$, *** $p < 0.002$.

References

1. Centers for Disease Control and Prevention. Healthy Places: Physical Activity. Available online: https://www.cdc.gov/healthyplaces/healthtopics/physactivity.htm (accessed on 3 July 2019).
2. Centers for Disease Control and Prevention. Healthy Schools: Physical Activity Facts. Available online: https://www.cdc.gov/healthyschools/physicalactivity/facts.htm (accessed on 3 July 2019).
3. Ferraro, K.F.; Kelley-Moore, J.A. Cumulative disadvantage and health: Long-term consequences of obesity? *Am. Sociol. Rev.* **2003**, *68*, 707–729. [CrossRef] [PubMed]
4. Robinson, L.E.; Stodden, D.F.; Barnett, L.M.; Lopes, V.P.; Logan, S.W.; Rodrigues, L.P.; D'Hondt, E. Motor competence and its effect on positive developmental trajectories of health. *Sports Med.* **2015**, *45*, 1273–1284. [CrossRef] [PubMed]
5. Centers for Disease Control and Prevention. Healthy Schools: Childhood Obesity Facts. Available online: https://www.cdc.gov/healthyschools/obesity/facts.htm (accessed on 3 July 2019).
6. Malina, R.M. Top 10 research questions related to growth and maturation of relevance to physical activity, performance, and fitness. *Res. Q. Exerc. Sport* **2014**, *85*, 157–173. [CrossRef] [PubMed]
7. International Physical Literacy Association. Homepage; International Physical Literacy Association. Available online: https://www.physical-literacy.org.uk/ (accessed on 3 July 2019).

8. Whitehead, M. *Physical Literacy: Throughout the Lifecourse*; Routledge: New York, NY, USA, 2010.
9. Whitehead, M. The history and development of physical literacy. *J. Sport Sci. Phys. Educ.* **2013**, *65*, 22–28.
10. Edwards, L.C.; Bryant, A.S.; Keegan, R.J.; Morgan, K.; Jones, A.W. Definitions, foundations and associations of physical literacy: A systematic review. *Sports Med.* **2017**, *47*, 113–126. [CrossRef] [PubMed]
11. Durden-Myers, E.J.; Green, N.R.; Whitehead, M.E. Implications for promoting physical literacy. *J. Teach. Phys. Educ.* **2018**, *37*, 262–271. [CrossRef]
12. Flemons, M.; Diffey, F.; Cunliffe, D. The role of PETE in developing and sustaining physical literacy informed practitioners. *J. Teach. Phys. Educ.* **2018**, *37*, 299–307. [CrossRef]
13. Stoddart, A.L.; Humbert, M.L. Physical literacy is … ? What teachers really know. *Revue PhénEPS/PHEnex J.* **2017**, *8*, 1–20.
14. Wartella, E.; Rideout, V.; Montague, H.; Beaudoin-Ryan, L.; Lauricella, A. Teens, health, and technology: A national survey. *Media Commun.* **2016**, *4*, 12–23. [CrossRef]
15. Madathil, K.C.; Rivera-Rodriguez, A.J.; Greenstein, J.S.; Gramopadhye, A.K. Healthcare information on YouTube: A systematic review. *Health Inform. J.* **2015**, *21*, 173–194. [CrossRef]
16. Murugiah, K.; Vallakati, A.; Rajput, K.; Sood, A.; Challa, N.R. YouTube as a source of information on cardiopulmonary resuscitation. *Resuscitation* **2011**, *82*, 332–334. [CrossRef] [PubMed]
17. Sood, A.; Sarangi, S.; Pandey, A.; Murugiah, K. YouTube as a source of information on kidney stone disease. *Urology* **2011**, *77*, 558–562. [CrossRef] [PubMed]
18. Stellefson, M.; Chaney, B.; Ochipa, K.; Chaney, D.; Haider, Z.; Hanik, B.; Chavarria, E.; Bernhardt, J.M. YouTube as a source of chronic obstructive pulmonary disease patient education: A social media content analysis. *Chronic Respir. Dis.* **2014**, *11*, 61–71. [CrossRef] [PubMed]
19. Paige, S.R.; Stellefson, M.; Chaney, B.H.; Alber, J.M. Pinterest as a resource for health information on Chronic Obstructive Pulmonary Disease (COPD): A social media content analysis. *Am. J. Health Educ.* **2015**, *46*, 241–251. [CrossRef]
20. Stellrecht, E. Pinterest interest: Converting a consumer health guide Wiki into a Pinterest page. *J. Consum. Health Internet* **2012**, *16*, 403–408. [CrossRef]
21. Paige, S.R.; Stellefson, M.; Chappell, C.; Chaney, B.H.; Chaney, J.D.; Alber, J.M.; Barry, A. Examining the relationship between online social capital and eHealth literacy: Implications for Instagram use for chronic disease prevention among college students. *Am. J. Health Educ.* **2017**, *48*, 264–277. [CrossRef]
22. Stellefson, M.; Paige, S.R.; Apperson, A.; Spratt, S. Social media content analysis of public diabetes Facebook groups. *J. Diabetes Sci. Technol.* **2019**, *13*, 428–438. [CrossRef]
23. Gagnon, K.; Sabus, C. Professionalism in a digital age: Opportunities and considerations for using social media in health care. *Phys. Ther.* **2015**, *95*, 406–414. [CrossRef]
24. Goodyear, V.A.; Armour, K.M. What young people tell us about health-related social media and why we should listen. In *Young People, Social Media and Health*; Goodyear, V.A., Armour, K.M., Eds.; Routledge: New York, NY, USA, 2019; pp. 1–20.
25. Frith, E. Social Media and Children's Mental Health: A Review of the Evidence. 2017. Available online: https://epi.org.uk/wp-content/uploads/2018/01/Social-Media_Mental-Health_EPI-Report.pdf (accessed on 2 September 2019).
26. Third, A.; Bellerose, D.; Oliveira, J.D.D.; Lala, G.; Theakstone, G. *Young and Online: Children's Perspectives on Life in the Digital Age*; Western Sydney University: Sydney, Australia, 2017.
27. Goodyear, V.A.; Armour, K.M.; Wood, H. Young people and their engagement with health-related social media: New perspectives. *Sport Educ. Soc.* **2019**, *24*, 673–688. [CrossRef]
28. Highfield, T.; Leaver, T. Instagrammatics and digital methods: Studying visual social media, from selfies and GIFs to memes and emoji. *Commun. Res. Pract.* **2016**, *2*, 47–62. [CrossRef]
29. Dudley, D.A.; Van Bergen, P.; McMaugh, A.; Mackenzie, E. The role of social media in developing young people's health literacy. In *Young People, Social Media and Health*; Goodyear, V.A., Armour, K.M., Eds.; Routledge: New York, NY, USA, 2019; pp. 147–161.
30. Cale, L. Young people, social media, physical activity, and health: Final thoughts on the work, the present, and the future. In *Young People, Social Media and Health*; Goodyear, V.A., Armour, K.M., Eds.; Routledge: New York, NY, USA, 2019; pp. 212–224.
31. Alfrey, L.; Cale, L.; Webb, L. Physical education teachers' continuing professional development in health related exercise. *Phys. Educ. Sport Pedagog.* **2012**, *17*, 477–491. [CrossRef]

32. Cale, L.; Harris, J.; Duncombe, R. Promoting physical activity in secondary schools. Growing expectations: Same old issues. *Eur. Phys. Educ. Rev.* **2016**, *22*, 526–544. [CrossRef]
33. Casey, A.; Goodyear, V.A.; Armour, K.M. Rethinking the relationship between pedagogy, technology and learning in health and physical education. *Sport Educ. Soc.* **2017**, *22*, 288–304. [CrossRef]
34. Yildirim, M.; Uslu, S. Investigation of reasons of social media usage of physical education and sports school students. *Int. J. High. Educ.* **2018**, *7*, 129–138. [CrossRef]
35. Sun, H.; Gao, Z.; Zeng, N. Overview: Promoting physical activity and health through emerging technology. In *Technology in Physical Activity and Health Promotion*; Gao, Z., Ed.; Routledge: London, UK, 2017; pp. 26–45.
36. Armour, K.M.; Casey, A.; Goodyear, V. A pedagogical cases approach to understanding digital technologies and learning in physical education. In *Digital Technologies and Learning in Physical Education: Pedagogical Cases*; Casey, A., Goodyear, V.A., Armour, K.M., Eds.; Routledge: New York, NY, USA, 2016; pp. 1–12.
37. Kirk, D. School physical education and learning about health: Pedagogical strategies for using social media. In *Young People, Social Media and Health*; Goodyear, V.A., Armour, K.M., Eds.; Routledge: New York, NY, USA, 2019; pp. 86–100.
38. Awidi, I.T.; Paynter, M.; Vujosevic, T. Facebook group in the learning design of a higher education course: An analysis of factors influencing positive learning experience for students. *Comput. Educ.* **2019**, *129*, 106–121. [CrossRef]
39. Barrot, J.S. Facebook as a learning environment for language teaching and learning: A critical analysis of the literature from 2010 to 2017. *J. Comput. Assist. Lear.* **2018**, *34*, 863–875. [CrossRef]
40. Espinosa, L.F. The use of Facebook for educational purposes in EFL classrooms. *Theor. Pract. Lang. Stud.* **2015**, *5*, 2206–2211. [CrossRef]
41. Zhang, N.; Tsark, J.; Campo, S.; Teti, M. Facebook for health promotion: Female college students' perspectives on sharing HPV vaccine information through Facebook. *Hawaii J. Med. Publ. Health* **2015**, *74*, 136–140.
42. Kite, J.; Foley, B.C.; Grunseit, A.C.; Freeman, B. Please like me: Facebook and public health communication. *PLoS ONE* **2016**, *11*, e0162765. [CrossRef]
43. Shaw, J.M.; Mitchell, C.A.; Welch, A.J.; Williamson, M.J. Social media used as a health intervention in adolescent health: A systematic review of the literature. *Digit. Health* **2015**, *1*, 1–10. [CrossRef]
44. Keelan, J.; Pavri-Garcia, V.; Tomlinson, G.; Wilson, K. YouTube as a source of information on immunization: A content analysis. *JAMA* **2007**, *298*, 2482–2484. [CrossRef] [PubMed]
45. Syed-Abdul, S.; Fernandez-Luque, L.; Jian, W.S.; Li, Y.C.; Crain, S.; Hsu, M.H.; Wang, Y.C.; Khandregzen, D.; Chuluunbaatar, E.; Nguyen, P.A.; et al. Misleading health-related information promoted through video-based social media: Anorexia on YouTube. *J. Med. Internet Res.* **2013**, *15*, e30. [CrossRef] [PubMed]
46. Akagi, C. YouTube? For health education? *Am. J. Health Educ.* **2008**, *39*, 58–60. [CrossRef]
47. Dogtiev, A. Business of Apps YouTube Revenue and Usage Statistics. Available online: http://www.businessofapps.com/data/youtube-statistics/ (accessed on 7 January 2019).
48. Maina, A. Small Business Trends 20 Popular Media Sites Right Now. Available online: https://smallbiztrends.com/2016/05/popular-social-media-sites.html (accessed on 6 June 2018).
49. Teens, Social Media and Technology 2018. Available online: https://www.pewinternet.org/2018/05/31/teens-social-media-technology-2018/ (accessed on 31 May 2018).
50. Social Media Use in 2018. Available online: http://www.pewinternet.org/2018/03/01/social-media-use-in-2018/ (accessed on 1 March 2018).
51. Liu, Y. Social media tools as a learning resource. *J. Educ. Technol. Dev. Exchang.* **2010**, *3*, 101–114. [CrossRef]
52. Petruscu, P. Google Organic Click-Through Rates in 2014. Available online: https://moz.com/blog/google-organic-click-through-rates-in-2014 (accessed on 1 October 2014).
53. Bernstam, E.V.; Shelton, D.M.; Walji, M.; Meric-Bernstam, F. Instruments to assess the quality of health information on the World Wide Web: What can our patients actually use? *Int. J. Med. Inform.* **2005**, *74*, 3–9. [CrossRef] [PubMed]
54. Fahy, E.; Hardikar, R.; Fox, A.; Mackay, S. Quality of patient health information on the Internet: Reviewing a complete and evolving landscape. *Australas Med. J.* **2014**, *7*, 4–8. [CrossRef]
55. Laversin, S.; Baujard, V.; Gaudinat, A.; Simonet, M.; Boyer, C. Improving the transparency of health information found on the internet through the HONcode: A comparative study. *Stud. Health Technol.* **2011**, *169*, 654–658.

56. Pletneva, N.; Cruchet, S.; Simonet, M.; Kajiwara, M.; Boyer, C. Results of the 10th HON survey on health and medical internet use. *Stud. Healt Technol.* **2011**, *169*, 73–77.
57. Gabarron, E.; Fernandez-Luque, L.; Armayones, M.; Lau, A.Y.S. Identifying measures used for assessing quality of YouTube videos with patient health information: A review of current literature. *Interact. J. Med. Res.* **2013**, *2*, e6. [CrossRef]
58. Lacy, S.; Riffe, D. Sampling error and selecting intercoder reliability samples for nominal content categories. *J. Mass Commun. Q.* **1997**, *73*, 963–973. [CrossRef]
59. McHugh, M.L. Interrater reliability: The kappa statistic. *Biochem. Med.* **2012**, *22*, 276–282. [CrossRef]
60. IBM Corp. *IBM SPSS Statistics for Windows, Version 25.0*; IBM Corp: Armonk, NY, USA, 2017.
61. Lin, L.I.-K. A concordance correlation coefficient to evaluate reproducibility. *Bioemtrics* **1989**, *45*, 255–268. [CrossRef]
62. Garcia-Granero, M. Lin's Concordance Correlation Coefficient (Correlation Coefficient with Small Sample). Available online: purabuana.wordpress.com/2009/02/20/lins-concordance-correlation-coefficient-correlation-coefficient-with-small-sample/ (accessed on 9 September 2019).
63. Lundvall, S. Physical literacy in the field of physical education—A challenge and a possibility. *J. Sport Health Sci.* **2015**, *4*, 113–118. [CrossRef]
64. Whitehead, M. Physical literacy: Philosophical considerations in relation to developing a sense of self, universality and propositional knowledge. *Sports Ethic Philos.* **2007**, *1*, 281–298. [CrossRef]
65. Roetert, E.P.; MacDonald, L.C. Unpacking the physical literacy concept for K—12 physical education: What should we expect the learner to master? *J. Sport Health Sci.* **2015**, *4*, 108–112. [CrossRef]
66. Gadbois, S.; Bowker, A.; Rose-Krasnor, L.; Findlay, L. A qualitative examination of psychologically engaging sport, non-sport, and unstructured activities. *Sport Psychol.* **2019**, *33*, 97–109. [CrossRef]
67. Herrington, S.; Brussoni, M. Beyond physical activity: The importance of play and nature-based play spaces for children's health and development. *Curr. Obes. Rep.* **2015**, *4*, 477–483. [CrossRef] [PubMed]
68. Sagas, M. *What Does the Science Say About Athletic Development in Children?* The Aspen Institute Sports & Society Program: Washington, DC, USA, 2013.
69. Murdoch, E.; Whitehead, M.E. Physical literacy, fostering the attributes and curriculum planning. In *Physical Literacy: Throughout the Lifecourse*; Whitehead, M.E., Ed.; Routledge: London, UK, 2010; pp. 175–188.
70. Hylton, K. Physical literacy, 'race' and the sociological imagination. *J. Sport Sci. Phys. Educ.* **2013**, *65*, 223–227.
71. Lounsbery, M.A.F.; McKenzie, T.L. Physically literate and physically educated: A rose by any other name? *J. Sport Health Sci.* **2015**, *4*, 139–144. [CrossRef]
72. Lynch, T.; Soukup, G.J. "Physical education", "health and physical education", "physical literacy" and "health literacy": Global nomenclature confusion. *Cogent Educ.* **2016**, *3*, 1217820. [CrossRef]
73. Corbin, C.B. Implications of physical literacy for research and practice: A commentary. *Res. Q. Exerc. Sport* **2016**, *87*, 14–27. [CrossRef] [PubMed]
74. Silverman, S.; Mercier, K. Teaching for physical literacy: Implications to instructional design and PETE. *J. Sport Health Sci.* **2015**, *4*, 150–155. [CrossRef]
75. Haydn-Davies, D. Physical literacy and learning and teaching approaches. In *Physical Literacy*; Whitehead, M., Ed.; Routledge: London, UK, 2010; pp. 185–194.
76. Lenhart, A. Teens, Social Media & Technology Overview 2015. Available online: https://www.pewinternet.org/2015/04/09/teens-social-media-technology-2015/ (accessed on 5 July 2019).
77. Tichavakunda, A.A.; Tierney, W.G. The "wrong" side of the divide: Highlighting race for equity's sake. *J. Negro Educ.* **2018**, *87*, 110–124. [CrossRef]
78. Hanif, F.; Read, J.C.; Goodacre, J.A.; Chaudhry, A.; Gibbs, P. The role of quality tools in assessing reliability of the internet for health information. *Inform. Health Soc. Care* **2009**, *34*, 231–243. [CrossRef] [PubMed]
79. Barker, S.; Charlton, N.P.; Holstege, C.P. Accuracy of internet recommendations for prehospital care of venomous snake bites. *Wilderness Environ. Med.* **2010**, *21*, 298–302. [CrossRef] [PubMed]
80. Parvizi, M.; Talai, N.N.; Parvizi, Z. Quality of healthcare information on the internet: The case of Apicectomies. *Oral Surg.* **2017**, *10*, e35–e39. [CrossRef]
81. Meric, F. Breast cancer on the World Wide Web: Cross sectional survey of quality of information and popularity of websites. *BMJ* **2002**, *934*, 577–581. [CrossRef] [PubMed]

82. Atkinson, N.; Saperstein, S.; Pleis, J. Using the Internet for health-related activities: Findings from a national probability sample. *J. Med. Internet Res.* **2009**, *11*, e4. [CrossRef] [PubMed]
83. Wimble, M. Understanding health and health-related behavior of users of Internet health information. *Telemed. J. E Health* **2016**, *22*, 809–815. [CrossRef]

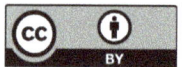

© 2019 by the authors. Licensee MDPI, Basel, Switzerland. This article is an open access article distributed under the terms and conditions of the Creative Commons Attribution (CC BY) license (http://creativecommons.org/licenses/by/4.0/).

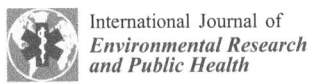

Article

Effect of Emotion, Expectation, and Privacy on Purchase Intention in WeChat Health Product Consumption: The Mediating Role of Trust

Ming-Yan Wang [1], Peng-Zhu Zhang [2,*], Cheng-Yang Zhou [1] and Neng-Ye Lai [1]

1. Department of Information Management, Management School, Shanghai University of Engineering Science, Shanghai 201620, China; wmycindy2020@126.com (M.-Y.W.); 13916826525@163.com (C.-Y.Z.); 15157107949@126.com (N.-Y.L.)
2. Department of Management Information System, AnTai College of Economics & Management, Shanghai Jiao Tong University, Shanghai 200030, China
* Correspondence: pzzhang@sjtu.edu.cn

Received: 4 August 2019; Accepted: 20 September 2019; Published: 12 October 2019

Abstract: With the aging of the population and the upgrading of the consumption structure of national health demand in China, it has become a new trend for the public to actively seek health products and services on social networks. Based on the theory of reasoned behavior and the theory of expectancy confirmation, this study aims to analyze the cognitive factors and their effects on WeChat users' purchase intention in the process of health product consumption. Considering that safety is a key feature of health products that distinguishes them from other consumer products, the "satisfaction" concept in the expectancy confirmation model is replaced by "trust" in this study. Two hundred and two (202) valid samples were collected by a questionnaire survey to analyze their intentions to buy health products on WeChat. Theoretical models and corresponding research hypotheses were verified by structural equation modeling. The research results show that emotional price and emotional experience are positively correlated with trust and purchase intention. There is an obvious negative correlation between privacy invasion and trust. Expectation confirmation is positively associated with trust. Moreover, the intermediary test shows that trust has completely mediated between emotional price and purchase intention, and trust also has a full intermediary effect on expectation confirmation and purchase intention.

Keywords: healthy consumption; purchase intention; trust; emotional support; expectation confirmation; privacy concern

1. Introduction

With the growth of urbanization and industrialization in China, the impacts on residents' lifestyle, ecological environment and food safety on health are gradually becoming apparent. Adolescent sub-health aging and chronic diseases have become urgent public health problems which could hinder the improvement of the health level of Chinese residents. Meanwhile, with the increase of disposable income of Chinese residents, the public's health awareness is also increasing, and the consumption and demand for health services are also gradually improving. How to meet the needs of public healthcare management and promote the development of the health industry has become an inevitable requirement for the sustainable and healthy development of the economy and society. According to the implementation of the "Healthy China Strategy", China's health care industry has been further promoted. In the new situation, the "Chinese-style health industry system" has been restructured, and the health care industry is the whole healthy chain guided by the new objective of improving people's health literacy, accepting scientific health guidance and reasonable health consumption. The health care industry involves many productions and service fields closely related to human health, and it has become an emerging industry with huge market opportunities. Consumption of health-related has become the mainstream consumption trend in China and the world. Conventional health products include medical products, health care products, nutrition products, healthcare management. A broader range of health products also includes functional food and nutritional food. The Chinese public is actively developing a healthy lifestyle and actively seeking health-related products and medical services through the Internet. With the development of mobile commerce, health products have been sold on the WeChat platform since 2014.

The combination of the Internet and the health care industry is an inevitable trend of today's development. Online health consumption could increase consumers' medical knowledge and more access to medical information, meanwhile, it also promotes health care quality [1,2]. Through network information technology, healthcare management services can be better provided for the public. Mobile commerce technology based on Web 2.0 plays a key role in the field of mobile health(m-health) and promotes the mobile socialization of healthcare management [3,4]. Digital media can provide users to find health information and potentially improve the chances of finding health content [5]. Users can obtain health information and purchase health products on the WeChat platform. According to the 39th report on China's Internet Network Information Center (CNNIC), as of December 2016, the scale of internet medical users was 195 million, accounting for 26.6% of online users, with an annual growth rate of 28.0% in China. Online counseling and online purchasing of health products and services account for about 6 percent of internet users [6].

The application of Internet and mobile application technology in healthcare management will have a great impact on consumers' health cognition and behavior. Consumers' health needs will affect their purchase intentions, emotional responses, and preferences of health products. Health-conscious consumers are more concerned about their healthy diet, so they actively change their health behaviors, for example, by being more willing to buy organic food [7]. Nowadays, social networks play an important role in health care. The web-based social health system can provide opportunities to expand medical knowledge and increase participation in individual healthcare management [8]. Health behaviors based on the social network are mainly health information seeking and health-related social support [9]. Health behaviors on social networks are related to emotional support and health self-efficacy, emotional support is the most common dimension in the Facebook environment [10]. Social relationships established in cyberspace can readily provide the public with self-managed medical staff, disease information and emotional support [11,12]. Emotional support is an emotional response to the experience of using products and services [13]. Customers' perception of service quality and service environment will have an impact on their emotional satisfaction, which will also change their beliefs and attitudes, and then affect their decisions [14,15]. Consumers' trust tendency, personal privacy concerns, website information quality, and brand reputation may all affect consumers' purchase intention of mobile commerce [16,17]. Health products such as nutritional supplement have a good reputation for corporate social responsibility, consumers will generate positive emotions and increase their willingness to buy healthy products [18,19].

The studies have clearly indicated that there is a relationship between the intention of buying health products and cognition of emotion. The process of changing consumers' attitudes towards products or brands also reflects their emotional reactions [20]. It is found that adding emotional attributes to brand marketing can increase consumers' participation and perceived differentiation, thus enhancing the stability of consumers' choice. Emotions in shopping online process of consumers include happiness, awakening, and domination, these emotions will have an impact on consumers' purchasing behavior before cognition [21]. If consumers can choose the product conveniently through the website functionality and have fun in the process of use and achieve the expected effect, these experience will stimulate their positive emotions, otherwise, it will cause negative effects [14,22]. Emotional design of products mainly starts from consumers' experience level and emotional needs. Emotional design is an important aspect of new product development, and it is also important to improve customer satisfaction with new products [23]. In the context of online consumption, sensory information generated by emotional design will have a significant impact on consumers' attitudes and preferences [24].

Trust seems to be a more critical factor of any high involvement in online consumption [25]. The online health community has become a valuable platform for patients to communicate and find support. However, health products of the network context cannot be tested online, so it would have a negative impact on trust in their purchasing decision [26]. Online consumers' perceived trust or risk can have a significant impact on their purchasing decisions, moreover, online consumers' perceived risks of products and web vendors have almost the same effect on trust [27]. Moreover, it is found that trust plays a fully mediating role in the relationship between perceived corporate reputation and purchase intention [28].

Many companies use information technology to process and mine consumer information to improve customer satisfaction, but sometimes these interventions can cause privacy concerns [29,30]. With the development of online healthcare management, social media could collect and store more information about users, the potential privacy threat brought by system insecurity is considered to be the invasion of users' privacy [31,32]. In recent years, a variety of mobile health apps have been installed on smartphones for users to use. Previous studies have found that users worry about apps collecting personal health and activity information [33,34]. People rarely share health information with their friends, they don't want health information to be accessed by third parties [35]. Moreover, privacy concerns can reduce trust and enhance risk awareness, thus indirectly affecting users' willingness to use information system [35,36].

Users will have initial expectations on products and services before a purchase. If perceived value and satisfaction increase, consumers' purchase intention will also increase [37]. Based on the expectation-confirmation theory, the positive expectation is positively correlated with satisfaction, and positive expectation will also increase the post-usage benefits [38]. Expectation confirmation could affect the willingness to use information system continuously through perceived availability and system satisfaction [39]. Perceived usefulness and perceived value will have an impact on mobile app stickiness and purchase intention, [40,41]. In the process of network business, if the perception of product experience or product usefulness is far lower than the expectation, then the satisfaction of consumers will be reduced [42,43].

WeChat has become the central hub of China's mobile network. WeChat is a network of strong emotional relationships, which could establish various relationships, such as classmates, colleagues, and friends. WeChat has become an emerging business platform for Chinese medical and health industry and even overseas purchasing and marketing of health products. Due to the strong relationship between users in social networks, the emotional and cognitive involvement of users in social networks will raise the purchase intention of recommended products in the circle of friends [44]. This shows that how to consider the emotional needs of consumers, increase the sense of trust, and promote the consumption of health products is a new problem worth studying in the WeChat strong relationship circle. In the pages that follow. This study will analyze how the cognitive behavior of Chinese users using WeChat affects their intention of healthy consumption. In this paper, health products on WeChat Commerce system studied in this article refer to the broad definition of the term, such as traditional Chinese and Western medicines (over the counter medicines), health therapy, health care underwear and weight loss, nutritional products, functional foods and so on. The emotional support involved in this paper is mainly the emotional response generated by users when they use WeChat social media service. Considering that the safety of health products is more important than other products, the trust might better express consumers' emotional cognition than satisfaction. Based on the Theory of Reasoned Action (TRA) and the Theory of Expectancy Confirmation (ECT), this paper establishes a cognition-trust-intention theoretical model. Data from the study were collected from WeChat users who had purchased health products. The theoretical model and corresponding research hypothesis are tested by structural equation modeling to explore the cognitive factors and influencing mechanism of users' purchase intention. It is hoped that this research will make a contribution to a deeper insight into the purchasing behavior of health products in social networks through empirical and theoretical research. It could improve the competitiveness of pharmaceutical enterprises to some extent and bring new impetus to the promotion of public healthcare management.

2. Research Hypothesis and Theoretical Model

2.1. Emotional Support and Purchase Intention

Rational and emotional factors for products or services play an important role in purchasing decision [45]. Emotional support in a social commerce environment allows consumers to actively overcome difficulties and seek answers to their inner perceptions of sellers, products or services, therefore, consumers may have a desire to purchase [46]. If consumers form emotional cognition in the social and business environment, it may have an impact on consumers' purchasing decisions [47]. Some studies found that the sensory design of products and brand experience will affect consumers' perception and will trigger participation in purchasing in decision-making [48,49]. In the online process of pharmaceutical sales, the main reasons for users to buy medicines online are price and convenience [50]. Moreover, consumers' pre-sale and after-sales service experience have a significant positive correlation with satisfaction and repurchase intention [51]. Emotional support can also influence the willingness to buy health products of WeChat. Based on the research reviewed, the study will attempt to verify this fact by the following hypotheses:

Hypotheses 1 a (H 1a.) *Emotion price is positively associated with purchase intention.*

Hypotheses 1 b (H 1b.) *Emotion product is positively associated with purchase intention.*

Hypotheses 1 c (H 1c.) *Emotion experience is positively associated with purchase intention.*

2.2. Emotional Support and Trust

Emotional support affects the formation of trust in social commerce [52,53]. Moreover, emotional support may significantly affect relationship satisfaction and trust [54]. The packaging design of products will affect consumers' health perception and judgment of product function and value [55,56]. Consumers' perception of the effectiveness and good experience in business systems will affect their attitudes and willingness to actively seek for disease information and accomplish healthcare management on the Internet [57,58]. Moreover, the response time, service content and interaction depth on the online medical platform will affect the trust and satisfaction of consumers on the online medical treatment [59]. Therefore, this study proposes the following hypotheses:

Hypotheses 2 a (H 2a.) *Emotion price is positively associated with trust.*

Hypotheses 2 b (H 2b.) *Emotion product is positively associated with trust.*

Hypotheses 2 c (H 2c.) *Emotion experience is positively associated with trust.*

2.3. Privacy Concern and Trust

Privacy is an important factor for users to accept using the information system for healthcare management services. Consumers regard disclosure of privacy without consent will decrease trust and make them no longer anonymous [60,61]. In particular, medical information is considered to be very sensitive personal information. Once private information is disclosed, it will threaten the data integrity and security of users, which may lead to malicious attacks on users [62]. Network users have certain expectations for network privacy, especially for the protection of information from unknown third parties [63,64]. In social networks, disclosure of private information will affect the trust of users, therefore, people will develop an attitude of resistance when they perceive that their privacy and freedom are controlled by others [65,66].

Consumer acceptance of mobile shopping applications can be affected by location sensitivity and risk [67]. Scholars have not conducted in-depth studies on the privacy factors of the WeChat. But "LBS+" opened a new model of WeChat marketing. The function of "find peoples nearby" may also be used by businesses to advertise for free, which may generate the disclosure of personal information at the same time. Based on previous research and the characteristics of privacy concern between the WeChat platform, this study defines that the privacy concern in the marketing process of WeChat health products is mainly affected by three factors: (1) Perceived monitoring refers to personal concerns that the WeChat system may monitor private information such as location or mobile phone; (2) Perceived intrusion refers to the concern of users that their privacy is received by too many business applications or illegally acquired by third-party platforms in the business process; (3) Information disclosure refers to user's concern that their privacy may be used for other business purposes without permission. Thus, the following three hypotheses were developed:

Hypotheses 3 a (H 3a.) *Perceived monitoring is negatively associated with trust.*

Hypotheses 3 b (H 3b.) *Perceived intrusion is negatively associated with trust.*

Hypotheses 3 c (H 3c.) *Perceived information disclosure is negatively associated with trust.*

2.4. Expectation Confirmation and Trust

Some studies show that when a trusted party demonstrates a level of reliability consistent with consumer expectations, consumers' trust will increase, moreover, consumers' willingness to buy products is mainly driven by perceived value, trust, and satisfaction [68,69]. Consumer trust is a prerequisite for establishing an online market for healthy products such as green products and nutrition, which have an important influence on purchasing decisions [70,71]. Consumers' perceived trust and expectation confirmation have an important impact on consumers' purchase intention, and a significant positive correlation is found between consumers' trust and expectation [72,73]. Based on the above discussions, hypothesis 4 is stated as:

Hypotheses 4 (H 4.) *Expectation confirmation is positively associated with trust.*

2.5. Trust and Purchase Intention

Based on the theory of organizational trust, the establishment of organizational trust in the context of e-commerce will affect purchase intention [74]. Organizational trust is meaningful to the establishment of economic relations between unfamiliar parties, which will maintain a significant supportive impact on consumers' purchase intention [75]. Trust in social networking sites (SNS) would increase the need for information seeking, which in turn increases the familiarity and social presence of the platform [76]. When consumers decide to provide private information on social media platforms, their trust mainly depends on the credibility of merchants [77]. Accordingly, this paper proposes that:

Hypotheses 5 (H 5.) *Trust in the process of consumers' purchase intention is positively associated with consumers' purchase intention.*

2.6. The Mediating Role of Trust Between Emotional Support and Purchase Intention

Network trust in e-commerce has a significant relationship with perceived privacy, perceived service quality and repurchase intention [78]. The enterprises could strengthen users' trust in their brands through emotional input, which had a positive impact on users' purchase intention [79]. In order to meet a higher level of consumer demand, emotional experience and product packaging play an increasingly effect on purchasing decisions [24]. At the same time, website content and website sex will have an impact on network user trust, and trust in the effectiveness of network marketing shows an intermediary function [80]. Product information, quality, and price in product attributes have a supportive effect on purchase intention [81]. So, the paper will verify the facts with the following hypotheses:

Hypotheses 6 a (H 6a.) *An intermediary effect of trust is shown between emotion price and its purchase intention.*

Hypotheses 6 b (H 6b.) *An intermediary effect of trust is shown between emotion product and its purchase intention.*

Hypotheses 6 c (H 6c.) *An intermediary effect of trust is shown between emotion experience and its purchase intention.*

2.7. Expectation Confirmation and Purchase Intention

Expectation confirmation plays important roles in purchasing behavior. Expectation confirmation and perceived value will significantly affect consumers' purchasing decisions [82]. When consumers buy a product for the first time, their purchase decision is based on the expectation created by the brand and packaging design of the product, or the previous experience of the relevant product [83,84]. By actively assuming social responsibilities, enterprises will improve consumers' expectation identification of enterprises and enhance their willingness to buy relevant products [85]. Accordingly, we propose that:

Hypotheses 7 (H 7.) *Expectation confirmation is positively corrected with consumers' purchase intention.*

2.8. The Mediating Role of Trust Between Expectation Confirmation and Purchase Intention

To improve online transactions, online retailers need to focus on measures to build and maintain consumer trust. The role of expectation shows a positive correlation with consumer trust [86,87]. In the electronic market, consumers make purchasing decisions based on trust and expectation of products or enterprises [70,88]. The quality of products and purchasing experience of online retailers will gain confidence in products and generate a sense of trust [89].

Referring to the preceding research, the following hypothesis is proposed for this study:

Hypotheses 8 (H 8.) *An intermediary effect of trust is shown between expectation confirmation and purchase intention.*

2.9. Proposed Model

The model of this study is proposed by referring to the theory of reasoned action and the theory of expectancy confirmation, which combines with previous studies and the definition of the above hypotheses. In this study, emotional support, privacy concern, expectation confirmation are taken as an independent variable, consumer trust is taken as an intermediary variable, and consumers' purchase intention is chosen as a dependent variable (Figure 1).

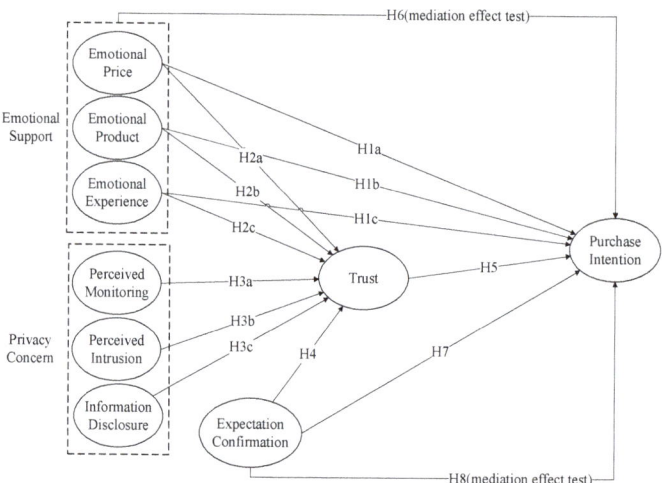

Figure 1. Theoretical model and hypotheses.

3. Method

3.1. Questionnaire Design and Analysis Method

This paper uses a 5-point Likert scale. In the design of the questionnaire survey. The verification of each variable should be measured using a minimum of three items to ensure the rationality of the questions [90]. Moreover, when factor analysis and structural equation model are carried out, the measurement items corresponding to each variable are less than 3, which may lead to unsatisfactory structural validity. The specific measurement questions about the questionnaire variables are summarized in Table 1. In the following research, variable names are abbreviated for ease of expression and calculation as shown in Table 1.

Table 1. Summary of specific measurement questions of questionnaire variables.

Variable/Abbreviation		Descriptive	Adapted From:
Emotional Support (ES)	Emotion Price (EP1)	Q1(EP1)- The product price is in line with my psychological price in online shopping.	Lee (2017) [81] Brijnath (2015) [50]
		Q2(EP1)- I will pay attention to promotions and discounts information in online shopping.	
		Q3(EP1)- I can discuss the product price with the seller in online shopping.	
	Emotion Product (EP2)	Q1(EP2)- The packaging and design of online products have a strong sensory impact on customers.	Pentus (2014) [24] Lee (2018) [49]
		Q2(EP2)- The packaging and design of online products deliver the value of the brand.	
		Q3(EP2)- Packaging and design of online products make me feel healthy.	
	Emotion Experience (EE)	Q1(EE)-The navigation of the application in the WeChat interface is clear and easy to understand.	Park (2012) [51] Hwang (2010) [47]
		Q2(EE)-The function of the WeChat enables me to accomplish a shopping task more quickly than other ways of shopping.	
		Q3(EE)- Customer services on WeChat are friendly and can solve my doubts.	
Privacy Concern (PC)	Perceived Monitoring (PM)	Q1(PM)- This system could monitor my location through my purchasing behavior.	Dienlin (2015) [91] Henke (2018) [92]
		Q2(PM)- The system could collect too much personal information from transactions.	
		Q3(PM)- This system could monitor the usage of my mobile phone. through my purchasing behavior.	
	Perceived Intrusion (PI1)	Q1(PI1)- I am afraid that others get more my privacy through this system than they are allowed.	James (2017) [93] Demmers (2018) [29]
		Q2(PI1)- I would be concerned that the information transmitted through online transactions could be intercepted by third parties.	
		Q3(PI1)- I would be worried about the security of the system by hackers login access to my personal data.	
	Information Disclosure (ID)	Q1(ID)- I could be concerned that the system may use private information for other purposes without authorization.	Kim (2008) [17] Yoonhyuk (2018) [61] Hallikainen (2018) [78]
		Q2(ID)- I could be concerned about the system selling private information to others without permission.	
		Q3(ID)- I could be worried that the system will share my private information with others without my authorization.	
	Expectation Confirmation (EC)	Q1(EC)- My experience in using this system was better than what I had expected.	Bhattacherjee (2001) [94]
		Q2(EC)- The product and service provided by this system were better than what I had expected.	
		Q3(EC)- Overall, most of my expectations from using this system were confirmed.	
	Trust (T)	Q1(T)- The interface design of the system is clear, professional and distinct, which will give customers a real feeling.	Kim (2012) [73] Oghuma (2016) [95]
		Q2(T)- Sellers actively maintain communication with customers, which reflects the importance of customers.	
		Q3(T)- WeChat system can share the information of buyers' feedback on products, which makes me feel credible.	
	Purchase Intention (PI)	Q1(PI)- I am likely to purchase the products on this business system.	Lankton (2014) [43] Fang (2014) [74]
		Q2(PI)- I am likely to recommend this bustiness system to my friends.	
		Q3(PI)-I am likely to make repurchase from this system.	

Structural equation modeling can estimate the relationships between multiple and interrelated variables. This method has the ability to deal with unobservable assumptions in the model, such as trust, expectation and other variables that cannot be directly measured. It can also analyze the structural relationships between potential factors. In this study, the method was used to examine the relationship between emotional support (ES), privacy concern (PC), expectation confirmation (EC), trust (T), and purchase intention (PI).

3.2. Profiling of the Sample

The main purpose of this study is to analyze the influence of individual purchase behaviors of health products on purchase intention in social networks. This study analyzes consumers with WeChat mobile network-shopping experience. A total of 212 questionnaires were collected in the form of paper and online questionnaires. There were 202 valid questionnaires, and the effective rate of questionnaires was 95.3%. A total of 89 male samples (44.1%) was collected from the survey and female samples were 113 (55.9%). From the age of the interviewed groups, users aged 20–31 accounted for 76.7% of the total number of surveyed users, and social media services have a higher penetration rate among the young user groups. In terms of education level, 96.5% of the respondents have a bachelor degree or above. The age distribution, education level and economic status of the population in this study can significantly reduce the number of variables introduced in the model, which is conducive to the establishment of a simplified analysis model.

4. Results

4.1. Reliability and Validity Test of the Questionnaire

According to the results of Table 2, the square root of AVE of the latent variables is higher than the correlation coefficient between various factors, which proves that the questionnaire about WeChat users' intention to buy health products has a good discriminant [96].

Table 2. Discriminant validity test.

Item	EP1	EP2	EE	PM	PI1	IL	EC	T	PI
EP1	0.742								
EP2	0.609	0.801							
EE	0.647	0.732	0.777						
PM	0.137	0.210	0.192	0.767					
PI1	0.019	0.090	0.141	0.568	0.805				
IL	0.165	0.219	0.243	0.621	0.735	0.871			
EC	0.616	0.632	0.584	0.024	−0.580	0.019	0.843		
T	0.705	0.626	0.584	−0.019	−0.019	−0.110	0.717	0.794	
PI	0.674	0.579	0.579	−0.027	−0.151	0.008	0.670	0.709	0.769

Note: Off-diagonal: correlation estimated between the factors. Diagonal (bold): square root of AVE. The abbreviations for variables are defined in Table 1.

Cronbach alpha coefficient was used to test the reliability of the questionnaire. According to the calculation, the Cronbach alpha coefficients of all variables were greater than 0.7, indicating that the reliability of the questionnaire was good (see the results in Table 3).

In terms of validity, we conducted an exploratory factor analysis on the questionnaire and found that KMO = 0.897 and sig = 0.000, which is suitable for factor analysis. We used AMOS25 for confirmatory factor analysis and found that the factor loads of all variables were greater than 0.5, CR > 0.7, and AVE > 0.5 indicating good validity of the questionnaire (see the results in Table 3).

Table 3. Reliability and validity test.

Variable	Cronbach α	Factor Loading	C.R.	AVE
EP1	0.781	0.699 0.842 0.719	0.7853	0.5504
EP2	0.835	0.880 0.666 0.842	0.8416	0.6423
EE	0.820	0.755 0.790 0.787	0.8208	0.6044
PM	0.804	0.672 0.865 0.750	0.8087	0.5876
PI1	0.801	0.871 0.861 0.667	0.8451	0.6483
ID	0.899	0.954 0.797 0.854	0.9034	0.7581
EC	0.829	0.807 0.877 0.825	0.8304	0.7104
T	0.889	0.732 0.817 0.830	0.8363	0.6307
PI	0.861	0.820 0.761 0.723	0.8124	0.5914

Note: AVE is the average variance extracted. C.R. is the composite reliability. The abbreviations for variables are defined in Table 1.

4.2. Model Fit

Table 4 shows that the indexes of the model meet the requirements, and the fitting is reasonable.

Table 4. Model fitting parameters.

Index	Model Value	Recommended Value	Acceptance
X^2/df	3.548	<3 good fit <5 reasonable fit	reasonable
RSMEA	0.091	<0.05 good fit, <0.1 reasonable fit	reasonable
SRMR	0.086	<0.05 good fit, <0.1 reasonable fit	reasonable
NFI	0.862	Close to 1	reasonable
CFI	0.928	Close to 1	good
IFI	0.831	Close to 1	reasonable
AIC	702.000	the smaller the better	reasonable
ECVI	7.852	the smaller the better	reasonable

Note: RMSEA is the root mean square error of approximation. SRMR is the standardized root mean square residual. NFI is the normed fit index. CFI is the comparative fit index. IFI is the incremental fit index. AIC is the Akaike information criterion. ECVI is the expected cross-validation index.

4.3. Second-Order Factor Analysis

The concept of Emotion Support (ES) in the social network services is constructed from three dimensions: Emotional Price (EP1), Emotional Product (EP2), and Emotional Experience (EE). The concept of Privacy Concern (PC) in the social network services is constructed from three dimensions: Perceived Monitoring (PM), Perceived Intrusion (PI1), and Information Disclosure (ID). Figures 2 and 3 show that all the factor load greater than 0.7, which means the constructions of Emotion Support (ES) and Privacy Concern (PC) are reasonable.

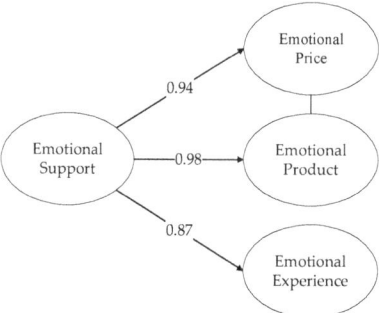

Figure 2. Emotion Support (ES).

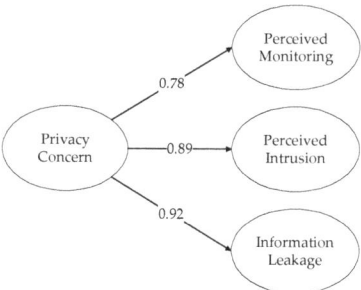

Figure 3. Privacy Concern (PC).

4.4. Structural Model Relationships Analysis

According to the Table 5, we found that emotional price and emotional experience can positively predict consumers' purchase intention, but the emotional product and purchase intention are negatively correlated, thus H1a and H1c are verified, and H1b is not supported. Then, emotional price and emotional experience can positively predict consumers' trust, but cannot show the relationship between emotional product and trust, thus H2a and H2c are verified, and H2b is not supported.

We also found that perceived intrusion is negatively associated with trust. The experiment shows that there is no significant influence between perceptual monitoring and trust. There was no positive effect between information disclosure and trust. Thus H3b is verified, and H3a and H3c are not supported. Studies have shown that expectation confirmation has a positive correlation with consumers' trust. However, it is not associated with consumers' purchase intention. Thus H4 is verified, and H8 is not supported. Finally, trust is positively associated with consumers' purchase intention, thus H5 is supported.

Table 5. Structural model relationships obtained.

Hypothesis	Estimate	C.R.	p-Value	Results
H1a:EP1 => PI	0.211	2.288	*	Supported
H1b:EP2 => PI	−0.153	−2.545	*	Not supported
H1c:EE => PI	0.173	2.448	*	Supported
H2a:EP1 => T	0.366	5.305	***	Supported
H2b:EP2 => T	0.083	1.619	0.106	Not supported
H2c:EE => T	0.142	2.407	*	Supported
H3a:PM => T	−0.021	−0.326	0.744	Not supported
H3b:PI1 => T	−0.276	−3.299	***	Supported
H3c:ID => T	−0.037	−0.645	0.519	Not supported
H4:EC => T	0.472	6.183	***	Supported
H5:T => PI	0.855	4.810	***	Supported
H7:EC => PI	0.100	0.946	0.344	Not supported

Note: * $p < 0.05$, ** $p < 0.01$, *** $p < 0.001$. C.R. is the composite reliability.

4.5. Mediation Test

We did the mediating test with Amos25, using 2500 resampling bootstrapping and the results are shown in Table 6. The indirect effects of emotional price on purchase intention via the trust are significant (0.313, $p = 0.008 < 0.01$), and the direct effects of emotional price on purchase intention are not significant (0.211, $p = 0.416 > 0.01$), which means that trust fully mediates the effect of emotional price on purchase intention. Thus, H6a is supported. The indirect effects of emotional products (0.071, $p = 0.449 > 0.01$) and emotional experience (0.122, $p = 0.140 > 0.01$) on purchase intention via the trust are not significant, which suggests they have no mediation effect. Thus, H6b and H6c are not supported. The indirect effects of expectation confirmation on purchase intention via trust are significant (0.403, $p = 0.014 < 0.05$), and the direct effects of expectation confirmation on purchase intention are not significant (0.100, $p = 0.584 > 0.01$), which means that trust fully mediates the effect of expectation confirmation on purchase intention. Thus, H8 is verified.

Table 6. Mediation test obtained.

Hypothesis	Indirect	Direct	Total	Mediation
H6a:EP1=> T => p	0.313 **	0.211 (NS)	0.525 ***	Supported (Fully mediation)
H6b:EP2=> T => p	0.071 (NS)	−0.153 (NS)	−0.082 (NS)	Not supported
H6c:EE=> T => p	0.122 (NS)	0.173 (NS)	0.195 (NS)	Not supported
H8:EC => T=> p	0.403 *	0.100 (NS)	0.504 **	Supported (Fully mediation)

Note: * $p < 0.05$, ** $p < 0.01$, *** $p < 0.001$.

4.6. Calculation Results of the Model

After calculation and arrangement, the model test diagram can be obtained (see the results in Figure 4).

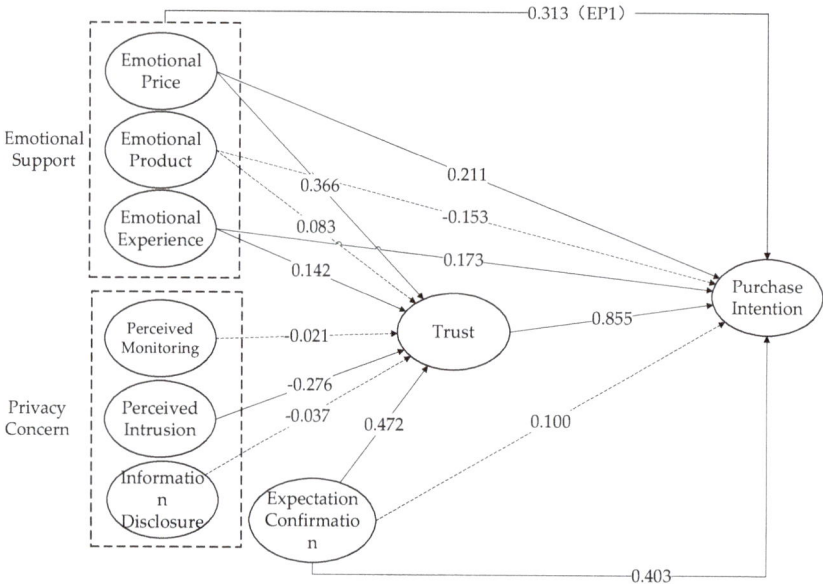

Figure 4. Model test diagram.

5. Discussion

According to the hypothesis test of WeChat emotional support on trust, the following conclusions are drawn. Firstly, WeChat emotional price and emotional experience have a significant positive correlation with consumer trust. The hypotheses H1a, H1c, H2a, and H2c are supported, which also confirm the previous studies which found the main reasons for users to buy medicines online are price and convenience [48,50,51]. These results suggest that a product price strategy might improve consumers' trust in products or enterprises. The improvement of product price strategy based on the WeChat platform could encourage consumers to establish a trust in enterprise product information, so as to enhance consumers' purchase intention. Consumers' emotional experience could also affect their purchase intention. Therefore, enterprises should improve the timeliness and effectiveness of WeChat system communication. At the same time, enterprises might strengthen the information quality of WeChat health products, optimize the operation interface of WeChat, and give full play to the emotional support effect of WeChat in healthcare management.

In the study, WeChat emotional products are negatively associated with purchase intention and it has nothing to do with consumer trust. It might mean that consumers' trust in products does not come from the exquisite packaging and design of products. Moreover, the better the packaging and design of products, the lower the purchase intention of consumers. This finding in the paper contradicts the results of previous research. Previous studies have shown that sensory experience of online products will affect purchasing behavior [37,38]. A previous study has also found that food packaging design will affect consumers' preferences and purchase intention [97]. One possible explanation is that the packaging design of products would have different effects on consumers' purchasing intentions due to the functions of different products. Moreover, the interviews and data of this research come from the purchasing experience of Chinese social network consumers. In recent years, health products including traditional Chinese medicine have also been sold on WeChat social network. Health products emphasize the special features of product safety and effectiveness. The packaging and design of products are not the focus of consumers buying health products online. Therefore, if enterprises invest too much in the packaging design of healthy products, it may cause the aversion of consumers.

Consumers may think that companies should spend less on improving the health and treatment effectiveness of their products. Therefore, this may lead to a decline in consumers' willingness to purchasing. This further suggests that Chinese consumers will be more willing to recognize and buy products from traditional Chinese medicine companies that are more than 100 years old, rather than emerging pharmaceutical companies. As a result, the new finding also indicates that the research result of this paper is a beneficial supplement to the research on the purchase intention behavior of network products.

The research finds that privacy invasion is negatively correlated with trust. It indicates that trust might reduce when users perceive the risk of invasion in the business system. After consumers register as system users, they hope that the information registered in the system can not release. This means that enterprises should strengthen security guarantees in health trading system to avoid personal information obtained by an unknown party. At the same time, the results of this paper show that perception monitoring and perception information disclosure will not affect the trust of users, which is contrary to the previous hypothesis. In China, the public might not be aware of the protection of personal privacy information and pays little attention to privacy. On the one hand, Chinese netizens might believe that private security comes more from the security guarantee provided by the registered business system. Therefore, the privacy invasion has a negative correlation with trust. On the other hand, in the use of mobile social services, people's positive perception of the usefulness of products and systems is much higher than their negative perception of privacy concerns. Hence, consumers would like to risk their privacy for a better online shopping experience.

Expectation confirmation is the perception that a user's expectations which is consistent with the reality of using social media services. If an individual expectation matches the actual performance of WeChat service, it would increase the trust of users and thus increase the purchase intention. In the study, the expectation confirmation has a significant positive effect on trust, and users with higher trust will have stronger purchase intention. The conclusion of this study might indicate that health services based on WeChat should also attach importance to the target of customer expectation, continuously improve user trust, and thus enhance user stickiness.

This paper verifies that trust fully mediates the relationship between emotional price and purchase intention. However, no evidence shows that trust plays a mediating role between emotional products and purchase intention. In the test, the mediating effect of trust between emotional experience and purchase intention is not verified. These results may be interpreted by the fact that the cognitive behavior of buying health products online is really different from other products. Because health products are very important to personal health and even life safety. So, buying health products on the WeChat platform, trust is particularly important for purchase intention. Meanwhile, trust plays a complete mediating role between expected confirmation and purchase intention. When consumers' expectation of products is consistent with reality, consumers' trust in products might be enhanced, and their purchase intention will also be enhanced. The findings confirm that consumers' trust in health products is also a psychological expectation, such as the efficacy, safety, and authority of health products. Therefore, emotional marketing will enhance the trust of consumers and enhance corporate reputation and brand identity.

6. Conclusions

In China, mobile social media has been widely used in the field of health product consumption, which has had an impact on netizens' healthy behaviors. Social media marketing of medical care products can play an active role in promoting public health. It can not only achieve precision marketing, improve the brand awareness of health products, but also play a positive role in personalized health care management. The social network platform represented by WeChat has a profound impact on public healthcare management. To sum up, this paper analyzes the status of China's health industry in the new media economic context. With a view to the emotional and cognitive needs of WeChat consumers, the influence model of purchase intention of health products was constructed. This study analyzes how emotional support, expectation confirmation, privacy concern, and trust have an effect on consumers' purchase intention in WeChat. It can be seen from this study that attaching importance to users' emotional support, providing a safe private environment and improving expectations for healthcare management is the basis for the long-term development of social media healthcare management on social media.

Firstly, the academic significance of this study lies in: the "satisfaction" in the expectancy confirmation model is replaced by "trust" because consumers buy health products, trust can better express the recognition of the quality and brand of health products than satisfaction. Moreover, the test of intermediate variables in this paper also proves that emotional input and meeting consumers' expectations for products will be conducive to the establishment of consumers' trust and thus affect their purchase intention. This also shows that trust as a mediator variable is appropriate in this article. In addition, the influence relationship between expectation confirmation and trust in this paper is consistent with that of previous scholars [72,73].

Secondly, this paper analyzes the influence of emotional price, emotional products and emotional experience on trust and purchase intention. It is worth noting that the results of emotional products of this study are different from previous studies. We find that emotional products are negatively correlated with purchase intention and it has no impact on consumer trust. The reasons for this contradiction may be as follows: (1) The research object of this paper is online health products sold on social media. Due to different characteristics from other online products of the previous study, respondents in this study could pay more attention to the treatment and health care effect of health products. Therefore, the design and packaging of health products have different influences on consumers' purchasing intention than other online products. (2) The purchase habits and social consumption culture of the respondents in the study are different. The respondents of this study are consumers of Chinese social network, who expect more effect of product treatment and health care than product packaging design.

Thirdly, this paper examines the sufficient mediating effect of trust in emotional price and purchase intention and the sufficient mediating effect of trust in expectation confirmation and purchase intention. The test of the intermediate variable also proves that enterprises' emotional input and meeting consumers' expectations for products are conducive to the establishment of consumer trust [79]. Therefore, the results of the study further verified the improved model in this paper that replacing the mediating variable with trust instead of satisfaction variable would be more in line with consumer' cognitive needs of buying health products online. Previous studies have shown that emotional experience and packaging design of products have an increasing influence on trust and purchase [24]. However, this paper finds that trust does not mediate between emotional products, emotional experience, and purchase intention. So, the results also show that the cognitive behavior of buying online health products is indeed different from other online products. Consumers may pay special attention to the expected efficacy of healthy products, and their purchase intention may be more influenced by the price and expectation of products (to some extent, the price represents the research and development investment of healthy products). In contrast, it is difficult to build consumer trust in healthy products of packaging design and emotional experience.

The study further verifies the applicability of privacy concern scale in China's mobile network. Another important finding is that Chines consumers seem not to pay that much attention to privacy concerns, only when they perceive that privacy information has been intruded will their trust in products be reduced. Previous studies have shown that privacy information disclosure will cause customer dissatisfaction and distrust [46,47]. We think there may be two reasons for this: (1) In China, netizens' awareness of privacy protection is not strong, which leads to the fact that even if personal information is leaked, people will not care too much about it. (2) The existence of the privacy paradox, when people want to obtain certain benefits, they can allow their private information to be disclosed [98]. Therefore, in order to buy health products and obtain better service experience, people are willing to accept a certain degree of privacy disclosure. On the whole, our research reflects Chinese netizens' attitudes towards privacy concerns.

Moreover, there are still other factors that could affect consumer behavior. Follow-up studies can further explore whether there are other mediating variables besides trust in WeChat healthy consumption, so as to have a more comprehensive understanding of healthy consumption behavior of consumers. In recent years, the online family health market in China has been developing rapidly. Meanwhile, the post-90s generation attaches more importance to their healthcare management [99]. Therefore, in the follow-up research, we try to take online family health consumers as the research object and use big data technology to accurately analyze the trend and group behavior characteristics of family health consumption. With the growth of the Internet, the post-90s generation has become the main force of online consumption, and they have a stronger sense of responsibility for themselves and their families. In the follow-up research, we can try to add responsibility as an intermediary variable to further fully understand the influence of online healthy consumers' rational cognition on consumption behavior.

Despite these inherent limitations, the healthcare industry will be the most important increment in China in the future. The medical and health industry constructed by social media has gradually formed an important environment for health communication and healthy consumption. In order for the public to fully enjoy the benefits of the digital health industry, health service providers must give priority to issues related to trust. Trust is a key way to promote public acceptance of health services and purchase of health products on the Internet.

Author Contributions: M.-Y.W.—Conceptualization, analysis, draft, revision, and approval of the final draft. P.-Z.Z.—Conceptualization, revision, and approval of the final draft. C.-Y.Z.—Investigation, analysis, data curation draft, revision. N.-Y.L.—Resources, analysis, draft, revision.

Funding: This research was funded by the National Social Science of China (17BGL159), as well as the NSFC grant (91646205).

Conflicts of Interest: The authors declare no conflict of interests.

References

1. Xiang, J.; Stanley, S.J. From online to offline: Exploring the role of e-health consumption, patient involvement, and patient-centered communication on perceptions of health care quality. *Comput. Hum. Behav.* **2017**, *70*, 446–452. [CrossRef]
2. Adibi, S. *Mobile Health: A Technology Road Map*; Springer Series in Bio-/Neuroinformatics; Springer International Publishing: Cham, Australia, 2015; Volume 5, ISBN 978-3-319-12816-0.
3. Hunt, D.; Koteyko, N.; Gunter, B. UK policy on social networking sites and online health: From informed patient to informed consumer? *Digit. Health* **2015**, *1*, 205520761559251. [CrossRef] [PubMed]
4. Silva, B.M.C.; Rodrigues, J.J.P.C.; de la Torre Díez, I.; López-Coronado, M.; Saleem, K. Mobile-health: A review of current state in 2015. *J. Biomed. Inform.* **2015**, *56*, 265–272. [CrossRef] [PubMed]
5. Dobransky, K.; Hargittai, E. Inquiring Minds Acquiring Wellness: Uses of Online and Offline Sources for Health Information. *Health Commun.* **2012**, *27*, 331–343. [CrossRef] [PubMed]
6. China Internet Network Information Center. *The 39th China Statistical Report on Internet Development in China*; China Internet Network Information Center: Beijing, China, 2017.
7. Rana, J.; Paul, J. Consumer behavior and purchase intention for organic food: A review and research agenda. *J. Retail. Consum. Serv.* **2017**, *38*, 157–165. [CrossRef]
8. Grosberg, D.; Grinvald, H.; Reuveni, H.; Magnezi, R. Frequent Surfing on Social Health Networks is Associated with Increased Knowledge and Patient Health Activation. *J. Med. Internet Res.* **2016**, *18*, e212. [CrossRef] [PubMed]
9. Kim, W.; Kreps, G.L.; Shin, C.-N. The role of social support and social networks in health information–seeking behavior among Korean Americans: A qualitative study. *Int. J. Equity Health* **2015**, *14*, 40. [CrossRef]
10. Oh, H.J.; Lauckner, C.; Boehmer, J.; Fewins-Bliss, R.; Li, K. Facebooking for health: An examination into the solicitation and effects of health-related social support on social networking sites. *Comput. Hum. Behav.* **2013**, *29*, 2072–2080. [CrossRef]
11. Benetoli, A.; Chen, T.F.; Aslani, P. Consumer Health-Related Activities on Social Media: Exploratory Study. *J. Med. Internet Res.* **2017**, *19*, e352. [CrossRef]

12. Allen, C.; Vassilev, I.; Kennedy, A.; Rogers, A. Long-Term Condition Self-Management Support in Online Communities: A Meta-Synthesis of Qualitative Papers. *J. Med. Internet Res.* **2016**, *18*, e61. [CrossRef]
13. Westbrook, R.A.; Oliver, R.L. The Dimensionality of Consumption Emotion Patterns and Consumer Satisfaction. *J. Consum. Res.* **1991**, *18*, 84. [CrossRef]
14. Ladhari, R.; Souiden, N.; Dufour, B. The role of emotions in utilitarian service settings: The effects of emotional satisfaction on product perception and behavioral intentions. *J. Retail. Consum. Serv.* **2017**, *34*, 10–18. [CrossRef]
15. Li, H.; Sarathy, R.; Xu, H. The role of affect and cognition on online consumers' decision to disclose personal information to unfamiliar online vendors. *Decis. Support. Syst.* **2011**, *51*, 434–445. [CrossRef]
16. Mohd Suki, N.; Mohd Suki, N. Modeling the determinants of consumers' attitudes toward online group buying: Do risks and trusts matters? *J. Retail. Consum. Serv.* **2017**, *36*, 180–188. [CrossRef]
17. Kim, D.J.; Ferrin, D.L.; Rao, H.R. A trust-based consumer decision-making model in electronic commerce: The role of trust, perceived risk, and their antecedents. *Decis. Support. Syst.* **2008**, *44*, 544–564. [CrossRef]
18. Coleman, K.L.; Miah, E.M.; Morris, G.A.; Morris, C. Impact of health claims in prebiotic-enriched breads on purchase intent, emotional response and product liking. *Int. J. Food Sci. Nutr.* **2014**, *65*, 164–171. [CrossRef] [PubMed]
19. Peloza, J.; Ye, C.; Montford, W.J. When Companies Do Good, Are Their Products Good for You? How Corporate Social Responsibility Creates a Health Halo. *J. Public Policy Mark.* **2015**, *34*, 19–31. [CrossRef]
20. Buchanan, L.; Kelly, B.; Yeatman, H. Exposure to digital marketing enhances young adults' interest in energy drinks: An exploratory investigation. *PLoS ONE* **2017**, *12*, e0171226. [CrossRef]
21. Richard, M.-O.; Chebat, J.-C. Modeling online consumer behavior: Preeminence of emotions and moderating influences of need for cognition and optimal stimulation level. *J. Bus. Res.* **2016**, *69*, 541–553. [CrossRef]
22. Albrechtsen, E. A qualitative study of users' view on information security. *Comput. Secur.* **2007**, *26*, 276–289. [CrossRef]
23. Jiang, H.; Kwong, C.K.; Park, W.Y.; Yu, K.M. A multi-objective PSO approach of mining association rules for affective design based on online customer reviews. *J. Eng. Des.* **2018**, *29*, 381–403. [CrossRef]
24. Pentus, K.; Mehine, T.; Kuusik, A. Considering Emotions in Product Package Design through Combining Conjoint Analysis with Psycho Physiological Measurements. *Procedia Soc. Behav. Sci.* **2014**, *148*, 280–290. [CrossRef]
25. Lee, J.; Pee, L.G. The Relationship between Online Trust and Distrust in Business: Testing Mutual Causality from a Cognitive-Affective Personality System Theory. *Asia Pac. J. Inf. Syst.* **2015**, *25*, 500–518. [CrossRef]
26. Ha, Y.; Lennon, S.J. Consumer Responses to Online Atmosphere: The Moderating Role of Atmospheric Responsiveness. *J. Glob. Fash. Mark.* **2011**, *2*, 86–94. [CrossRef]
27. Pappas, N. Marketing strategies, perceived risks, and consumer trust in online buying behaviour. *J. Retail. Consum. Serv.* **2016**, *29*, 92–103. [CrossRef]
28. Kim, H.; Hur, W.-M.; Yeo, J. Corporate Brand Trust as a Mediator in the Relationship between Consumer Perception of CSR, Corporate Hypocrisy, and Corporate Reputation. *Sustainability* **2015**, *7*, 3683–3694. [CrossRef]
29. Demmers, J.; van Dolen, W.M.; Weltevreden, J.W.J. Handling Consumer Messages on Social Networking Sites: Customer Service or Privacy Infringement? *Int. J. Electron. Commer.* **2018**, *22*, 8–35. [CrossRef]
30. Smith, H.J.; Milberg, S.J.; Burke, S.J. Information Privacy: Measuring Individuals' Concerns about Organizational Practices. *MIS Q.* **1996**, *20*, 167. [CrossRef]
31. Zhang, X.; Liu, S.; Chen, X.; Wang, L.; Gao, B.; Zhu, Q. Health information privacy concerns, antecedents, and information disclosure intention in online health communities. *Inf. Manag.* **2018**, *55*, 482–493. [CrossRef]
32. Anastasopoulou, K.; Kokolakis, S.; Andriotis, P. Privacy Decision-Making in the Digital Era: A Game Theoretic Review. In *Human Aspects of Information Security, Privacy and Trust*; Tryfonas, T., Ed.; Springer International Publishing: Cham, Switzerland; Vancouver, BC, Canada, 2017; Volume 10292, pp. 589–603. ISBN 978-3-319-58459-1.
33. Kotz, D.; Gunter, C.A.; Kumar, S.; Weiner, J.P. Privacy and Security in Mobile Health: A Research Agenda. *Computer* **2016**, *49*, 22–30. [CrossRef]
34. Dehling, T.; Gao, F.; Schneider, S.; Sunyaev, A. Exploring the Far Side of Mobile Health: Information Security and Privacy of Mobile Health Apps on iOS and Android. *JMIR mHealth uHealth* **2015**, *3*, e8. [CrossRef] [PubMed]

35. Prasad, A.; Sorber, J.; Stablein, T.; Anthony, D.; Kotz, D. Understanding sharing preferences and behavior for mHealth devices. In Proceedings of the 2012 ACM workshop on Privacy in the electronic society-WPES '12, Raleigh, NC, USA, 15 October 2012; p. 117.
36. Yang, Q.; Pang, C.; Liu, L.; Yen, D.C.; Michael Tarn, J. Exploring consumer perceived risk and trust for online payments: An empirical study in China's younger generation. *Comput. Human Behav.* **2015**, *50*, 9–24. [CrossRef]
37. Hsu, C.-L.; Lin, J.C.-C. What drives purchase intention for paid mobile apps?—An expectation confirmation model with perceived value. *Electron. Commer. Res. Appl.* **2015**, *14*, 46–57. [CrossRef]
38. Venkatesh, V.; Thong, J.Y.L.; Chan, F.K.Y.; Hu, P.J.-H.; Brown, S.A. Extending the two-stage information systems continuance model: Incorporating UTAUT predictors and the role of context: Context, expectations and IS continuance. *Inf. Syst. J.* **2011**, *21*, 527–555. [CrossRef]
39. Lai, T.L. Service Quality and Perceived Value's Impact on Satisfaction, Intention and Usage of Short Message Service (SMS). *Inf. Syst. Front.* **2004**, *6*, 353–368. [CrossRef]
40. Wu, B.; Chen, X. Continuance intention to use MOOCs: Integrating the technology acceptance model (TAM) and task technology fit (TTF) model. *Comput. Human Behav.* **2017**, *67*, 221–232. [CrossRef]
41. Hsu, C.-L.; Lin, J.C.-C. Effect of perceived value and social influences on mobile app stickiness and in-app purchase intention. *Technol. Forecast. Soc. Chang.* **2016**, *108*, 42–53. [CrossRef]
42. Brown, S.A.; Venkatesh, V.; Goyal, S. Expectation Confirmation in Technology Use. *Inf. Syst. Res.* **2012**, *23*, 474–487. [CrossRef]
43. Lankton, N.; McKnight, D.H.; Thatcher, J.B. Incorporating trust-in-technology into Expectation Disconfirmation Theory. *J. Strateg. Inf. Syst.* **2014**, *23*, 128–145. [CrossRef]
44. Park, M.-S.; Shin, J.-K.; Ju, Y. The Effect of Online Social Network Characteristics on Consumer Purchasing Intention of Social Deals. *Glob. Econ. Rev.* **2014**, *43*, 25–41. [CrossRef]
45. Khan, S.N.; Mohsin, M. The power of emotional value: Exploring the effects of values on green product consumer choice behavior. *J. Clean. Prod.* **2017**, *150*, 65–74. [CrossRef]
46. Zhu, D.H.; Sun, H.; Chang, Y.P. Effect of social support on customer satisfaction and citizenship behavior in online brand communities: The moderating role of support source. *J. Retail. Consum. Serv.* **2016**, *31*, 287–293. [CrossRef]
47. Hwang, K.O.; Ottenbacher, A.J.; Green, A.P.; Cannon-Diehl, M.R.; Richardson, O.; Bernstam, E.V.; Thomas, E.J. Social support in an Internet weight loss community. *Int. J. Med Inform.* **2010**, *79*, 5–13. [CrossRef] [PubMed]
48. Schifferstein, H.N.J.; Fenko, A.; Desmet, P.M.A.; Labbe, D.; Martin, N. Influence of package design on the dynamics of multisensory and emotional food experience. *Food Qual. Prefer.* **2013**, *27*, 18–25. [CrossRef]
49. Lee, S.; Jeong, M.; Oh, H. Enhancing customers' positive responses: Applying sensory marketing to the hotel website. *J. Glob. Sch. Mark. Sci.* **2018**, *28*, 68–85. [CrossRef]
50. Brijnath, B.; Antoniades, J.; Adams, J. Investigating Patient Perspectives on Medical Returns and Buying Medicines Online in Two Communities in Melbourne, Australia: Results from a Qualitative Study. *Patient* **2015**, *8*, 229–238. [CrossRef] [PubMed]
51. Park, I.; Cho, J.; Rao, H.R. The effect of pre- and post-service performance on consumer evaluation of online retailers. *Decis. Support. Syst.* **2012**, *52*, 415–426. [CrossRef]
52. Liang, T.-P.; Ho, Y.-T.; Li, Y.-W.; Turban, E. What Drives Social Commerce: The Role of Social Support and Relationship Quality. *Int. J. Electron. Commer.* **2011**, *16*, 69–90. [CrossRef]
53. Chong, A.Y.L.; Lacka, E.; Boying, L.; Chan, H.K. The role of social media in enhancing guanxi and perceived effectiveness of E-commerce institutional mechanisms in online marketplace. *Inf. Manag.* **2018**, *55*, 621–632. [CrossRef]
54. Hajli, M.N. The role of social support on relationship quality and social commerce. *Technol. Forecast. Soc. Chang.* **2014**, *87*, 17–27. [CrossRef]
55. Karnal, N.; Machiels, C.J.A.; Orth, U.R.; Mai, R. Healthy by design, but only when in focus: Communicating non-verbal health cues through symbolic meaning in packaging. *Food Qual. Prefer.* **2016**, *52*, 106–119. [CrossRef]
56. Krishna, A.; Cian, L.; Aydınoğlu, N.Z. Sensory Aspects of Package Design. *J. Retail.* **2017**, *93*, 43–54. [CrossRef]
57. Kauppinen-Räisänen, H. The impact of extrinsic and package design attributes on preferences for non-prescription drugs. *Manag. Res. Rev.* **2010**, *33*, 161–173. [CrossRef]
58. Yun, E.K.; Park, H.-A. Consumers' disease information-seeking behaviour on the Internet in Korea: Internet disease information-seeking behaviour. *J. Clin. Nurs.* **2010**, *19*, 2860–2868. [CrossRef] [PubMed]

59. Yang, Y.; Zhang, X.; Lee, P.K.C. Improving the effectiveness of online healthcare platforms: An empirical study with multi-period patient-doctor consultation data. *Int. J. Prod. Econ.* **2019**, *207*, 70–80. [CrossRef]
60. Calero Valdez, A.; Ziefle, M. The users' perspective on the privacy-utility trade-offs in health recommender systems. *Int. J. Human Comput. Stud.* **2019**, *121*, 108–121. [CrossRef]
61. Jung, Y.; Park, J. An investigation of relationships among privacy concerns, affective responses, and coping behaviors in location-based services. *Int. J. Inf. Manag.* **2018**, *43*, 15–24. [CrossRef]
62. Meingast, M.; Roosta, T.; Sastry, S. Security and Privacy Issues with Health Care Information Technology. In Proceedings of the 2006 International Conference of the IEEE Engineering in Medicine and Biology Society, New York, NY, USA, 15 December 2006; pp. 5453–5458.
63. Martin, N.; Rice, J.; Martin, R. Expectations of privacy and trust: Examining the views of IT professionals. *Behav. Inf. Technol.* **2016**, *35*, 500–510. [CrossRef]
64. Househ, M. Sharing sensitive personal health information through Facebook: The unintended consequences. *Stud. Health Technol. Inf.* **2011**, *169*, 616–620.
65. Bansal, G.; Zahedi, F.M.; Gefen, D. The role of privacy assurance mechanisms in building trust and the moderating role of privacy concern. *Eur. J. Inf. Syst.* **2015**, *24*, 624–644. [CrossRef]
66. James, T.L.; Wallace, L.; Warkentin, M.; Kim, B.C.; Collignon, S.E. Exposing others' information on online social networks (OSNs): Perceived shared risk, its determinants, and its influence on OSN privacy control use. *Inf. Manag.* **2017**, *54*, 851–865. [CrossRef]
67. Hubert, M.; Blut, M.; Brock, C.; Backhaus, C.; Eberhardt, T. Acceptance of Smartphone-Based Mobile Shopping: Mobile Benefits, Customer Characteristics, Perceived Risks, and the Impact of Application Context: Acceptance of smartphone-based mobile shopping. *Psychol. Mark.* **2017**, *34*, 175–194. [CrossRef]
68. Hong Kong Polytechnic University; Lam, A.Y.C.; Lau, M.M.; Hong Kong Polytechnic University; Cheung, R.; University of South Australia. Modelling the Relationship among Green Perceived Value, Green Trust, Satisfaction, and Repurchase Intention of Green Products. *CMR* **2016**, *12*, 47–60. [CrossRef]
69. Akter, S.; Ray, P.; D'Ambra, J. Continuance of mHealth services at the bottom of the pyramid: The roles of service quality and trust. *Electron. Mark.* **2013**, *23*, 29–47. [CrossRef]
70. Grabner-Kraeuter, S. The Role of Consumers' Trust in Online-Shopping. *J. Bus. Ethics* **2002**, *39*, 43–50. [CrossRef]
71. Sullivan, Y.W.; Kim, D.J. Assessing the effects of consumers' product evaluations and trust on repurchase intention in e-commerce environments. *Int. J. Inf. Manag.* **2018**, *39*, 199–219. [CrossRef]
72. Kim, Y.; Peterson, R.A. A Meta-analysis of Online Trust Relationships in E-commerce. *J. Interact. Mark.* **2017**, *38*, 44–54. [CrossRef]
73. Kim, D.J. An investigation of the effect of online consumer trust on expectation, satisfaction, and post-expectation. *Inf. Syst. e-Bus. Manag.* **2012**, *10*, 219–240. [CrossRef]
74. Fang, Y.; Qureshi, I.; Sun, H.; McCole, P.; Ramsey, E.; Lim, K. Trust, Satisfaction, and Online Repurchase Intention: The Moderating Role of Perceived Effectiveness of E-Commerce Institutional Mechanisms. *MIS Q.* **2014**, *38*, 407–427. [CrossRef]
75. Clemons, E.K.; Wilson, J.; Matt, C.; Hess, T.; Ren, F.; Jin, F.; Koh, N.S. Global Differences in Online Shopping Behavior: Understanding Factors Leading to Trust. *J. Manag. Inf. Syst.* **2016**, *33*, 1117–1148. [CrossRef]
76. Hajli, N.; Sims, J.; Zadeh, A.H.; Richard, M.-O. A social commerce investigation of the role of trust in a social networking site on purchase intentions. *J. Bus. Res.* **2017**, *71*, 133–141. [CrossRef]
77. Belanger, F.; Hiller, J.S.; Smith, W.J. Trustworthiness in electronic commerce: The role of privacy, security, and site attributes. *J. Strateg. Inf. Syst.* **2002**, *11*, 245–270. [CrossRef]
78. Hallikainen, H.; Laukkanen, T. National culture and consumer trust in e-commerce. *Int. J. Inf. Manag.* **2018**, *38*, 97–106. [CrossRef]
79. Liu, L.; Lee, M.K.O.; Liu, R.; Chen, J. Trust transfer in social media brand communities: The role of consumer engagement. *Int. J. Inf. Manag.* **2018**, *41*, 1–13. [CrossRef]
80. Rahimnia, F.; Hassanzadeh, J.F. The impact of website content dimension and e-trust on e-marketing effectiveness: The case of Iranian commercial saffron corporations. *Inf. Manag.* **2013**, *50*, 240–247. [CrossRef]
81. Lee, W.-I.; Cheng, S.-Y.; Shih, Y.-T. Effects among product attributes, involvement, word-of-mouth, and purchase intention in online shopping. *Asia Pac. Manag. Rev.* **2017**, *22*, 223–229. [CrossRef]

82. Napolitano, F.; Braghieri, A.; Piasentier, E.; Favotto, S.; Naspetti, S.; Zanoli, R. Effect of information about organic production on beef liking and consumer willingness to pay. *Food Qual. Prefer.* **2010**, *21*, 207–212. [CrossRef]
83. Diddi, S.; Niehm, L.S. Corporate Social Responsibility in the Retail Apparel Context: Exploring Consumers' Personal and Normative Influences on Patronage Intentions. *J. Mark. Channels* **2016**, *23*, 60–76. [CrossRef]
84. Kytö, E.; Virtanen, M.; Mustonen, S. From intention to action: Predicting purchase behavior with consumers' product expectations and perceptions, and their individual properties. *Food Qual. Prefer.* **2019**, *75*, 1–9. [CrossRef]
85. Sánchez-Torres, J.A.; Arroyo-Cañada, F.J.; Varon-Sandoval, A.; Sánchez-Alzate, J.A. Differences between e-commerce buyers and non-buyers in Colombia: The moderating effect of educational level and socioeconomic status on electronic purchase intention. *DYNA* **2017**, *84*, 175–189. [CrossRef]
86. Arcia, P.L.; Curutchet, A.; Costell, E.; Tárrega, A. Influence of Expectations Created by Label on Consumers Acceptance of Uruguayan Low-Fat Cheeses: Influence of Expectations Created by Label. *J. Sens. Stud.* **2012**, *27*, 344–351. [CrossRef]
87. Xu, J.; Cenfetelli, R.T.; Aquino, K. Do different kinds of trust matter? An examination of the three trusting beliefs on satisfaction and purchase behavior in the buyer–seller context. *J. Strateg. Inf. Syst.* **2016**, *25*, 15–31. [CrossRef]
88. Hong, I.B. Understanding the consumer's online merchant selection process: The roles of product involvement, perceived risk, and trust expectation. *Int. J. Inf. Manag.* **2015**, *35*, 322–336. [CrossRef]
89. Lin, C.; Wei, Y.-H.; Lekhawipat, W. Time effect of disconfirmation on online shopping. *Behav. Inf. Technol.* **2018**, *37*, 87–101. [CrossRef]
90. Atkins, L.; Francis, J.; Islam, R.; O'Connor, D.; Patey, A.; Ivers, N.; Foy, R.; Duncan, E.M.; Colquhoun, H.; Grimshaw, J.M.; et al. A guide to using the Theoretical Domains Framework of behaviour change to investigate implementation problems. *Implement. Sci.* **2017**, *12*, 77. [CrossRef]
91. Dienlin, T.; Trepte, S. Is the privacy paradox a relic of the past? An in-depth analysis of privacy attitudes and privacy behaviors: The relation between privacy attitudes and privacy behaviors. *Eur. J. Soc. Psychol.* **2015**, *45*, 285–297. [CrossRef]
92. Henke, J.; Joeckel, S.; Dogruel, L. Processing privacy information and decision-making for smartphone apps among young German smartphone users. *Behav. Inf. Technol.* **2018**, *37*, 488–501. [CrossRef]
93. James, T.L.; Warkentin, M.; Collignon, S.E. A dual privacy decision model for online social networks. *Inf. Manag.* **2015**, *52*, 893–908. [CrossRef]
94. Bhattacherjee, A. An empirical analysis of the antecedents of electronic commerce service continuance. *Decis. Support. Syst.* **2001**, *32*, 201–214. [CrossRef]
95. Oghuma, A.P.; Libaque-Saenz, C.F.; Wong, S.F.; Chang, Y. An expectation-confirmation model of continuance intention to use mobile instant messaging. *Telemat. Inform.* **2016**, *33*, 34–47. [CrossRef]
96. Fornell, C.; Larcker, D.F. Evaluating Structural Equation Models with Unobservable Variables and Measurement Error. *J. Mark. Res.* **1981**, *18*, 39–50. [CrossRef]
97. ST Wang, E. The influence of visual packaging design on perceived food product quality, value, and brand preference. *Int. J. Retail. Distrib. Mgt.* **2013**, *41*, 805–816. [CrossRef]
98. Kokolakis, S. Privacy attitudes and privacy behaviour: A review of current research on the privacy paradox phenomenon. *Comput. Secur.* **2017**, *64*, 122–134. [CrossRef]
99. China Business Network Business Data 2019 Chinese Family Medical and Health Consumption Trend Report. Available online: https://www.cbndata.com/report/1355/detail (accessed on 26 February 2019).

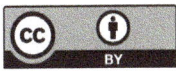

© 2019 by the authors. Licensee MDPI, Basel, Switzerland. This article is an open access article distributed under the terms and conditions of the Creative Commons Attribution (CC BY) license (http://creativecommons.org/licenses/by/4.0/).

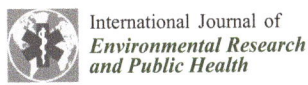

Article

Finding Users' Voice on Social Media: An Investigation of Online Support Groups for Autism-Affected Users on Facebook

Yuehua Zhao [1], Jin Zhang [2] and Min Wu [3],*

[1] School of Information Management, Jiangsu Key Laboratory of Data Engineering and Knowledge Service, Nanjing University, Nanjing 210023, China; yuehua@nju.edu.cn
[2] School of Information Studies, University of Wisconsin Milwaukee, Milwaukee, WI 53211, USA; jzhang@uwm.edu
[3] College of Health Sciences, University of Wisconsin Milwaukee, Milwaukee, WI 53211, USA
* Correspondence: wu@uwm.edu; Tel.: +1-414-229-4778

Received: 7 November 2019; Accepted: 27 November 2019; Published: 29 November 2019

Abstract: The trend towards the use of the Internet for health information purposes is rising. Utilization of various forms of social media has been a key interest in consumer health informatics (CHI). To reveal the information needs of autism-affected users, this study centers on the research of users' interactions and information sharing within autism communities on social media. It aims to understand how autism-affected users utilize support groups on Facebook by applying natural language process (NLP) techniques to unstructured health data in social media. An interactive visualization method (pyLDAvis) was employed to evaluate produced models and visualize the inter-topic distance maps. The revealed topics (e.g., parenting, education, behavior traits) identify issues that individuals with autism were concerned about on a daily basis and how they addressed such concerns in the form of group communication. In addition to general social support, disease-specific information, collective coping strategies, and emotional support were provided as well by group members based on similar personal experiences. This study concluded that Latent Dirichlet Allocation (LDA) is feasible and appropriated to derive topics (focus) from messages posted to the autism support groups on Facebook. The revealed topics help healthcare professionals (content providers) understand autism from users' perspectives and provide better patient communications.

Keywords: consumer health informatics; natural language processing (NLP); online support groups; autism

1. Introduction

Today, in the Web 2.0 era, social media are pervasive, rapidly evolving, and increasingly influencing people's daily life and their health behavior. With the access to information on the social media platforms, people find useful information more effectively and personally than traditional information retrieval through search engines.

According to survey results from parents across the United States, 1 in 40 children (2.5%) have autism spectrum disorder (ASD), representing an estimated 1.5 million children ages 3 to 17 years [1]. Autism is a developmental disorder that appears in the first 3 years of life. It is characterized by substantial deficits in communication and social functioning, as well as restrictive, repetitive, and stereotyped behavior [2]. People with autism experience diverse social and emotional difficulties, such as struggles with social skills and communication impairment [3]. Previous studies have revealed that the special challenges faced by autism patients are associated with social communication, social integration, and social imagination [4,5].

When it comes to adults with autism, the majority of them used social networking sites to seek social connections [3]. Researchers have suggested that social media use appears to be beneficial for individuals with autism in communicating and engaging with others in a comfortable way [3]. Support groups on Facebook provide an efficient platform for autism patients and their caregivers where they can ask for help and advice from other users, make contributions to others, receive assistance from the group members, and share their experiences in the community.

Across different social media platforms, social and informational supports were emphasized as some of the most critical benefits of obtaining health information from online support groups. Through interviews with 14 participants who used support groups on Facebook for weight loss and diabetes management, it was unveiled that participants used Facebook support groups in pursuit of emotional support, motivation, accountability, and advice [6]. Findings from previous studies have identified that informational and emotional supports occupied a significant proportion of the total interaction among users [7].

The topics/focus in social media groups varied time to time. There have been few studies that systematically explore what kind of information is being shared for autism-affected users in social media and how users interact with each other. In this study, data in support groups for autism-affected users on Facebook within a six-month period were collected and analyzed through natural language process (NLP) techniques and the findings were presented by a visualization tool.

The online activities conducted by group members in autism support groups on Facebook produce rich textual content in addition to the interaction connections between users. In this study, the textual content mainly consists of two parts: the original posts submitted by group members, and the comments made by other members. The content created by users in the process of the group interactions reveals the concerns, interests, and other potential information behind the information sharing actions among group members. The content-based analysis uncovers the topics that emerge from group discussions. It provides knowledge regarding the information need of autism-affected users.

The primary research problem of this study is to investigate the content-based characteristics describing the content pattern derived from the communication. The research objects are the autism support groups on Facebook. The autism support groups on Facebook refer to any existing Facebook groups dedicated to autism-related topics. The autism support groups consist of autism patients, their relatives, caregivers, researchers, and physicians. Based on the primary problem, this study aims to address the following research question: *What are the topics that emerged from the discussions and communications posted in autism support groups on Facebook?* The discussions and communications that appeared in the autism support groups were in the form of posts and comments posted by group members.

This study is an investigation of online support groups for autism-affected users on Facebook and the contribution of this study is to find users' voice on social media, using NLP methods (e.g., Latent Dirichlet Allocation (LDA)) to systematically derive topics (focus) from messages posted to the autism support groups on Facebook. The revealed topics will help healthcare professionals (content providers) understand autism from users' perspectives and provide better patient communications.

2. Materials and Methods

2.1. Sampling and Data Collection

2.1.1. Sampling Strategy

The purpose of this study was to investigate the autism support groups on Facebook, thus the screening strategy focused on finding the appropriate Facebook groups. Based on the definition from PubMed Health [8], autism is also called autistic spectrum disorder (ASD) and pervasive developmental disorder (PDD). In order to reach broad data sources, the following autism-related terms were used to search the groups on Facebook: "autism", "autistic", "asperger", "aspie", and "pervasive developmental disorder". The search was restricted to Facebook groups. To be included in the study, the groups had to meet the following criteria: (1) the group was related to autism, (2) the group possessed more than 50 group members, and (3) the group operated in English. The first criterion ensured that the sampled groups could be related to the research problem and research questions. The second criterion ensured the conduction of further social network analysis and inferential analysis, while the third criterion ensured the process of content analysis of information shared in the group. For each group identified in the search results, the researcher manually checked the purpose and the operation language of the group through the group title and group description, and recorded the number of group members via group profile. In total, 341 Facebook groups met the requirements.

Through a thorough analysis of the group purposes, all appropriate groups were categorized into ten categories. Table 1 summarizes the categories and the sub-categories of the autism-related Facebook groups.

Table 1. Categories and sub-categories of the autism-related Facebook groups.

Category	Sub-category	Category	Sub-category
Autism patient group	Women Teenager Christian Adults Youth Islam LGBT (Lesbian, Gay, Bisexual, and Transgender)	Autism with other related diseases	Sensory Processing Disorder Ehlers Danlos Syndrome/ Hypermobility Syndrome Neurological/behavioral challenge Down Syndrome Type 1 Diabetes Dyslexia
Care support group	Mother General family members and caregivers Partner (wife/spouse) Parents	Society and education	Awareness Fundraising and charity Art Education Non-profit organization
Treatment and therapy	Essential Oils Chlorine dioxide MAPS (Medical Academy of Pediatric Special Needs) Treatment	Patient and society	Friend seeking Relationship Job Protest
Specific autism type	Severe autism High-functioning autism	Commercial and research	Consumer group Consultancy services Research
Scope	Local support National support Global support	Special discussion	Buying and selling Gift

2.1.2. Group Data Collection Procedure

To achieve sufficient information, the researcher tended to choose the largest and comparative active groups that were available. Five public Facebook autism support groups, each selected from a distinct category (i.e., awareness (under the society and education category), treatment (under the treatment and therapy category), parents (under the care support group category), research (under the commercial and research category), and local support (under the scope category)), became the data sources. According to Facebook, anyone can access the posts in public groups. After joining the groups, a flyer was posted in the groups notifying the process of this study. The comparably largest and most active groups in which group members showed no uncomfortable feelings to the study were selected as the sample groups. In addition, the author intentionally chose groups focusing on diverse topics.

After identifying the sampled groups, data collection for this study centered on the extraction of the interactions and content that appeared in each group. To ensure the fair comparativeness among the groups, a 6-month period was set as the time range of data collection. Data from the sampled public groups on Facebook was collected using NodeXL (The Social Media Research Foundation, Redwood City, USA). NodeXL, produced by Microsoft Research, is an extendible toolkit for network overview, discovery, and exploration [9]. The data import features support data collection from Facebook [9], and export the data into an Excel spreadsheet. To begin the data extraction, we need to go to the

"Import" dropdown menu and select "From Facebook Groups". NodeXL enables the capture of some pertinent aspects of Facebook (e.g., posts, likes, shares, comments). However, due to the limits of Facebook API (Application programming interface), NodeXL can only collect data from the public groups on Facebook.

Data from each of the sampled groups was collected and then saved in Excel spreadsheets for further analysis. On the home page of each group, all of the wall posts created by group members were accessed. Each post included the following information: the Facebook user who created the post, the content of the post, the tag(s) within the post, the post time, the total likes it received, the Facebook user(s) who liked the post, the total share-outs it received, the Facebook user(s) who shared the post, the total number of comments it received, and the content of each comment. For each comment replied to in an original post, it possessed the following components: the Facebook user who made the comment, the content of the comment, the specific time when it was made, the total likes it received, and the Facebook user(s) who liked the comment.

Data from the sampled public groups on Facebook was gathered on December 12–15, 2017. The data collection window was set from April 1, 2017, to September 30, 2017, which covered six months. The time span was flexible to be expanded if there were not sufficient data for data analysis procedures when the final data collection was conducted.

2.2. Topic Modeling

2.2.1. Text Preparation Process

Text preparation process refers to a series of steps to prepare the raw text before more in-depth natural language processing, e.g., topic model training. Text preparation commonly consists of the selection, cleansing, and preprocessing of text [10]. In this study, the text preparation process was operated by Python scripts using NLTK toolkits [11].

2.2.2. Latent Dirichlet Allocation (LDA)

Latent dirichlet allocation (LDA) was proposed as a particular generative model for topic discovery [10]. LDA assumes a latent structure consisting of a set of topics, and the words that appear in a paper reflect the particular set of topics [12].

Following the methods introduced by previous researchers, in this study, the LDA model was implemented in the Python with gensim package using the Gibbs sampling inference method [13]. The hyperparameters α was set to 50/K (K is the number of topics) while β equals 0.01. The number of iterations was set as 500. The settings of α and β were based on the suggestion of a previous study where they found it worked well with many different text collections [12].

2.2.3. LDA Model Evaluation

Model evaluation is of importance to the topic modeling methods. The pre-specified numbers of topics influence the performance of the topic model training. The topics discovered by the LDA capture the correlations between words in documents, but the LDA cannot generate the correlations among the captured topics [14]. Too few topics do not allow authors to be distinguished, whereas too many may cause relationships to be weaker [15]. Ideally, topics identified from the documents are supposed to be distinctive from each other. One way to evaluate the LDA model is through the interactive visualization supporting rapid experimentation for interpretive hypotheses [16].

LDAvis handles the model checking problem to aid topic interpretation by displaying the ranking of terms within topics and the relevance among topics [17]. It presents topic–word and topic–topic relationships alongside composition information. In this study, the pyLDAvis package was implemented in Python to visualize the topics generated from the group discussions, as well as assist the modeling checking process. Different values of K, or numbers of topics, were tested. The authors assessed the outcomes and decided the most reasonable outcomes based on the data.

To identify the optimal number of topics as the K parameter, which is the number of topics in the model training process, interactive visualization methods (pyLDAvis package imported in Python) were employed to evaluate produced models. Using the methods applied in a previous study [18], the number of LDA topics was tuned until it reached a set of non-overlapping clusters that had sufficient distance between each other. The parameter of K was given for a series of descending numbers to train the model until the circles representing the topics became separated without any significant overlapping. For example, given the K parameter as five, three of the five resulted topics represented as the circles in the inter-topic distance map overlapped with each other (see the left part in Figure 1). When the value of K was lowered from five to four, the resulted four topics appeared to be split (see the right part in Figure 1), which meant the generated topics were distinctive to each other. The authors stopped searching for the optimal number of the topics when the circles did not overlap anymore. The size of the circles represents the popularity of the topic within the overall set of topics [18].

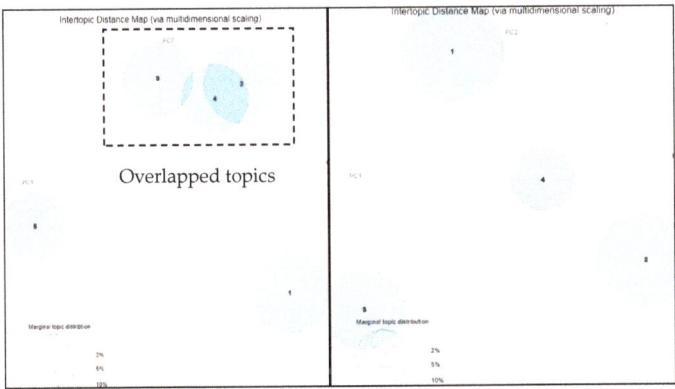

Figure 1. Topic visualization results for different values of K parameter.

All five investigated groups were explored through the model training and evaluation process. After producing the appropriate LDA models, the revealed topics in each group were labeled manually according to the top terms in the topic-term distributions. Labelling topics makes it possible to interpret the corpus to see which concepts are prevalent [19]. The interpretation of a topic can be achieved by examining a ranked list of the most probable terms in that topic [17].

3. Results

3.1. Description of the Collected Data

As a result, five Facebook autism support groups, each selected from a distinct category, were collected on December 12–15, 2017. All of the group wall posts and group interactions were downloaded by NodeXL. Table 2 presents the basic descriptions of the sampled groups and the collected data. The names of the groups were not revealed for the privacy concerns.

Table 2. Descriptive statistics for the five collected autism support groups.

Group	Category	Members	Involved Members	Posts and Comments
Group 1	Awareness	5902	299	314
Group 2	Treatment	1577	297	259
Group 3	Parents	1513	523	924
Group 4	Research	2603	156	88
Group 5	Local support	2847	438	756

Group 1 is the largest group among the five selected groups, where only 5.1% of the group members participated in the six-month data collection period. Group 3, created for parents, family, and friends of autism patients, had 34.6% of group members engaged in the group discussions. Among the five groups, group 3 had the most group members involved in the group discussions, while group 5 provided the support for people living in a state. After the text preparation process, group 3 remained with the most posts and comments (924 records). In order to protect the user privacy, the Facebook usernames are replaced by serial numbers.

3.2. Discussion Topics of Autism Support Groups

3.2.1. Discussion Topics of Group 1 (Awareness Group)

The modeling evaluation process indicated that four topics emerged from the posts and comments in group 1. The inter-topic distance map of the four topics (represented by the four circles) is visualized in Figure 2. The right part of Figure 2 lists the top 20 terms and the associated probabilities of the terms to each topic. The four topics that emerged from the discussions in group 1 were *parenting, behavioral traits, diagnosis,* and *video sharing*. The parenting topic was related to discussions on parents of autistic children sharing their children's daily life. People shared their children's accomplishments and sometimes expressed the frustrating issues which happened with their children. Along with talking about the parenting challenges, group members also shared their own behavior traits as patients or their kids' behaviors. There was a post saying, "*Can anyone tell me if this lining up of toys is a trait of Autism Spectrum Disorder?*" This question raised a number of replies from other group members. Some comments expressed similar observations: "*Our son who has autism LOVES to line up his toys*". Some stated other opinions: "*Not in of itself. It depends on the age of the child and how the child uses these toys and other toys in other play activities*". Since autism often appears in early ages of children, parents sometimes struggled with the diagnosis process: "*We keep pushing but the pediatrician just won't commit to a diagnosis and it's been 2 1/2 to 3 years now*". Video sharing topics were contributed mainly by one of the group members, user a41, who posted 30 original messages in the group and was identified as one of the most active users in group 1. After checking with the post content from User a41, he/she has declared himself/herself as a professional speaker with autism. He/she regularly uploaded videos regarding stories about real autism patients and their parents, basic knowledge about autism, how to communicate with people who have autism, school bulling problems for children with autism, etc.

Topic 1 Parenting		Topic 2 Behavioral traits		Topic 3 Diagnosis		Topic 4 Video sharing	
autism	0.02	autism	0.046	well	0.009	autism	0.014
son	0.013	son	0.015	happy	0.009	get	0.013
need	0.009	like	0.008	like	0.008	autist	0.01
thank	0.008	autist	0.007	son	0.008	vlog	0.009
children	0.007	vlog	0.007	look	0.008	go	0.008
get	0.007	thing	0.006	need	0.007	like	0.007
time	0.007	people	0.006	feel	0.007	son	0.007
use	0.006	help	0.006	get	0.007	well	0.006
thing	0.006	look	0.006	year	0.006	new	0.006
keep	0.006	year	0.006	autism	0.006	great	0.006
take	0.006	see	0.006	people	0.006	kid	0.006
well	0.005	know	0.005	birthday	0.006	help	0.006
child	0.005	toy	0.005	person	0.006	got	0.006
ashley	0.005	love	0.004	sometime	0.006	thing	0.005
see	0.005	disorder	0.004	know	0.005	time	0.005
way	0.005	line	0.004	autist	0.005	work	0.005
someone	0.005	life	0.004	parent	0.005	hope	0.005
good	0.005	today	0.004	skill	0.005	want	0.005
great	0.005	say	0.004	pediatrician	0.005	come	0.005
autist	0.005	differ	0.004	read	0.005	every	0.005

Figure 2. Topic map of four discussion topics in group 1 (awareness group) and top 20 terms and the associated probabilities of the terms to each topic.

3.2.2. Discussion Topics of Group 2 (Treatment Group)

Figure 3 gives the global overview of the relationship between the topics based on the established topic-document relationship. Three distinct topics emerged from the discussions in group 2, including *EMF (electromagnetic field) pollution, home decoration,* and *wireless safety* (as shown in the right part of Figure 3). The main discussion topic was about the EMF pollution, since the group founder described this group as follows: "Exploring the emerging link between autism and EMF/wireless, and helping ASD families to heal their children by providing information and resources for reducing their exposure". On several occasions, group members shared their advocacy of reducing the EMF pollution. Another discussion theme was regarding home decorations that may reduce or enlarge the EMF (electromagnetic field) pollution. In addition, a number of posts and comments were related to smart meters, including how to install smart meter shields and specific products that can replace the smart meters. Wireless (wifi) networks are one type of sources of EMF according to the National Institute of Environmental Health Sciences [20]. People discussed concerns about a variety of wireless products in the group, such as "Does anyone still have a child using a Fitbit, Apple watch, or location tracker? Those are all big wireless emitters and can really increase stimming in the kids".

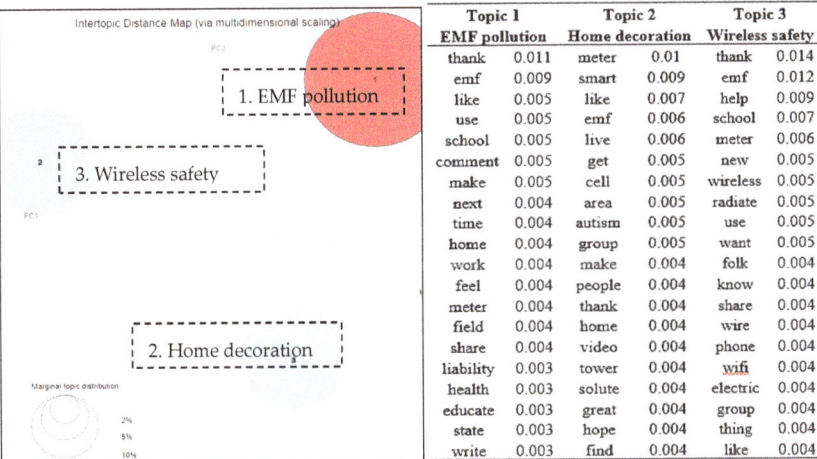

Figure 3. Topic map of three discussion topics in group 2 (treatment group) and top 20 terms and the associated probabilities of the terms to each topic.

3.2.3. Discussion Topics of Group 3 (Parents Group)

The five discussion topics drawn from group 3 are shown in Figure 4, while the top terms associated with each topic are listed in the right part of Figure 4. As a group created for parents, *family support,* and *parenting* were not unexpected to be three of the major discussion themes.

Group members shared the stories and experiences about their family members (e.g., brother, son, daughter) in the group, such as "I was brought to this group because I wanted to connect with people whose lives have been affected by autism. The person in the photo is my baby brother . . . .". People also brought up specific questions in being parents of autistic children, such as "R there any summer camp for my 11-year-old son with autism that in Memphis TN please I need help". Another topic, *experiences,* included posts and comments regarding some videos shared by group members. These videos explained the way people on the autism spectrum saw the world and the social difficulties they experienced in real life. With respect to the fourth topic, *education,* people asked questions about how to educate autistic children, such as "I'm in need of a provider for my 17-year-old girl. . . . I need someone who can deal with autism. Please help". The comments they received provided informational support with methods that might work for their kids, such as "As a person who has a hyperactive body type, I can emphatically state that heavy *work, stretching, and music are all helpful in regulating me"*. In addition to all the discussions regarding specific information needs, both group administrators and other group members posted *welcome messages* (the fifth topic), which showed the welcoming environment of the group to new members.

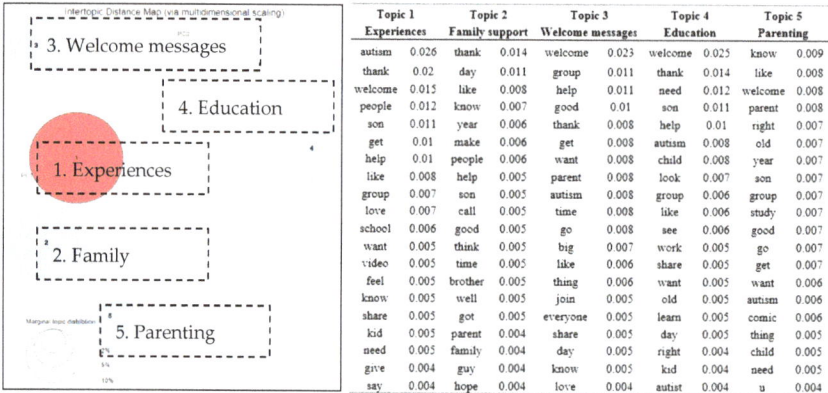

Figure 4. Topic map of five discussion topics in group 3 (parents group) and top 20 terms and the associated probabilities of the terms to each topic.

3.2.4. Discussion Topics of Group 4 (Research Group)

As described on the group main page, group 4 was described as "plays a leading role—locally, nationally and internationally—in developing an improved understanding of the biological and psychosocial basis of autism". Figure 5 shows that three distinct topics emerged from group 4, while the right part of Figure 5 lists the top 20 terms associated with each topic. The three major topics which appeared in group 4 were related to the *therapies*, the *trainings* and *workshops*, and the *events* and *visits*. Group members talked about various types of therapy for autism patients, such as *"Play therapy builds on the natural way that children learn about themselves and their relationships in the world around them"*. Information regarding trainings and workshops was also shared in the group, such as *"We are excited to announce that our new Online Certification Programme on Play Therapy for Children with Special Needs will launch this August!"* The trainings and workshops discussed in the group were not only for professional therapists but also for parents of autistic kids. User C2 posted most frequently (27 messages) in the group and contributed most to the topic of events and visits. User C2 is the group administrator and serves as an occupational therapist as identified in his/her posts. He/she often updated his professional visits at different places and events he and his colleagues arranged.

3.2.5. Discussion Topics of Group 5 (Local Support Group)

The posts and comments in group 5 focused on four topics, as shown in Figure 6. These were *greetings, support, conferences,* and *help requests*. The word "MM" appeared to be among the top words for both the first and the third topic. "MM" is the name of the group founder's daughter who has autism. A pseudonym was used to protect the privacy of subject. The group founder, user D14, was the most active person in the group, who posted 49 messages and provided 140 comments. He posted photos and daily updates about his daughter. Those posts usually received compliments like *"She is so beautiful love u mia grace!!!"*. As shown in Figure 6, the first two topics were comparatively close to each other. People posted greetings on special days such as on Mother's Day and someone's birthday. The third discussion topic was related to an adult autism conference. One of the group members kept posting information regarding the conference, such as the call for presentation flyers, the conference agendas, and the photos of conference presentations. Another discussion topic was questions and answers regarding specific help inquiries, such as *"I am new to this group. I have an amazing 3-year-old* son who has recently been given an ASD diagnosis ... So I ask, what has been other mom's or family's experience with obtaining SSI Disability benefits?". Such specific help request tended to receive informational replies from others, such as "I filed with copy of diagnosis and 4 weeks later start getting payments on child".

Topic 1		Topic 2		Topic 3	
Therapies		Trainings and workshops		Events and visits	
therapy	0.022	share	0.017	autism	0.021
learn	0.014	autism	0.013	children	0.018
autism	0.014	parent	0.01	therapy	0.013
children	0.012	program	0.01	karthikeyan	0.013
center	0.011	special	0.008	visit	0.011
toy	0.011	respect	0.008	minister	0.011
occupation	0.011	workshop	0.008	day	0.011
seat	0.011	early	0.008	tamilnadu	0.011
visit	0.011	id	0.008	special	0.011
therapist	0.009	like	0.008	parent	0.011
special	0.009	dear	0.007	therapist	0.011
today	0.009	learn	0.006	occupationaltherapi	0.01
play	0.009	aware	0.006	occupation	0.008
online	0.009	friend	0.006	iotg	0.008
support	0.009	educate	0.006	participate	0.008
good	0.006	day	0.006	sai	0.008
time	0.006	child	0.006	dr	0.008
experience	0.006	sensory	0.006	respect	0.008
make	0.006	research	0.006	expense	0.006
early	0.006	children	0.006	social	0.006

Figure 5. Topic map of three discussion topics in group 4 (research group) and top 20 terms and the associated probabilities of the terms to each topic.

Topic 1		Topic 2		Topic 3		Topic 4	
Greetings		Support		Conferences		Help requests	
love	0.016	get	0.014	autism	0.015	autism	0.021
autism	0.013	thank	0.013	get	0.015	help	0.011
go	0.009	like	0.013	try	0.008	son	0.008
work	0.008	autism	0.011	take	0.008	autist	0.007
like	0.008	go	0.009	true	0.008	make	0.006
get	0.008	know	0.008	love	0.007	child	0.006
mia	0.008	son	0.007	conference	0.006	share	0.006
help	0.007	help	0.007	mm	0.006	love	0.006
great	0.007	month	0.006	adult	0.006	year	0.006
child	0.006	sure	0.006	thank	0.005	try	0.006
day	0.006	need	0.006	day	0.005	give	0.005
know	0.006	time	0.006	think	0.005	get	0.005
good	0.006	everyone	0.006	that	0.005	old	0.005
take	0.006	beauty	0.006	kid	0.005	new	0.005
need	0.005	look	0.005	keep	0.004	family	0.005
thank	0.005	great	0.005	always	0.004	free	0.005
want	0.005	happy	0.005	he	0.004	people	0.005
time	0.005	make	0.005	need	0.004	hope	0.004
children	0.005	year	0.005	go	0.004	asd	0.004
start	0.004	work	0.005	know	0.004	he	0.004

Figure 6. Topic map of four discussion topics in group 5 (Local support group) and top 20 terms and the associated probabilities of the terms to each topic.

4. Discussion

4.1. Social and Informational Exchange in Support Groups on Facebook

Through interviews with 14 participants who used support groups on Facebook for weight loss and diabetes management, it was unveiled that participants used Facebook support groups in pursuit of emotional support, motivation, accountability, and advice [6]. Sugimoto identified informational and emotional supports as the common type of support exchanged in depression online support groups [7]. Sugimoto then summarized findings from previous studies that informational and emotional supports occupied a significant proportion of the total interaction among users [7].

Similar with other support groups on Facebook, social support was also found in the investigated autism support groups. Group members often received comments from others with similar situations and experiences (e.g., "*I can relate entirely and feel this way every day I drop my brave boy at pre-school. Xx*"). Although people may not receive actual information regarding their information needs, the social support they acquired may help with emotional relief.

In addition to general social support, disease-specific information was also exchanged in the support groups on Facebook. Online health communities offer the opportunity for patients to seek and share disease-related information with others who may have similar experiences [21]. A previous study examined online health communities related to arthritis and discovered medication was one of the most popular topics discussed within the community [22]. For individuals in Facebook support groups for presumed ocular histoplasmosis syndrome (POHS), issues regarding diagnosis, treatment, adjustment, and emotional distress were discussed. In the five investigated autism support groups of this study, the following autism-related topics were shared in the Facebook groups: "parenting", "behavior traits", "diagnosis", "home decorations", "education", and "therapies".

As a beneficial result of membership, collective coping strategies were identified as well as timely medical advice based on personal experience, research resources, linkage to services, compassionate support, camaraderie, and social interaction [23]. In this study, it was noticed that group members brought up questions regarding the coping strategies and received multiple suggestions from others with the similar experiences. For example, a mother asked in one of the investigated autism groups: "*what has been other mom's or family's experience with obtaining SSI Disability benefits?*". The post obtained 11 comments including information from others with similar experiences, e.g., "*I filed with copy of diagnosis and 4 weeks later start getting payments on child*". Another group member replied to the post and expressed the willingness to provide personal help: "*Pm me! I'm happy to help!!!*". As demonstrated by a previous study, such health communities provide access to experience-based information about particular situations, which many users find more relevant or accessible than information obtained from professionals [6].

Previous studies argued that, unlike face-to-face support groups, instrumental or tangible support was either absent or very rare in online depression support groups [7]. However, it was noticed that group members offered tangible responses when people asked specific questions in the autism support groups in this study. For example, one group member brought up a question: "*I am thinking of purchasing this EMF meter for our home. . . . Are any of you familiar with this product or have a recommendation for a different meter?*". Several instrumental and tangible comments replied by others included "*For about the same price, you can get this one: http://www.electricsense.com/10786/cornet-ed88t-emf-meter/*" and "*Tue Cornet is way better for a similar price.*". In this case, the product recommendations can be considered as informational and useful support for people who did not have such experiences.

Disseminating information with others about upcoming events was identified as one of the most popular things to do on Facebook [24]. In both group 4 (research group) and group 5 (local support group), there was information about a variety of events and conferences shared in the groups. These types of information were also noticed in other Facebook support groups [25]. It suggested that one of the benefits of being involved in support groups on Facebook is to gain access to beneficial information like available events and conferences. It helps group members feel connected and supported, since they could stay current and up-to-date with the groups they choose to be a part of [25].

4.2. Emotional Exchange in Facebook Support Groups

The results of this study are consistent with prior studies indicating that that venting is one of the purposes for people who use Facebook groups to fulfill a need to share feelings [26]. Members in online health communities preferred to talk to strangers online about their illness experience than with their offline contacts [27]. In this study, for all of the five investigated autism support groups on Facebook, a prominent theme that conveyed negative emotions can be classified into the venting category (e.g., "*Yes its a very scaring feeling my son is 3 an he takes off on me...My heart sinks*"). It suggested that Facebook groups, similar with other online health communities for long-term conditions [27,28], could serve as not only a place to seek informational and emotional help but also a venue that people could feel free to express the negative feelings.

There are contrasting and possibly conflicting views on the pros and cons to participating in online support communities [26]. In four self-injury groups on Facebook, it was revealed that 3.6% of the total posts were praising or thanking the group [26]. In contrast to the self-injury groups, as shown in Figures 3, 4 and 6, "thank" appeared to be one of the most frequently occurring keywords in three of the five autism support groups. It implied that autism support groups offered a more supportive emotional atmosphere for group members than those of the self-injury groups.

From Figures 2–6, many positive words (e.g., "well", "like", "thank", "happy", "love", "good", and "great") appeared to be the most relevant terms to the discussion topics revealed in the groups. These findings were consistent to a reported healthy and continuous communication loop uncovered in a stutter support group on Facebook [13]. Raj identified that the sense of family which came from the Facebook group helped to diminish feelings of loneliness or isolation for people who had communication barriers [25].

4.3. Active Users Lead the Discussions in the Support Groups

As presented above, user A41 in group 1 contributed most in the discussion topic of *video sharing*. User C2 in group 4 shared most of the posts related to the topic of *events and visits*. Part of the posts and comments of the *greetings* topic and the *support* topic were generated by user D14 in group 5. Based on the group interactions, the above three users served as the influential users in their respective group. This suggests that influential users took significant roles in controlling or leading the discussions in their groups.

4.4. Limitations

Like most of research studies, there are certain limitations in this study. The first and most obvious one of all the limitations to this study concerns the sampling and data collection. Facebook groups were the only social community on social media addressed in this study. In addition, due to ethical considerations, only public Facebook groups were investigated in this study. Furthermore, the sampled Facebook groups might not be representative of all autism-related support groups on Facebook. Also, this data collection period was six months. The limited time window might be unable to provide a whole picture of the group behaviors.

Another limitation is related to the research methods adopted in this study. This study identified and examined only the quantitative aspect of the autism support groups on Facebook. Understanding the motivations behind the group interactions and group posts could shed insight on the meanings and purposes of the autism-related social communities on social media. However, this study did not interview group members that participated in the support groups on Facebook. The inclusion of interviews or questionnaires was not considered in this study but should be conducted in the future study.

5. Conclusions

This study concluded that latent dirichlet allocation (LDA) is feasible and appropriated to derive topics (focus) from messages posted to the autism support groups on Facebook. An interactive visualization method (pyLDAvis) was employed to evaluate produced models and visualize the inter-topic distance maps.

As a result, distinct discussion topics were summarized and labeled in each group. Each group had certain distinctive discussion topics that related to the purposes of the groups. Parenting was a common theme in group 1 and group 3. In addition, several time-sensitive topics appeared during the group discussions. Group members greeted about Mother's Day during May.

Theoretically, the results of this study align with previous studies that have demonstrated the significance of social media for autism users. The unique implication of this study is to identify autism support groups on Facebook as a source of informational, social, and emotional support for autism-related users. This observation suggested new opportunities of using Facebook to help users who suffer from autism. The findings regarding discussion topics appearing in the autism support groups on Facebook revealed the information needs of autism-related users. In addition, it examined that the informational support, such as specific strategies to deal with autistic kids, was provided in those support groups on Facebook.

This study examined topics derived from messages posted to the autism support groups on Facebook. These topics can also be used as the road map for the design of autism websites and the creation of subject directories for social media information organization. In addition, the revealed topics help professionals understand autism from users' perspectives. The keywords can be used to assist the thesaurus and subject headings. In addition, the symptom-related content (e.g., lining toys, reading comic books) which emerged from the group discussions aids the screening for parents who wonder whether their children show autism symptoms. The relationships between keywords and topics identified through topic modeling may also be used to build recommendation mechanisms for the Facebook group platform and social question and answer (Q &A) websites.

These focus and overviews of autism-related users in this study can be used to improve the design of autism websites and the creation of subject directories for social media information organization and increases the usage of the digital content. In addition, the revealed topics help healthcare professionals (content providers) understand autism from users' perspectives and provide better patient communications.

Author Contributions: Y.Z. conducted the research design, data collection, data analysis and wrote the majority of the paper. J.Z. led the research design and part of data analysis. M.W. gave guidance throughout the whole research process.

Funding: This research was supported by Jiangsu Province Social Science Foundation (#19TQC005).

Acknowledgments: The authors wish to thank the anonymous reviewers for their highly constructive and helpful comments.

Conflicts of Interest: The authors declare no conflict of interest.

References

1. Kogan, M.D.; Vladutiu, C.J.; Schieve, L.A.; Ghandour, R.M.; Blumberg, S.J.; Zablotsky, B.; Perrin, J.M.; Shattuck, P.; Kuhlthau, K.A.; Harwood, R.L.; et al. The Prevalence of Parent-Reported Autism Spectrum Disorder Among US Children. *Pediatrics* **2018**, *142*, e20174161. [CrossRef] [PubMed]
2. Volker, M.A.; Lopata, C. Autism: A review of biological bases, assessment, and intervention. *Sch. Psychol. Q.* **2008**, *23*, 258–270. [CrossRef]
3. Mazurek, M.O. Social media use among adults with autism spectrum disorders. *Comput. Hum. Behav.* **2013**, *29*, 1709–1714. [CrossRef]
4. Roffeei, S.H.M.; Abdullah, N.; Basar, S.K.R. Seeking social support on Facebook for children with Autism Spectrum Disorders (ASDs). *Int. J. Med. Inf.* **2015**, *84*, 375–385. [CrossRef] [PubMed]
5. Rump, K.M.; Giovannelli, J.L.; Minshew, N.J.; Strauss, M.S. The Development of Emotion Recognition in Individuals with Autism. *Child. Dev.* **2009**, *80*, 1434–1447. [CrossRef] [PubMed]
6. Newman, M.W.; Lauterbach, D.; Munson, S.A.; Resnick, P.; Morris, M.E. It's Not That I Don'T Have Problems, I'M Just Not Putting Them on Facebook: Challenges and Opportunities in Using Online Social Networks for Health. In Proceedings of the ACM 2011 Conference on Computer Supported Cooperative Work, CSCW '11, New York, NY, USA, 19–23 March 2011; ACM: New York, NY, USA, 2011; pp. 341–350.
7. Sugimoto, S. Support Exchange on the Internet: A Content Analysis of an Online Support Group for People Living with Depression. Ph.D. Thesis, University of Toronto, Toronto, ON, Canada, November 2013.
8. Board, ADAME. Autism. Available online: http://www.ncbi.nlm.nih.gov/pubmedhealth/PMH0002494/ (accessed on 13 March 2019).

9. Smith, M.A.; Shneiderman, B.; Milic-Frayling, N.; Rodrigues, E.M.; Barash, V.; Dunne, C.; Capone, T.; Perer, A.; Gleave, E. Analyzing (Social Media) Networks with NodeXL. In Proceedings of the Fourth International Conference on Communities and Technologies, University Park, PA, USA, 25–27 June 2009; pp. 255–264.
10. Liddy, E.D. Text Mining. *Bull. Am. Soc. Inf. Sci. Technol.* **2000**, *27*, 13–14. [CrossRef]
11. Bird, S.; Klein, E.; Loper, E. *Natural Language Processing with Python: Analyzing Text with the Natural Language Toolkit*; O'Reilly Media, Inc.: Sevastopol, CA, USA, 2009.
12. Griffiths, T.L.; Steyvers, M. Finding scientific topics. *Proc. Natl. Acad. Sci. USA* **2004**, *101* (Suppl. 1), 5228–5235. [CrossRef]
13. Řehůřek, R.; Sojka, P. Software Framework for Topic Modelling with Large Corpora. In Proceedings of the LREC 2010 Workshop on New Challenges for NLP Frameworks, Valletta, Malta, 22 May 2010; pp. 45–50.
14. Cao, J.; Xia, T.; Li, J.; Zhang, Y.; Tang, S. A Density-Based Method for Adaptive LDA Model Selection. *Neurocomputing* **2009**, *72*, 1775–1781. [CrossRef]
15. Lu, K.; Wolfram, D. Measuring Author Research Relatedness: A Comparison of Word-Based, Topic-Based, and Author Cocitation Approaches. *J. Am. Soc. Inf. Sci. Technol.* **2012**, *63*, 1973–1986. [CrossRef]
16. Murdock, J.; Allen, C. Visualization Techniques for Topic Model Checking. In Proceedings of the Twenty-Ninth AAAI Conference on Artificial Intelligence, AAAI'15, Austin, TX, USA, 25–30 January 2015; AAAI Press: Austin, TX, USA, 2015; pp. 4284–4285.
17. Sievert, C.; Shirley, K.E. LDAvis: A method for visualizing and interpreting topics. In Proceedings of the Workshop on Interactive Language Learning, Visualization, and Interfaces, Baltimore, MD, USA, 27 June 2014.
18. Ellmann, M.; Oeser, A.; Fucci, D.; Maalej, W. Find, Understand, and Extend Development Screencasts on YouTube. In Proceedings of the 3rd ACM SIGSOFT International Workshop on Software Analytics, Paderborn, Germany, 4 September 2017.
19. Saeidi, A.M.; Hage, J.; Khadka, R.; Jansen, S. ITMViz: Interactive Topic Modeling for Source Code Analysis. In Proceedings of the 2015 IEEE 23rd International Conference on Program Comprehension, Piscataway, NJ, USA, 16–24 May 2015; pp. 295–298.
20. Electric & Magnetic Fields. Available online: http://www.niehs.nih.gov/health/topics/agents/emf/index.cfm (accessed on 14 March 2019).
21. Willis, E. Applying the Health Belief Model to Medication Adherence: The Role of Online Health Communities and Peer Reviews. *J. Health Commun.* **2018**, *23*, 743–750. [CrossRef] [PubMed]
22. Willis, E.; Royne, M.B. Online Health Communities and Chronic Disease Self-Management. *Health Commun.* **2017**, *32*, 269–278. [CrossRef] [PubMed]
23. Thompson, L.A. A Descriptive Case Study of Individuals with Presumed Ocular Histoplasmosis Syndrome Utilizing a Facebook Support Group. Ph.D. Thesis, University of Arkansas, Fayetteville, AK, USA, December 2015.
24. Cheung, C.M.K.; Chiu, P.-Y.; Lee, M.K.O. Online social networks: Why do students use facebook? *Comput. Hum. Behav.* **2011**, *27*, 1337–1343. [CrossRef]
25. Raj, E. Online Communities for People Who Stutter: An Ethnographic Study of A Facebook Social Networking Support Group. Ph.D. Thesis, Wayne State University, Detroit, MI, USA, January 2015.
26. Niwa, K.D.; Mandrusiak, M.N. Self-Injury Groups on Facebook. *Can. J. Couns. Psychother. Rev. Can. Couns. Psychothérapie* **2012**, *46*, 972.
27. Allen, C.; Vassilev, I.; Kennedy, A.; Rogers, A. Long-Term Condition Self-Management Support in Online Communities: A Meta-Synthesis of Qualitative Papers. *J. Med. Internet Res.* **2016**, *18*, e61. [CrossRef] [PubMed]
28. Zhang, J.; Li, F.; Lin, Y.; Sheng, Q.; Yu, X.; Zhang, X. Subjective Sleep Quality in Perimenopausal Women and Its Related Factors. *J. Nanjing Med. Univ.* **2007**, *21*, 116–119. [CrossRef]

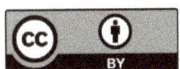

© 2019 by the authors. Licensee MDPI, Basel, Switzerland. This article is an open access article distributed under the terms and conditions of the Creative Commons Attribution (CC BY) license (http://creativecommons.org/licenses/by/4.0/).

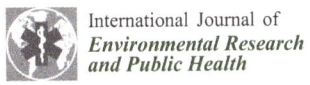

Article

Facebook Groups on Chronic Obstructive Pulmonary Disease: Social Media Content Analysis

Avery Apperson [1], Michael Stellefson [1,*], Samantha R. Paige [2], Beth H. Chaney [1], J. Don Chaney [1], Min Qi Wang [3] and Arjun Mohan [4]

1. Department of Health Education and Promotion, East Carolina University, Greenville, NC 27858, USA
2. STEM Translational Communication Center, University of Florida, Gainesville, FL 679205, USA
3. Department of Behavioral and Community Health, University of Maryland, College Park, MD 20742, USA
4. Division of Pulmonary, Critical Care and Sleep Medicine, Department of Internal Medicine, East Carolina University Brody School of Medicine, Greenville, NC 27858, USA
* Correspondence: stellefsonm17@ecu.edu

Received: 31 August 2019; Accepted: 4 October 2019; Published: 9 October 2019

Abstract: Facebook Groups facilitate information exchange and engagement for patients with chronic conditions, including those living with Chronic Obstructive Pulmonary Disease (COPD); however, little is known about how knowledge is diffused throughout these communities. This study aimed to evaluate the content that is available on COPD-related Facebook Groups, as well as the communication (self-disclosures, social support) and engagement (agreement, emotional reaction) strategies used by members to facilitate these resources. Two researchers independently searched the "Groups" category using the terms "COPD", "emphysema", and "chronic bronchitis". Twenty-six closed ($n = 23$) and public ($n = 3$) COPD Facebook Groups were identified with 87,082 total members. The vast majority of Group members belonged to closed ($n = 84,684$; 97.25%) as compared to open ($n = 2398$; 2.75%) groups. Medications were the most commonly addressed self-management topic ($n = 48$; 26.7%). While overall engagement with wall posts was low, the number of "likes" (an indicator of agreement) was significantly greater for wall posts that demonstrated social support as compared to posts that did not ($p < 0.001$). Findings from this study showed that COPD Facebook group members share specific disease-related experiences and request information about select self-management topics. This information can be used to improve the quality of self-management support provided to members of popular COPD Facebook groups.

Keywords: COPD; Facebook; social media; online community; self-management; social support

1. Introduction

Chronic Obstructive Pulmonary Disease (COPD) refers to a group of respiratory diseases, including chronic bronchitis and emphysema, characterized by airflow blockage and a progressive worsening of breathing [1]. Airflow limitation is caused by thickening and inflammation of the airway lining and destruction of the tissues that allow for gas exchange to occur. As COPD progresses, symptoms often worsen and become disabling during the everyday lives of people living with the condition [2]. COPD is currently the fourth leading cause of death in the United States [3]. This debilitating chronic condition is also responsible for killing more than three million people worldwide every year [4]. There are currently 16 million people diagnosed with COPD in the United States (U.S.) [5], and approximately 12 million adults are likely living with COPD but remain undiagnosed [6]. COPD is commonly underdiagnosed in people who are not current or past smokers and young adults who have minimal breathing limitations [7]. By 2030, the World Health Organization (WHO) anticipates that COPD will become the third leading cause of mortality and seventh leading cause of morbidity worldwide [8].

In the U.S., annual healthcare expenses attributable to COPD and its sequelae cost is in excess of $32 billion dollars. However, these costs could be even higher due to the large amount of people likely to be living with COPD who remain undiagnosed. Medical costs associated with COPD are projected to approach $49 billion dollars by 2020 [9]. An estimated 16.4 million days of missed work are caused by COPD, causing annual indirect costs associated with lost productivity due to COPD to be approximately $3.9 billion dollars [10]. As annual healthcare expenditures attributable to COPD continue to rise, secondary and tertiary prevention, including screening for COPD via spirometry and successful smoking cessation will be increasingly important to help manage medical costs related to COPD [10].

Symptoms of COPD often include wheezing, productive cough, shortness of breath, and chest tightness [5]. These symptoms often worsen over time, which can be disabling for many people diagnosed with the condition. A worsening, or flare up, of these symptoms is known as an exacerbation. An exacerbation of symptoms is usually due to an infection of the lungs or airways; however, sometimes the cause of an exacerbation is unknown. Inhaling irritating pollutants and allergies can sometimes be the cause of symptom exacerbations [11]. In 2008, there were 822,500 documented hospital stays attributed to COPD in the U.S. among people 40 years of age and older [12]. Hospitalization rates for acute exacerbations of COPD were higher in the Midwest and South, particularly in rural and low-income areas [12]. The average length of stay for a hospital visit was 4.8 days, and the average cost of a COPD-related hospital stay was $7500 [12].

Prolonged exposure to tobacco smoke is by far the most significant risk factor for COPD. Cigarette smoking produces many toxins that destroy lung tissues, cause inflammation in airways, and weaken the ability of the lungs to prevent infections [13]. Other risk factors for COPD include poor indoor air quality, second-hand smoke, exposure to toxins, older age, and genetic factors including Alpha-1 antitrypsin deficiency [14]. COPD is diagnosed based on symptoms, degree of airflow limitation, risk for exacerbations, and identifiable comorbidities. Common comorbidities associated with COPD include cardiovascular disease, diabetes, anemia, obstructive sleep apnea, gastroesophageal reflux disease, anxiety, and depression [15].

Although there is currently no cure for COPD, treatment can slow the progression and control symptoms [5]. Common types of medications used to treat COPD are bronchodilators, oral steroids, inhaled steroids, antibiotics, and combination inhalers. Bronchodilators, such as albuterol, work to relieve coughing and shortness of breath by relaxing the muscles around the airways. Inhaled steroids and oral steroids help prevent and relieve exacerbations by reducing airway inflammation, while combination inhalers use a mixture of inhaled steroids and bronchodilators. Respiratory infections can worsen COPD symptoms and are treated with antibiotics such as azithromycin [16]. Poor medication adherence among patients with COPD often results in adverse health outcomes, reduced quality of life, higher hospitalization rates, and increased healthcare expenditures [17].

While COPD treatments such as pulmonary rehabilitation, bronchodilators, nutritional counseling, and smoking cessation can alleviate symptoms and decrease exacerbations [1], many patients receive poor information on lifestyle changes and ways to manage their disease [18]. People living with chronic diseases are increasingly using the Internet to gain knowledge of specific diseases and their treatments [19]. Studies show that patients with COPD are moderately confident making health decisions based on information gained from the Internet [20]. However, patients with COPD are less confident in their ability to distinguish between low and high-quality sources of health information [21]. The introduction of technology into disease management has generated mixed perceptions from patients. Some see the benefits—such as early detection of exacerbations and awareness of symptoms—while others believe it creates a divide between the patient and health care professional [22].

Social media platforms provide an online space for Internet users to create user profiles, make connections with other users, and engage in online discussions [23]. Social media is used by 69% of Americans today. Although young adults continue to be the largest users of social media, older adults have become more accustomed to using social technologies. In 2016, 80% of 30- to 49-year old and

64% of 50- to 64-year old adults were using at least one type of social media. Among the major social media platforms, Facebook is the most widely used [24]. Sixty-eight percent of U.S. adults report using Facebook, with approximately 75% of these users visiting the site daily [25].

People with chronic diseases are now using online social networks to seek advice and obtain evidence-based health information to help with self-managing their conditions [19]. According to Allen, Vassilev, Kennedy and Roger [26], "social ties forged in online spaces provide the basis for performing relevant self-management work that can improve an individual's illness experience, tackling aspects of self-management that are particularly difficult to meet offline." (p. e61). Free social networking sites, such as micro-blogs (e.g., Twitter), Facebook, Pinterest, and discussion boards, allow users to share and obtain information through user-friendly platforms. In addition, these sites could be useful for reaching specific, intended audiences; for example, a social media content analysis of Pinterest found that this social networking website is highly marketed to women as a resource for living with COPD [27]. Therefore, the research suggests that the use of certain social media websites, in this case—Pinterest, may be useful for disseminating health information to specific audiences, thus allowing for audience segmentation.

New media tools, like social networks, are also re-engineering the way doctors, patients, and their caregivers interact with each other. Results of a systematic review investigating social media use among health professionals suggest that health care providers perceive social media platforms to be useful tools in facilitating chronic disease self-management with patients [28]. Social networks allow greater accessibility to health-related information and provide an outlet for communication between people living with a similar chronic disease(s) [29]. Research shows that social media has been used for diagnostic purposes, patient education, and disease management [30]. Moreover, there has been an increase in the number of social media-based health management systems used to deliver more convenient health care services. Gu and colleagues [31] found that a patient's personality (openness to new experiences) impacts their use of social media-based health management systems. However, research on the use of social networks for disease prevention and management is limited. Patel and colleagues [30], note that although it is evident technology has the potential to improve public health, it is necessary to conduct further research on how patients and technology interact to improve disease management and outcomes.

Facebook is a popular online social network that allows users to share photos, posts, and engage in discussions [32]. With over one billion active daily users [33], Facebook has a broad reach for sharing information related to chronic disease. Sixty percent of state health departments report using social media, with fifty-six percent having a Facebook account [34]. When patients access health-related information on Facebook, their main motives are social support, exchange of advice, and increasing knowledge [35]. Facebook "Groups" are unique forums used by Facebook users who share common interests. These Groups allow Facebook users to communicate about a common organization, event, or issue in a variety of formats (e.g., photos, text) [36]. Content is communicated through self-disclosures and support-reciprocating topics and engaged in the form of agreements and contributions (e.g., comments) [36]. Disease-specific information exchanges now occur within Facebook Groups.

Past studies have shown Facebook Groups to be a communication tool used by patients seeking information or support for breast cancer [37], depression [38], and diabetes [39]; however, there are no studies examining what self-management content is communicated on COPD-related Facebook groups and how the content is engaged among its members. Users communicate content through self-disclosures and support, whereas, this content is engaged through reactions (e.g., agreement and expression, comments). Exploring how Facebook Groups host COPD self-management information content will inform researchers and practitioners about what content is available and diffused within online COPD communities. To this end, three research questions (RQ) were proposed.

RQ1: What (a) self-management content areas, (b) communication strategies, and (c) engagement metrics are available on COPD Facebook Groups?

RQ2: Are certain communication strategies more common on COPD Facebook Group wall posts that mention (a) generic self-management, (b) medication management, and (c) hospitalization/doctor visits?

RQ3: Which communication strategies yield most user engagement on COPD Facebook Group wall posts?

2. Materials and Methods

2.1. Theoretical Framework

Understanding the processes and variables involved in health behavior, lifestyle change, and self-management allows for better communication of health enhancing messages [40]. The Common-Sense Model of Illness Self-Regulation (CSM) examines the perceptual, behavioral, and cognitive responses that patients often have when self-managing their health threats [40]. The beliefs and expectations people have about an illness, or illness representations, is the key construct in this model [41]. These expectations inform the ways in which patients navigate their responses to the illness, including what decisions patients make for managing the illness. Major beliefs involved in illness representations of COPD include comorbid identities (i.e., asthma), causes (i.e., cigarette smoking), consequences (i.e., mental health disorders), and curability (i.e., rescue medications, pursed lipped breathing techniques). Relationships among these beliefs tend to guide how patients cope with and treat their own chronic illness(es). Social media is one mechanism for providing self-management support for coping and treating chronic illness(es) [30]; however, research on how concepts of CSM can be utilized on this platform for the promotion of successful self-management of chronic illness(es) is limited [40]. Therefore, a better understanding of how social media is being used to motivate and engage users, as a way to self-manage a health threat, and communicate content regarding chronic illness(es) is warranted.

2.2. Search Procedures

Two researchers individually searched the "Groups" category of Facebook using the terms "COPD", "emphysema", and "chronic bronchitis" to locate existing both public and closed COPD groups. Closed Facebook groups are defined as groups requiring approval from an administrator or current member to join before Group content can be viewed. Public groups are those that can be joined by any Facebook user with a valid account; any Facebook user can view group wall post content of public groups, even if they are not a member of group. Both public and closed Facebook groups allow all Facebook members to view the group title, description, members, and post activity, even if they are not a member of the group. For closed Facebook groups, administrators are contacted to gain access to the group's wall post content. Closed groups commonly have questions that accompany a request to join, such as asking about the Facebook user's reason for joining the group. These questions were answered by each member of the research team by responding in the following manner: "Please see message in private inbox before accepting this request. Thank you". The message sent to each group administrator's private inbox (Appendix A) was approved by East Carolina University's Institutional Review Board (IRB).

2.3. Inclusion/Exclusion Criteria

The analysis was restricted to all public and closed Facebook Groups related to COPD with content posted content in English. Secret Facebook groups, or those that did not show up in Facebook group searches, were excluded from the analysis because only individual Facebook users who have been invited by the Secret group administrator or a current Facebook member have the ability to see the group title, description, members, and wall post content. Any closed Group that did not accept the researchers' request to join the Facebook Group by the beginning of data collection was excluded because wall posts can only be viewed by Facebook group members. However, we were able to record general membership data about closed groups, as this information is publicly accessible to anyone with a valid Facebook account.

2.4. Data Collection

Institutional Review Board (IRB) approval was obtained from the researchers' university prior to collecting data from Facebook. Twenty-six closed (n = 23) and public (n = 3) COPD Facebook Groups were identified after accounting for inclusion and exclusion criteria as described in Figure 1. Fifteen Facebook groups were initially excluded (n = 15) because they focused on other pulmonary diseases and disorders other than COPD. After excluding these groups, 26 were retained for further analysis. Of these, 17 were excluded due to group administrators not responding to our request to join their group (n = 15) or disallowing our request to join (n = 2). The two COPD Facebook group administrators who declined investigator requests to join their group did not provide a specific reason for doing so. Upon accounting for exclusion criteria, researchers recorded membership statistics and coded wall posts from three public and six private COPD Facebook groups.

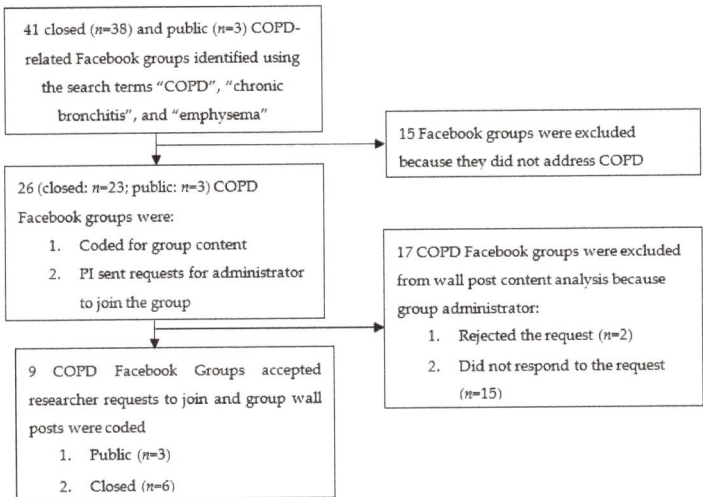

Figure 1. Flowchart depicting Chronic Obstructive Pulmonary Disease (COPD) Facebook group selection process.

Two researchers independently reviewed these nine COPD Facebook groups and coded publicly-accessible group information such as group title, number of members, and wall post activity. Member accessibility to Facebook Groups (closed or public) was noted by the researchers. Based on prior social media content analysis research [37,38,40] a coding and classification scheme was applied to the 20 most recent wall posts within nine closed (n = 6) and public (n = 3) Facebook COPD groups. This resulted in 180 unique wall posts considered for analysis.

2.5. Measures

Demographics of each COPD Facebook Group and wall post were examined. For the groups, post activity included the number of members gained or lost in the last 30 days, number of new daily posts, and number of posts made in the last 30 days. In addition, researchers recorded the privacy setting (closed or public), intended audience (patient, caregiver, health care provider), and number of months each COPD Facebook group was in existence. For COPD Facebook Group wall posts, reach (number of members in each group) and engagement (wall post activity) metrics were recorded. Group wall posts were also coded to determine the type of media modality (i.e., text, video, photo, and infographics).

Table 1 shows the categories and definitions for each code in the analysis. Group titles and descriptions were coded to determine the purpose of the group related to the following categories: (1) building awareness/sharing information, (2) providing support, (3) fundraising purpose, (4) marketing/promoting a product or service, or (5) other. Wall posts were coded based on self-management content areas: (1) mental health, (2) medication management, (3) hospitalizations, (4) asthma, (5) cigarette smoking, (6) breathing techniques, (7) nutrition, and (8) physical activity. Communication strategies were recorded using the following categories: (1) self-disclosures about the disease; (2) referrals; (3) information-providing, (3) requests for information, (4) demonstrations of support, (5) product/service promotion, and (6) other (See Table 1 for definitions of group purpose codes). Engagement metrics such as number of reactions (i.e., likes, emojis for love, funny, surprise, sad, and anger), comments, and shares of wall posts were recorded. Use of emoticons or "emojis" to evaluate user reactions may not accurately reflect all user attitudes about Facebook content, but these visual communication tools can serve as a useful proxy for assessing user reactions to health care content found on social media [41].

Table 1. Facebook group content analysis codes, definitions, and code sources.

Code	Definition	Code Source	Illness Self-Regulation Representation [a]
Group Purpose			
Building Awareness/Sharing Information	Created to bring attention to the importance of COPD and share COPD-related information	Bender et al. [37]	Comorbid identities, causes, curability, consequences
Providing Support	Created to meet the emotional needs of COPD patients and their caregivers	Bender et al. [37]	Comorbid identities, causes, curability, consequences
Fundraising	Created to attract financial resources for COPD	Bender et al. [37]	N/A
Marketing/Promoting a Product/Service	Created to promote a COPD-related product or service	Bender et al. [37]	Curability
Media Modality			
Text	Text included in the post	Neiger et al. [42]	N/A
Video	Video included in the post	Neiger et al. [42]	N/A
Photo	Photo included in the post	Neiger et al. [42]	N/A
Infographic	Infographic included in the post	Neiger et al. [42]	N/A
Communication Strategies			
Self-Disclosures	Information was self-disclosed about personal experiences with COPD	Lerman et al. [38]	Comorbid identities, causes, curability, consequences
Referrals	Providing information about COPD through links to external websites, pages, groups, or documents	Lerman et al. [38]	Comorbid identities, causes, curability, consequences
Information Providing	COPD-related information was shared in the post	Greene et al. [43]	Comorbid identities, causes, curability, consequences
Information Requesting	COPD-related queries were posed to the group	Greene et al. [43]	Comorbid identities, causes, curability, consequences
Demonstrating Support	Emotional support was provided to the group	Greene et al. [43]	Comorbid identities, causes, curability, consequences
Product/Service Promotion	A product or service was promoted	Greene et al. [43]	Curability
Self-Management Content Area			
Mental Health	Mentions mental health issues such as depression, anxiety, etc.	CDC [44]	Comorbid identities, Consequences
Medications	Mentions medications such as antibiotics, inhalers, etc.	CDC [44]	Curability
Hospitalizations/Doctor Visits	Mentions hospitalization or doctors visit related to COPD	GOLD [45]	Consequences
Asthma	Mentions asthma specifically	GOLD [45]	Comorbid identities
Smoking	Mentions smoking such as cigarette smoking, vaping, e-cigarette use, etc.	GOLD [45]	Causes
Breathing Techniques	Mentions specific breathing techniques to cope with exacerbations	CDC [44]	Curability
Nutrition	Mentions nutrition such as recipes and health eating habits	CDC [44]	Curability
Physical Activity	Mentions physical activity such as walking, stair climbing, etc.	CDC [44]	Curability, Consequences

Table 1. Cont.

Code	Definition	Code Source	Illness Self-Regulation Representation [a]
Engagement			
Like	Number of times members reacted to the post by pressing the thumbs up icon	Neiger et al. [42]	N/A
Love	Number of times members reacted to the post by pressing the heart emoji	Neiger et al. [42]	N/A
Sad	Number of times members reacted to the post by pressing the sad emoji	Neiger et al. [42]	N/A
Angry	Number of times members reacted to the post by pressing the angry emoji	Neiger et al. [42]	N/A
Laugh	Number of times members reacted to the post by pressing the haha emoji	Neiger et al. [42]	N/A
Surprised	Number of times members reacted to the post by pressing the wow emoji	Neiger et al. [42]	N/A
Comment	Number of times members reacted to the post by replying with text, gif, etc.	Neiger et al. [42]	N/A
Share	Number of times members reacted to a post by sharing it	Neiger et al. [42]	N/A

[a] Illness self-regulation representations were coded based on information from Leventhal et al. [40] and Hale et al. [46].

2.6. Coder Training

A codebook was developed based on existing social media content analysis research [37,38,40] and relevant COPD self-management guidelines [44,45]. Two researchers met before data collection to discuss the coding methods operationalized in the codebook and resolved discrepancies in how codes were to be interpreted. Subsequently, each researcher independently extracted data from COPD Facebook groups and recorded the data. Intercoder reliability of applied codes was determined using Cohen's Kappa Statistic [47]. The Kappa statistic was selected, because it serves as a robust measure of intercoder reliability in research that involves the coding of behavior-related variables [48], including those measured on social media. A subset of 10–25% of the total sample was sufficient for determining inter-rater reliability of codes; therefore, a sub-sample of 5 Facebook groups was independently coded by each researcher. The cut-off value for acceptable intercoder reliability was set at 0.70 [49].

2.7. Data Analysis

The user analytic data was exported to Statistical Package for Social Sciences (SPSS) v24.0 for further analyses. Frequency and descriptive statistics were computed to determine the group purpose, membership levels, wall post activity, and group member engagement activity within COPD Facebook groups. Nonparametric data led to reporting medians (±IQR). Descriptive median (±IQR) statistics were used to determine average engagement (likes, comments, etc.) metrics for wall posts addressing various aspects of self-management (mental health, medication management, etc.). Chi-square analyses were conducted to determine if the number of wall post communication strategies (self-disclosure, referral, information providing, information requesting, offering support, and product/service promotion) varied based on whether or not (a) general self-management, (b) medication management or (c) hospitalizations were specifically addressed. A series of Mann-Whitney U tests were conducted to examine the extent to which wall post communication strategies (i.e., providing information, requesting information, and/or demonstrating support) were associated with group member engagement (i.e., number of wall post likes, sad emojis, and comments).

3. Results

3.1. Data Reliability

Kappa agreement between coders ranged from 0.66–0.99 (M = 0.90, SD = 0.15) for the self-management content areas (Table 2). Kappa estimates for wall post characteristics ranged from 0.66–0.99 (M = 0.91, SD = 0.12). All Kappa statistics were at or near the cut-off value used to establish adequate intercoder reliability (0.70).

Table 2. Intercoder reliability scores for self-management content areas and characteristics of Chronic Obstructive Pulmonary Disease (COPD) group wall posts ($n = 40$).

Self-Management Content Area	Cohen's Kappa
Mental Health	>0.99
Medications	>0.99
Hospitalizations/Doctor Visits	0.91
Asthma	>0.99
Smoking	>0.99
Breathing Techniques	0.66
Nutrition	>0.99
Physical Activity	0.66
Mean	0.90
SD	0.15
Wall Post Characteristics	**Cohen's Kappa**
Post Included Text	0.66
Post Included Video	>0.99
Post Included Photo	0.87
Post Included Infographic	>0.99
Information Providing	>0.99
Information Requesting	0.95
Demonstrating Support	0.75
Personal Self-Disclosure	0.95
Referral to Other Resources	>0.99
Product/Service Promotion	>0.99
Mean	0.91
SD	0.12

3.2. Group Characteristics

The purpose of most COPD Facebook groups was to provide support (19/26, 73.1%), while the remaining groups (7/26, 26.9%) built awareness or shared health information. None of the groups had a primary purpose of fundraising or marketing/promoting a product or service. The median time in existence for both public and closed groups was 60 months (IQR= 30 months to 90 months), or about five years. There were no statistically significant differences in the median number of members, growth in members over the past 30 days, new daily posts, and number of wall posts in the past 30 days based on group purpose.

3.3. Group Size

Table 3 describes the general characteristics and membership statistics for the 26 COPD Facebook groups analyzed in this content analysis. In total, 87,082 members were identified as members of these groups. The vast majority of members belonged to closed ($n = 84,684$; 97.25%), as opposed to open ($n = 2398$; 2.75%) groups. The number of members ranged from 153 members in the smallest group ("Chronic Bronchitis Support & Awareness") to 12,337 members in the largest group ("Ultimate Pulmonary Wellness: COPD, PF, Pulmonary Hypertension and Others"). The largest group was closed, had a group purpose of providing support, and was in operation for 36 months or approximately 3 years.

Table 3. General characteristics and membership in 26 COPD Facebook groups as of March 2019.

Group Name	Privacy Setting	Group Purpose	Number of Members	Number of New Members in Past 30 Days	Number of Posts in Past 30 Days	Months in Operation
Ultimate Pulmonary Wellness: COPD, PF, Pulmonary Hypertension and Others	Closed	Providing Support	12,337	245	632	36
COPD Warriors Hope, Support, Love & Laughter	Closed	Providing Support	10,451	692	2764	60
COPD/Emphysema/Pulmonary Disease- I have COPD- COPD does not have me!	Closed	Building Awareness/Sharing Information	7952	0	367	60
COPD- GET EDUCATED!	Closed	Providing Support	6837	0	277	24
(COPD) Emphysema/Chronic Bronchitis Support Group	Closed	Providing Support	5537	0	67	120
COPD Information and Support	Closed	Building Awareness/Sharing Information	5028	294	1087	48
Let's Talk COPD Support Group	Closed	Providing Support	4139	213	672	24
Support Group for People with COPD, Emphysema, Asthma, Bronchitis	Closed	Providing Support	3938	192	233	84
Emphysema	Closed	Providing Support	3794	84	243	96
COPD Xplained- USA	Closed	Building Awareness/Sharing Information	3748	90	291	108
COPD Support Group	Closed	Providing Support	3049	229	551	36
COPD/ A WARM LOVING PLACE TO HANG OUT	Closed	Providing Support	3027	97	1998	48
COPD Breathing Buddies	Closed	Providing Support	2776	0	660	60
Lift Up- COPD Support Group	Closed	Providing Support	2438	282	381	12
COPD- New Treatments and Advice	Closed	Building Awareness/Sharing Information	2238	0	34	48
COPD/COAD Support	Closed	Building Awareness/Sharing Information	2223	0	125	96
COPD/ALPHA 1	Public	Providing Support	1273	4	59	60
COPD- A BREATH OF FRESH AIR	Closed	Providing Support	974	0	272	48
COPD-Emphysema-Chronic Bronchitis	Closed	Providing Support	886	0	6	96
COPD Tackling it Together	Closed	Providing Support	868	0	103	132
COPD Service	Public	Providing Support	830	0	0	60
COPD CRAZINESS AND SUPPORT	Closed	Providing Support	810	0	301	120
Chronic Obstructive Pulmonary Disease	Closed	Providing Support	781	0	7	96
C.O.P.D Warriors	Closed	Building Awareness/Sharing Information	700	0	343	24
Support & Awareness for COPD, Emphysema and Chronic Bronchitis	Public	Building Awareness/Sharing Information	295	0	6	132
Chronic Bronchitis Support & Awareness	Closed	Providing Support	153	0	0	12

3.4. Wall Post Content and Characteristics

The most common communication strategy used in wall posts was self-disclosure (80/180, 44.4%), followed by referrals to external web sources of information (53/180 or 29.4%). Forty-five (25%) wall posts provided information related to COPD, while 69 (38%) requested information about COPD. Wall posts that offered messages of support comprised 14.4% (26/180) of total group wall posts, while only 2.7% (5/180) of wall posts promoted a product or service.

Specific self-management content areas most often included in group wall posts were medication management (48/180, 26.7%) and hospitalizations/doctor visits (28/180, 15.6%). Other generic aspects of self-management, including mental health (14/180, 7.8%), cigarette smoking (10/180, 5.6%), physical activity (8/180, 4.4%), asthma (5/180, 3.3%), breathing techniques (5/180, 2.8%), and nutrition (1/180, 0.6%), received less attention.

3.5. Group Wall Post Engagement

There was low overall engagement on wall posts. The median number of wall post "likes" was four (IQR = 8.5), while the median number of comments was five (IQR = 12). Love emojis, sad emojis, angry emojis, "haha" emojis, wow emojis, and shares of wall posts were virtually non-existent ($Mdn = 0$, $IQR = 0$).

3.6. Wall Post Communication Strategy and Self-Management

Wall posts that addressed self-management were more likely to include a self-disclosure (62.5%), as compared to posts that did not address self-management (28%), $\chi^2(df = 1) = 21.54$, $p < 0.001$ (Table 4). A greater proportion of self-management posts posed questions to other members (60.9%), $\chi^2(df = 1) = 14.01$, $p < 0.001$, but a lesser proportion provided support to fellow group members (7.7%), $\chi^2(df = 1) = 15.72$, $p < 0.001$. These estimates are compared to self-management posts that did not request information (32.4%) but provided support (49.4%) to fellow group members. Self-management posts were also less likely to refer members to external web sources (24.5% vs. 51.2%), $\chi^2(df = 1) = 10.82$, $p < 0.05$.

Table 4. Frequency of wall post content ($n = 180$) of 26 COPD Facebook Groups according to whether or not wall post addressed any self-management topics.

Wall Post Communication Strategies	Posts Addressing COPD Self-Management n (%)	Posts Not Addressing COPD Self-Management n (%)	p Value
Self-Disclosure			
Yes ($n = 80$)	50 (62.5) **	30 (37.5)	0.0001
No ($n = 100$)	28 (28)	72 (72)	
Referral to External Information Source			
Yes ($n = 53$)	13 (24.5) *	40 (75.5)	0.001
No ($n = 127$)	65 (51.2)	62 (48.8)	
Information Provided			
Yes ($n = 45$)	19 (42.2)	26 (57.8)	0.862
No ($n = 135$)	59 (43.7)	76 (56.3)	
Information Requested (i.e., Asks a Question)			
Yes ($n = 69$)	42 (60.9) **	27 (39.1)	0.0001
No ($n = 111$)	36 (32.4)	75 (67.6)	
Offers Support			
Yes ($n = 26$)	2 (7.7) **	24 (92.3)	0.0001
No ($n = 154$)	76 (49.4)	78 (50.6)	
Product/Service Promotion			
Yes ($n = 5$)	3 (60)	2 (40)	0.446
No ($n = 175$)	75 (42.9)	100 (57.1)	

* $p < 0.05$, ** $p < 0.001$.

3.6.1. Wall Post Communication Strategy and Medication Management

Medication management was the most common self-management topic included within wall posts (48/180, 26.7%) (Table 5). Medication management posts were less likely to include a self-disclosure (40.0%), as compared to posts that did not (16.0%), $\chi^2(df = 1) = 13.09$, $p < 0.001$. A lower proportion of medication management posts referred group members to an external web source (13.2%, as compared to the posts that did include this service (32.3%), $\chi^2(df = 1) = 6.96$, $p < 0.05$. Medication management posts were also more likely to request information from other online users, $\chi^2(df = 1) = 16.17$, $p < 0.001$.

Table 5. Frequency of communication strategies used in COPD Facebook group wall posts according to whether or not post addressed medication management ($n = 48$).

Communication Strategy	Post Addressed Medication Management n (%)	Post Did Not Address Medication Management n (%)	p Value
Self-Disclosure			
Yes ($n = 80$)	32 (40) **	48 (60)	0.0001
No ($n = 100$)	16 (16)	84 (84)	
Referral to External Information Source			
Yes ($n = 53$)	7 (13.2) *	46 (86.8)	0.008
No ($n = 127$)	41 (32.3)	86 (67.7)	
Information Provided			
Yes ($n = 45$)	10 (22.2)	35 (77.8)	0.436
No ($n = 135$)	38 (28.1)	97 (71.9)	
Information Requested (i.e., Asks a Question)			
Yes ($n = 69$)	30 (43.5) **	39 (56.5)	0.0001
No ($n = 111$)	18 (16.2)	93 (83.8)	
Offers Support			
Yes ($n = 26$)	0 (0) *	26 (100)	0.001
No ($n = 154$)	48 (31.2)	106 (68.8)	
Product/Service Promotion			
Yes ($n = 5$)	1 (20)	4 (80)	0.732
No ($n = 175$)	47 (26.9)	128 (73.1)	

* $p < 0.05$, ** $p < 0.001$.

3.6.2. Wall Post Communication Strategy and Hospitalizations/Doctor Visits

Hospitalizations/doctor visits were the second most common self-management topic included in group wall posts (28/180, 15.6%) (Table 6). Posts highlighting a hospitalization or doctor's visit were more likely to include self-disclosures (33.8%) than to withhold personal information (1.0%), $\chi^2(df = 1) = 36.29$, $p < 0.001$. None of the wall posts that addressed hospitalizations/doctor visits referred group members to an external web source. Finally, posts that did not address hospitalizations/doctor visits (97.8%) were far more likely to provide information as compared to posts that did not (2.2%), $\chi^2(df = 1) = 8.12$, $p < 0.05$.

Table 6. Frequency of communication strategies used in COPD Facebook group wall posts based on whether or not post addressed hospitalizations/doctor visits ($n = 28$).

Type of Communication Strategy	Post Addressed Hospitalizations/Doctor Visits n (%)	Post Did Not Address Hospitalizations/Doctor Visits n (%)	p Value
Self-Disclosure			
Yes ($n = 80$)	27 (33.8) **	53 (66.2)	0.0001
No ($n = 100$)	1 (1)	99 (99)	
Referral to External Information Source			
Yes ($n = 53$)	0 (0) **	53 (100)	0.0001
No ($n = 127$)	28 (22.0)	99 (78.0)	

Table 6. Cont.

Type of Communication Strategy	Post Addressed Hospitalizations/Doctor Visits n (%)	Post Did Not Address Hospitalizations/Doctor Visits n (%)	p Value
Information Provided			
Yes (n = 45)	1 (2.2) *	44 (97.8)	0.004
No (n = 135)	27 (20)	108 (80)	
Information Requested (i.e., Asks a Question)			
Yes (n = 69)	15 (21.7)	54 (78.3)	0.071
No (n = 111)	13 (11.7)	98 (88.3)	
Offers Support			
Yes (n = 26)	2 (7.7)	24 (92.3)	0.232
No (n = 154)	26 (16.9)	128 (83.1)	
Product/Service Promotion			
Yes (n = 5)	0 (0)	5 (100)	0.330
No (n = 175)	28 (16)	147 (84)	

* $p < 0.05$, ** $p < 0.001$.

3.7. Engagement with COPD Wall Posts according to Communication Strategy

Results from the Mann-Whitney U Test showed that the number of likes on COPD group wall posts was significantly greater for posts that did not provide information about COPD (Mdn = 4) compared to posts that did provide information about COPD (Mdn = 2), U = 1996.00, p = 0.001. In addition, the number of comments on group wall posts was significantly greater for posts that did not provide information about COPD (Mdn = 7) as compared to posts that did (Mdn = 1), U = 1256.5, $p < 0.001$. The number of likes for wall posts requesting information about COPD was significantly greater for posts that did not request information about COPD (Mdn = 4) as compared to posts that did (Mdn = 3), U = 2843.5, p = 0.004. In addition, the number of comments on wall post requests for information was significantly greater for posts that did request information about COPD (Mdn = 7) as compared to posts that did not (Mdn = 2), U = 8813.5, $p < 0.001$. The number of likes was significantly greater for wall posts that demonstrated peer-to-peer (social) support (Mdn = 9.5) as compared to posts that did not demonstrate social support (Mdn = 3), U = 985.50, $p < 0.001$.

4. Discussion

The current study explored online content and communication strategies used among members of COPD Facebook groups. This content analysis investigated how wall post communication strategies varied based on the presence of self-management topics in wall posts, specifically medication management and hospitalizations/doctor visits. The study also noted variability in engagement metrics according to the communication strategies used by members. To our knowledge, this is the first study to assess the content and group member communication strategies used in Facebook groups related to COPD.

COPD Facebook groups were intended to exchange social support, rather than for the purposes of awareness building or fundraising. This finding is inconsistent with prior research examining the purpose of chronic disease self-management groups on social media. Bender and colleagues [37], for example, found that most Facebook groups related to breast cancer were created for awareness and fundraising purposes. Further, Greene and colleagues [43] reported that sharing information was the predominant communication strategy on diabetes-related social media communities. The differential prevalence of communication strategies used across chronic disease online forums highlights the value of developing and sustaining disease-specific, rather than generic chronic disease, communities. Future research should explore the discrete types of social support (emotional, appraisal, information, instrumental) provided within online communities, such as Facebook Groups, dedicated to COPD.

The most common communication strategy used in COPD-related Facebook wall posts was self-disclosure (i.e., information was revealed about personal experiences with COPD), followed by making referrals to external web sources for additional information on topics of interest. Further examination of posts found that personal self-disclosures about the COPD experience and requests for information were more likely to be used as communication strategies in self-management posts (e.g., medication management, hospitalizations/doctor's visits). As such, COPD Facebook Group members are exhibiting a form of communication competence, by contextualizing their question with information about the COPD experience, presumably to increase the relevance and accuracy of responses from other members. The high reliance on self-disclosures in this context may help to explain the substantial disparity between the number of members in closed (n = 84,684) versus public COPD Facebook groups (n = 2398), as social support and self-disclosures usually include more sensitive information being shared, and thus are more likely to occur in private groups. Research is needed to understand the social circumstances under which patients with COPD are more or less likely to disclose personal information on the Internet.

Results of this study also demonstrate that referring patients to an external web source was a common communication strategy across the groups; however, referrals were less common in self-management posts. External web sources, especially those developed by reputable health-related organizations and agencies (e.g., NIH, CDC, WHO), provide evidence-based health information; therefore, information being shared within COPD Facebook groups may not be valid or accurate based on the latest scientific research. This is particularly concerning given that patients with COPD are only moderately confident when making health decisions based on information gained from the Internet [20]. Patients with COPD also report a low degree of health literacy [50]. To optimize content evaluation and site navigation, plain language standards recommend against directing an online user to an outside website as a universal health literacy precaution [51]. It is promising that self-management posts did not include these external website referrals; however, their prevalence across COPD Facebook Groups brings attention for the need to determine what exactly members are being directed toward outside of the online community.

In this study, COPD Facebook Group members requested information about self-management. Users who addressed medication management were more likely to request health information. Due to the importance of medication adherence in COPD, there may be a need for physicians, pharmacists, and patient/health educators to collaborate on novel ways to support patient use of medications via COPD Facebook Groups. Posts that addressed medication management specifically rarely included member referrals to reliable sources of health information. This was likely due to the "closed" (private) nature of the vast majority of COPD Facebook groups identified in this cross-sectional study. While information sharing seems to occur primarily within the "group walls", which may limit the dissemination of inaccurate information, the restricted nature of resource sharing limits what can be learned by Group members. Facebook group administrators should consider instituting policies that require moderators to post content from reputable governmental and non-profit sources based on the latest discussions and questions posted by group members.

Discussions around hospitalizations or doctor visits were the second most common self-management topic discussed within group wall posts. Wall posts that included mentions of hospitalizations or doctor visits were more likely to include personal self-disclosures about the COPD experience, but they were less likely to include informational resources or provide external website resources. In other words, these posts were generally intended as a personal recount of the hospitalization or doctor visit experience. Despite the health communication potential of social media platforms such as Facebook groups, there may be a need for health care providers to also direct patients with COPD to their personal electronic health record to facilitate meaningful information exchange [52]. Facebook group administrators should configure processes that will alert group members that certain self-management topics are best broached within primary care through private patient-provider communication channels.

COPD Facebook Groups are very purposeful; they provide support from an emotional and informational perspective. While overall member engagement with wall posts was quite low, supportive posts, even those that did not provide any additional health information, were more often "liked" than informative posts that lacked any encouraging messages. Likewise, posts whose initiator requested information about COPD from other members were met with a greater number of comments from the community. The few members "engaged" with wall post content seemed to gravitate to posts without self-management information about COPD, which insinuates that "information heavy" posts should be avoided in favor of encouragement and motivational support about how patients can live their best life with COPD. Future primary research with actual patients who live with COPD should seek to confirm or disconfirm patient preferences for using social media platforms such as Facebook groups.

Limitations

This study had several limitations. First, this study only included COPD Facebook groups that posted content in English. "Secret" Facebook groups, where users cannot view group content unless invited by an administrator or current member, were excluded from this study. The increased privacy of these groups could have resulted in different communication strategies and discussion of different self-management topics. In addition, this study was cross-sectional in nature, which could have resulted in missing seasonal effects of COPD self-management covered within Facebook Groups. For example, collecting information during fall or winter may have resulted in more discussion about flu/pneumococcal vaccinations, which are strongly recommended for patients with COPD. Also, the group search was limited to the terms of "COPD", "emphysema", and "chronic bronchitis". Therefore, the search may have excluded COPD Facebook groups that did not include these specific search terms in the group title. Furthermore, rather than identifying self-management topics through a qualitative approach, this study adopted pre-defined codes to identify and categorize wall post content. This non-grounded-theory approach did not account for the wide range of topics that could potentially be discussed within COPD Facebook Groups. Use of theory-based text mining or machine learning algorithms may help identify the broad array of communication patterns that may occur on group walls.

5. Conclusions

Researchers have stated the need for further research regarding peer support groups on Facebook and their impact on chronic disease self-management [53]. In the current study, results show that COPD Facebook group members are utilizing Facebook groups to share their experience managing their condition. The findings of this study support several important implications for practice among health education specialists and health care providers; including, the potential of COPD Facebook groups for establishing social support networks among patients living with COPD, as the groups were found to primarily serve that purpose. COPD Facebook Groups are very purposeful from an emotional and informational support perspective; however, in the context of the CSM [40], understanding more about the interactions among users on the COPD Facebook Groups could potentially help practitioners understand patient processes involved in managing illness threats such as dyspnea triggers. Additional research with patients living with COPD should evaluate the dynamics of these behavioral processes underlying patient motivations and uses of social media sites for disease management and emotional support.

In addition, given most of the communication on the Facebook wall posts involved patient self-disclosures, patient privacy protections need to be considered by practitioners who use Facebook groups as a platform for self-management education. In a similar vein, as COPD Facebook Group members request information about self-management, specifically medication management, it is important that physicians, pharmacists, and patient health education specialists work collaboratively to best use this platform to support the medication compliance and adherence needs that surfaced. While many COPD Facebook group members request information about self-management, there is a need for more informational and motivational support on these platforms to adequately support members in addressing their needs. Further research should explore the quality and safety of self-management information exchanged among patients with COPD on this popular social media platform. In addition, further research is needed to explore additional online user behaviors that quantify how COPD patients are utilizing information found within chronic disease self-management Facebook Groups, including those that are private. Patient dependence on social media tools for self-management, as opposed to reliance on their health care provider(s) for support, should also be explored further. This research will help produce a better understanding of unique patient preferences and motives for utilizing social media for COPD self-management.

Author Contributions: Conceptualization, A.A., M.S. and S.R.P.; Data curation, A.A.; Formal analysis, A.A. and M.S.; Funding acquisition, A.A. and M.S.; Investigation, A.A.; Methodology, A.A., M.S., S.R.P. and M.Q.W.; Project administration, A.A. and M.S.; Resources, M.S.; Supervision, M.S., J.D.C. and M.Q.W.; Validation, A.A., S.R.P. and B.H.C.; Visualization, A.A. and M.S.; Writing—original draft, A.A. and M.S.; Writing—review & editing, M.S., S.R.P., B.H.C., J.D.C., M.Q.W. and A.M.

Funding: This research was funded by an Undergraduate Research and Creative Activity Award from East Carolina University's Division of Research, Economic Development and Engagement (REDE).

Conflicts of Interest: The authors declare no conflict of interest.

References

1. Centers for Disease Control and Prevention. Chronic Obstructive Pulmonary Disease. 2017. Available online: https://www.cdc.gov/copd/index.html (accessed on 5 July 2019).
2. American Lung Association. What is COPD? Available online: http://www.lung.org/lung-health-and-diseases/lung-disease-lookup/copd/learn-about-copd/what-is-copd.html (accessed on 5 July 2019).
3. COPD Foundation. Is COPD the Third of Fourth Leading Cause of Death? Available online: https://www.copdfoundation.org/COPD360social/Community/COPD-Digest/Article/1399/Is-COPD-the-Third-or-Fourth-Leading-Cause-of-Death.aspx (accessed on 5 July 2019).
4. Rabe, K.; Watz, H. Chronic obstructive pulmonary disease. *Lancet* **2017**, *389*, 1931–1940. [CrossRef]
5. National Heart, Lung and Blood Institute. What is COPD? Available online: https://www.nhlbi.nih.gov/health/health-topics/topics/copd/# (accessed on 5 July 2019).
6. National Institutes of Health. Chronic Obstructive Pulmonary Disease (COPD). 2013. Available online: https://report.nih.gov/nihfactsheets/ViewFactSheet.aspx?csid=77&key=C#C (accessed on 5 July 2019).
7. Lamprecht, B.; Soriano, J.; Studnicka, M.; Kaiser, B.; Vanfleteren, L.; Gnatiuc, L.; Burney, P.; Miravitlles, M. Determinants of underdiagnosis of COPD in national and international surveys. *Chest* **2015**, *148*, 971–985. [CrossRef] [PubMed]
8. Sobnath, D.D.; Philip, N.; Kayyali, R.; Nabhani-Gebara, S.; Pierscionek, B.; Vaes, A.W.; Spruit, M.A.; Kaimakamis, E. Features of a mobile support app for patients with chronic obstructive pulmonary disease: Literature review and current applications. *JMIR* **2017**, *5*. [CrossRef] [PubMed]
9. Koutnik-Fotopoulos, E. COPD: Challenges and Consequences for Stakeholders. Available online: https://www.managedhealthcareconnect.com/article/copd-challenges-and-consequences-stakeholders (accessed on 5 July 2019).
10. Ford, E.; Murphy, L.; Khavjou, O.; Giles, W.; Holt, J.; Croft, J. Total and state-specific medical and absenteeism costs of COPD among adults aged 18 years in the United States for 2010 and projections through 2020. *Chest* **2015**, *147*, 31–45. [CrossRef] [PubMed]
11. American Thoracic Society. Exacerbation of COPD. *Am. J. Respir. Crit. Care Med.* **2014**, *189*, 11–12. [CrossRef] [PubMed]
12. Wier, L.M.; Elixhauser, A.; Pfuntner, A.; Au, D.H. Agency for Healthcare Research and Quality. Overview of Hospitalizations among Patients with COPD, 2008. HCUP Statistical Brief #106. Agency for Healthcare Research and Quality. Available online: http://www.hcup-us.ahrq.gov/reports/statbriefs/sb106.pdf (accessed on 5 July 2019).

13. American Lung Association. What Causes COPD. Available online: http://www.lung.org/lung-health-and-diseases/lung-disease-lookup/copd/symptoms-causes-risk-factors/what-causes-copd.html (accessed on 5 July 2019).
14. National Institutes of Health. Alpha-1 Antitrypsin Deficiency. Available online: https://ghr.nlm.nih.gov/condition/alpha-1-antitrypsin-deficiency (accessed on 5 July 2019).
15. Martinez, C.; Miguel, D.; Mannino, D. Defining COPD-related comorbidities. *Chronic Obstr. Pulm. Dis.* **2014**, *1*, 51–63. [CrossRef] [PubMed]
16. Mayo Clinic. COPD. 2017. Available online: https://www.mayoclinic.org/diseases-conditions/copd/diagnosis-treatment/drc-20353685 (accessed on 5 July 2019).
17. DiMatteo, M. Variations in patients' adherence to medical recommendations: A quantitative review of 50 years of research. *Med. Care* **2004**, *42*, 200–209. [CrossRef] [PubMed]
18. Jones, R.C.M.; Hyland, M.; Hanney, K.; Erwin, J. A qualitative study of compliance with medication and lifestyle modification in chronic obstructive pulmonary disease (COPD). *Prim. Care Respir. J.* **2004**, *13*, 149–154. [CrossRef] [PubMed]
19. Fox, S.; Purcell, K. Chronic Disease and the Internet. Available online: http://www.pewinternet.org/files/old-media/Files/Reports/2010/PIP_Chronic_Disease_with_topline.pdf (accessed on 5 July 2019).
20. Stellefson, M.; Chaney, B.; Chaney, D.; Paige, S.; Payne-Purvis, C.; Tennant, B.; Walsh-Childers, K.; Sriram, P.S.; Alber, J. Engaging community stakeholders to evaluate the design, usability, and acceptability of a chronic obstructive pulmonary disease social media resource center. *JMIR Res. Protoc.* **2015**, *4*, e17. [CrossRef] [PubMed]
21. Stellefson, M.; Shuster, J.; Chaney, B.; Paige, S.; Alber, J.; Chaney, D.; Sriram, P. Web-based health information seeking and eHealth literacy among patients living with chronic obstructive pulmonary disease (COPD). *Health Commun.* **2017**, *33*, 1410–1424. [CrossRef] [PubMed]
22. Williams, V.; Price, J.; Hardinge, M.; Tarassenko, L.; Farmer, A. Using a mobile health application to support self-management in COPD: A qualitative study. *Br. J. Gen. Pract.* **2014**, *64*, 392–400. [CrossRef]
23. Health Information National Trends Survey. U.S. Social Media Use and Health Communication. Available online: https://permanent.access.gpo.gov/gpo59550/HINTS_Brief_19.pdf (accessed on 5 July 2019).
24. Pew Research Center. Social Media Fact Sheet. 2017. Available online: http://www.pewinternet.org/fact-sheet/social-media/ (accessed on 5 July 2019).
25. Pew Research Center. Social Media Use in 2018. Available online: http://assets.pewresearch.org/wp-content/uploads/sites/14/2018/03/01105133/PI_2018.03.01_Social-Media_FINAL.pdf (accessed on 5 July 2019).
26. Allen, C.; Vassiley, I.; Kennedy, A.; Rogers, A. Long-term condition self-management support in online communities: A meta-synthesis of qualitative papers. *J. Med. Internet Res.* **2016**, *18*, e61. [CrossRef] [PubMed]
27. Paige, S.R.; Stellefson, M.; Chaney, B.H.; Alber, J.M. Pinterest as a resource for health information on chronic obstructive pulmonary disease (COPD): A social media content analysis. *Am. J. Health Educ.* **2015**, *46*, 241–251. [CrossRef]
28. Angelis, G.D.; Wells, G.A.; Davies, B.; King, J.; Shallwni, S.M.; McEwan, J.; Cavallo, S.; Brosseau, L. The use of social media among health professionals to facilitate chronic disease self-management with their patients: A systematic review. *Digit. Health* **2018**, *4*. [CrossRef] [PubMed]
29. Moorhead, S.A.; Hazlett, D.E.; Harrison, L.; Carroll, J.K.; Irwin, A.; Hoving, C. A new dimension of health care: Systematic review of the uses, benefits, and limitations of social media for health communication. *JMIR* **2013**, *15*, e85. [CrossRef]
30. Patel, R.; Chang, T.; Greysen, S.R.; Chopra, V. Social media use in chronic disease: A systematic review and novel taxonomy. *Am. J. Med.* **2015**, *128*, 1335–1350. [CrossRef] [PubMed]
31. Gu, D.; Guo, J.; Liang, C.; Lu, W.; Zhao, S.; Liu, B.; Long, T. Social media-based health management systems and sustained health engagement: TPB perspective. *Int. J. Environ. Res. Public Health* **2019**, *16*, 1495. [CrossRef]
32. Krivak, T. Information Today. *Facebook 101: Ten Things You Need to Know About Facebook*. 2008. Available online: http://www.infotoday.com/IT/mar08/Krivak.shtml (accessed on 7 September 2019).
33. Facebook. Statistics. 2017. Available online: https://newsroom.fb.com/company-info/ (accessed on 5 July 2019).
34. Thackeray, R.; VanWagenen, S.; Koch Smith, A.; Neiger, B.; Prier, K. Adoption and use of social media among state health departments. *BMC Public Health* **2011**, *12*, 242. [CrossRef]

35. Antheunis, M.; Tates, K.; Nieboer, T. Patients' and health professionals' use of social media in health care: Motives, barriers and expectations. *Patient Educ. Couns.* **2013**, *92*, 426–431. [CrossRef]
36. Facebook. Facebook tips. *What's the Difference Between a Facebook Page and Group?* 2010. Available online: https://www.facebook.com/notes/facebook/facebook-tips-whats-the-difference-between-a-facebook-page-and-group/324706977130/ (accessed on 5 July 2019).
37. Bender, J.L.; Jimenez-Marroquin, M.C.; Jadad, A.R. Seeking support on facebook: A content analysis of breast cancer groups. *JMIR* **2011**, *13*, e16. [CrossRef]
38. Lerman, B.; Lewis, S.; Lumley, M.; Grogan, G.; Hudson, C.; Johnson, E. Teen depression groups of facebook: A content analysis. *J. Adolesc. Res.* **2016**, *32*, 719–741. [CrossRef]
39. Zhang, Y.; He, D.; Sang, Y. Facebook as a platform for health information and communication: A case study of a diabetes group. *J. Med. Syst.* **2013**, *37*, 9942. [CrossRef] [PubMed]
40. Leventhal, H.; Phillips, A.; Burns, E. The common sense model of self-regulation (CSM): A dynamic framework for understanding illness self-management. *J. Behav. Med.* **2016**, *39*, 935–946. [CrossRef] [PubMed]
41. Skiba, D.J. Face with tears of joy is word of the year: Are emoji a sign of things to come in health care? *Nurs. Educ. Perspect.* **2002**, *37*, 56–57. [CrossRef]
42. Neiger, B.; Thackeray, R.; Van Wagenen, S.; Hanson, C.; West, J.; Barnes, M.; Fagen, M. Use of social media in health promotion: Purposes, key performance indicators, and evaluation metrics. *Health Promot. Pract.* **2012**, *13*, 159–164. [CrossRef]
43. Greene, J.; Choudhry, N.; Kilabuk, E.; Shrank, W. Online social networking by patients with diabetes: A qualitative evaluation of communication with facebook. *J. Gen. Intern. Med.* **2011**, *26*, 287–292. [CrossRef] [PubMed]
44. Centers for Disease Control and Prevention (CDC). Managing Chronic Obstructive Pulmonary Disease (COPD). Available online: https://www.cdc.gov/learnmorefeelbetter/programs/copd.htm (accessed on 5 July 2019).
45. Global Initiative for Chronic Obstructive Lung Disease (GOLD). Global Strategy for the Diagnosis, Management, and Prevention of Chronic Obstructive Pulmonary Disease. Available online: https://goldcopd.org/wp-content/uploads/2018/11/GOLD-2019-v1.7-FINAL-14Nov2018-WMS.pdf (accessed on 5 July 2019).
46. Hale, E.D.; Treharne, G.J.; Kitas, G.D. The common-sense model of self-regulation of health and illness: How can we use it to understand and respond to our patients' needs? *Rheumatology* **2007**, *46*, 904–906. [CrossRef]
47. Brennan, R.L.; Prediger, D.J. Coefficient kappa: Some uses, misuses, and alternatives. *Educ. Psychol. Meas.* **1981**, *41*, 687–699. [CrossRef]
48. Bakeman, R. Behavioral observation and coding. In *Handbook of Research Methods in Social and Personality Psychology*, 2nd ed.; Reis, H.T., Judge, C.M., Eds.; Cambridge University Press: New York, NY, USA, 2000; pp. 138–159, ISBN 978-110-760-075-1.
49. Lombard, M.; Snyder-Duch, J.; Bracken, C. Content analysis in mass communication: Assessment and reporting of intercoder reliability. *Hum. Commun. Res.* **2002**, *28*, 587–604. [CrossRef]
50. Roberts, N.J.; Ghiassi, R.; Partridge, M.R. Health literacy in COPD. *Int. J. Chron Obstruct. Pulmon. Dis.* **2008**, *3*, 499–507.
51. Write Effective Links. Available online: https://www.plainlanguage.gov/guidelines/web/write-effective-links/ (accessed on 1 October 2019).
52. Lyles, C.; Fruchterman, J.; Youdelman, M.; Schillinger, D. Legal, practical, and ethical considerations for making online patient portals accessible for all. *Am. J. Public Health* **2017**, *107*, 1608–1611. [CrossRef] [PubMed]
53. Partridge, S.R.; Gallagher, P.; Freeman, B.; Gallagher, R. Facebook Groups for the management of chronic diseases. *J. Med. Internet Res.* **2018**, *20*, e21. [CrossRef] [PubMed]

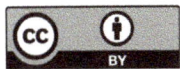

© 2019 by the authors. Licensee MDPI, Basel, Switzerland. This article is an open access article distributed under the terms and conditions of the Creative Commons Attribution (CC BY) license (http://creativecommons.org/licenses/by/4.0/).

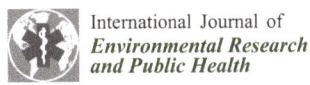

Article

How Health Communication via Tik Tok Makes a Difference: A Content Analysis of Tik Tok Accounts Run by Chinese Provincial Health Committees

Chengyan Zhu [1], Xiaolin Xu [1], Wei Zhang [2,*], Jianmin Chen [2] and Richard Evans [3]

[1] College of Public Administration, Huazhong University of Science and Technology, Wuhan 430030, China; 2016512018@hust.edu.cn (C.Z.); xiaolin@hust.edu.cn (X.X.)
[2] School of Medicine and Health Management, Huazhong University of Science and Technology, Wuhan 430030, China; m201975543@hust.edu.cn
[3] College of Engineering, Design and Physical Sciences, Brunel University London, Kingston Lane, Uxbridge, Middlesex UB8 3PH, UK; richard.evans@brunel.ac.uk
* Correspondence: weizhanghust@hust.edu.cn; Tel.: +86-13397110378

Received: 7 November 2019; Accepted: 25 December 2019; Published: 27 December 2019

Abstract: During the last two decades, social media has immersed itself into all facets of our personal and professional lives. The healthcare sector is no exception, with public health departments now capitalizing on the benefits that social media offers when delivering healthcare education and communication with citizens. Provincial Health Committees (PHCs) in China have begun to adopt the micro-video sharing platform, Tik Tok, to engage with local residents and communicate health-related information. This study investigates the status quo of official Tik Tok accounts managed by PHCs in mainland China. In total, 31 PHC accounts were analyzed during August 2019, while the top 100 most liked micro-videos were examined using content analysis. Coding included three major aspects: Quantified Impact, Video Content, and Video Form. 45.2% (n = 14) of PHCs had official Tik Tok accounts. A limited number of accounts (n = 2) were yet to upload a micro-video, while most (n = 9) had uploaded their first micro-video during 2019. For the top 100 most liked micro-videos, a sharp difference was observed in terms of number of Likes, Comments and Reposts. Videos containing cartoons or documentary-style content were most frequently watched by citizens. Similarly, content that promoted professional health or provided knowledge of diseases was frequently viewed. Content containing original music, formal mandarin language, subtitles, and which lasted less than 60 s, were most frequently followed. It is considered a missed opportunity that most PHCs struggle to take advantage of the Tik Tok platform, especially given its growing popularity and daily increase in account creation.

Keywords: micro-video; Provincial Health Committee; healthcare; Tik Tok; social media; China

1. Introduction

1.1. Social Media Use by Healthcare Departments

Since the inception of social media in the late 1990s, it has had an unprecedented influence on our personal and professional lives, impacting the way we communicate, stay connected, and share information. By July 2019, the number of worldwide active social media users reached 3.534 billion, with a penetration rate of 46% [1]. Undoubtedly, the popularity and ease in adoption of social media has changed the ways in which public services are delivered and communicated. An increasing number of government agencies have realized the importance of actively participating on social media for citizen engagement, relationship building, and citizen compliance [2–6]. One recently introduced social media platform is Tik Tok, a micro-video sharing platform that allows users to create short videos, lasting from several seconds to several minutes, and then share it with the wider Tik Tok community. Founded in 2017, it is the fastest growing social media application in the world, topping the chart for 'Most Downloaded' in the USA in 2018, and now being available in over 150 countries. It is claimed that Tik Tok has more than 500 million active users with more than 1 billion downloads [7]. By contrast with other social media platforms, Tik Tok is characterized by short micro-videos with simple-to-use editing and music-inclusion functions [8,9]. The application provides a non-complicated user interface for creating videos, with users being able to embed their preferred music choices and special effects into their recorded video, easily [9].

In the healthcare sector, the adoption of social media is not new [10,11]. Social media has been widely adopted by patients, care-givers, and healthcare professionals, with numerous studies reporting its usefulness in patient empowerment, health promotion, patient–physician relationship building, public health surveillance, and quality improvement [12–17]. On the contrary, other studies have focused on revealing the dark side of social media in healthcare; for example, examining how unverified content leads to the sharing of misleading information [18], patients becoming overconfident in their own medical decision making [19,20], and privacy violation [18,21]. Scholars have also noted the level of diffusion of social media among healthcare departments [22], observing differences in content shared and patient interactions [23]. Since healthcare departments concern the quality in medical care delivered to citizens, their adoption of social media is often cautious and can lag behind other public-facing sectors.

1.2. The Use of Tik Tok by Government Agencies in China

In October 2016, the State Council of China established the Healthy China 2030 Strategy, aimed at promoting healthier lifestyles, improving health literacy and mental health. In the process of developing the strategy, health communication was viewed as critical for providing access to public health information, education and health literacy improvement. In July 2019, the Healthy China Promotion Committee of the State Council strengthened the importance of establishing and improving the "Two databases and one mechanism" for public health education. The two databases refer to the database of national and provincial experts in public health education and the database of national public health education resources. One mechanism refers to a holistic media perspective on public health education and communications, denoting that health communication via integrated media forms has garnered national attention.

In China, social media usage is the most popular online activity, with most citizens now focusing their attention on creating and watching micro-videos. According to the 44th report of Internet development in China, produced by CNNIC (China Internet Network Information Center), the number of mobile internet users has reached 817 million, with the number of micro-video users now exceeding 648 million, showing a penetration rate of 75.8% by June 2019 [24]. The popularity of Tik Tok has also attracted local government attention. In China, government organizations have begun to use Tik Tok to engage with local citizens, enabling them to clarify public concerns and keep citizens informed [25,26]. Tik Tok has also penetrated local health authorities in China, although at a much-reduced rate compared with the large-scale adoption witnessed by local governments. This study explores this emerging phenomenon in China where local health committees are utilizing the micro-video sharing platform to provide health information to the general public. It examines how Chinese citizens are participating on the platform, analyzing the top 100 most liked videos from PHCs to determine the most common features and communication strategies favored by the general public. The results of our study will enrich the understanding of social media use by PHCs, drawing comparisons against previous social media types and providing guidance for the future operation of Tik Tok accounts.

2. Materials and Method

2.1. Data Collection

In this study, 31 provincial level health committees in mainland China were examined. Data was captured on 20 August 2019. All PHCs were classified based on their provincial economic development capacity and geographic location, including the Western, Central and Eastern regions. To begin, we searched the Tik Tok platform for the official accounts of all PHCs in China by using the official name of the health committee and abbreviations of their name. If no result was found, we located the official website of the committee and checked if there were any links to their official Tik Tok account [27]. To ensure that all Tik Tok accounts were official, we analyzed only those that were verified accounts on the Tik Tok platform, represented by a blue check mark (verified badge).

2.2. Analysis of Tik Tok Accounts

A Microsoft Excel worksheet was constructed to store the data extracted from the official Tik Tok accounts. The extraction was completed by one person, the third author. The data was cross-sectional in nature and included: (1) established time of the account i.e., date since the first uploaded Tik Tok video, (2) number of videos posted, (3) number of likes received, (4) number of video reposts, and (5) number of comments received.

To further analyze the content of uploaded micro-videos, content analysis of the top 100 most liked micro-videos among all PHCs was conducted. Content analysis is widely used when analyzing video-based health communication [28–31], e.g., obesity videos [32] and e-cigarettes [33]. However, many studies that have adopted content analysis mainly examined videos lasting from several minutes to hours. Their coding usually includes content types, subtitles, valence, and specifically designed codes based on topics being studied. In our study, the coding scheme for micro-videos produced by healthcare departments on Tik Tok is still immature; therefore, we followed the codes of common practice for video-based health communication and piloted the coding scheme with an initial analysis of 20% (20/100) of the selected micro-videos. We then made amendments as further videos were processed [16,34]. The final coding scheme consisted of three dimensions: Quantified Impact, Video Content, and Video Form. Each dimension had several sub-dimensions.

The Quantified Impact does not intend to measure the effect of watching a micro-video on an individual's health literacy or their health-related behavioral change. Instead, we record the index observable via Tik Tok, for example how many people watched it, how many people liked it after watching it, and how many people shared it. We did not aggregate the index into one due to the difficulty in compiling a formula to evaluate their impact. Video Content concerns the video type, major themes, embedded emotions, and the characters involved in the video. Specifically, video theme refers to the topic referred to in the video, including disease knowledge, daily diet, health professionals' image promotion, healthcare, and health reform. Disease knowledge features specific information on types and causes of disease e.g., the cause of hypertension and treatment available to the patient. Daily diet provides insight into developing healthy eating habits. Videos on health professionals image promotion center on stories of good doctors, nurses, hospital managers, administrators and others employed in healthcare field, which highlight the individuals positive image rather than specific medical knowledge e.g., a cardiovascular surgeon saved a patient experiencing a sudden heart attack on a high-speed train. Healthcare information refers to healthy lifestyles, including diet and exercise activities. Health reform views the topic of health from a wider perspective, the policy dimension, referring to e.g., policies surrounding family doctors. Finally, emotion refers to the major emotion presented within the video, rather than the emotion triggered by watching the video. We created four sub-dimensions based on a previous classification on the emotions involved in Tik Tok, and made this fit the health communication setting [26]. Video Form concerns the style, language, and special techniques used. Specifically, the background music relates to how the music is selected, with original music being defined as the music being made by the uploader themselves, rather than them selecting a piece of music from the Tik Tok music library.

In total, 12 codes were merged. Specifically, the Quantified Impact dimension had three sub-dimensions: Number of Likes, Comments and Reposts. The video content dimension had four sub-dimensions: Video type, Theme, Emotion, and Characters. The video form dimension included five sub-dimensions: Background Music, Language Feature, Emphasized Theme in the ending, Length of video, and Subtitles. The final coding scheme is presented in Figure 1 and Table 1. Two graduate students studying Health Informatics were trained before coding the micro-videos separately, with their inter-reliability rate being 0.94 [6,35], deeming the coding scheme effective.

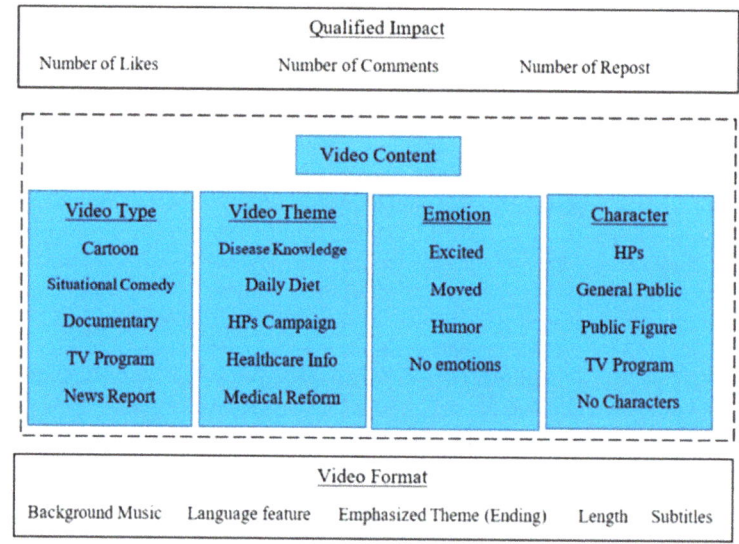

Figure 1. The coding framework for the top 100 most liked micro-videos run by Provincial Health Committees (PHCs).

Table 1. The coding scheme for video analysis.

Index	Explanation
Number of Likes	Total number of Likes by 20 August 2019
Number of Comments	Total number of Comments received by 20 August 2019
Number of Reposts	Total number of Reposts by 20 August 2019
Video Type	Refers to the different types of health communication, divided into five categories, including: cartoon, documentary, situation comedy, excerpt from TV program, excerpt from news report.
Video Theme	Refers to the major topic involved in the micro-video, encompassing disease knowledge, daily diet, health professionals' image promotion, healthcare info, and health reforms.
Emotion	Refers to the major emotion involved; classified as excited, moved, humor or no specific emotion.
Character	Refers to the character playing the leading role or being shown most during the micro-video; divided into health professionals, public figures and general public (with patients included).
Background Music	Refers to the background music used, including no music, music selected from the Tik Tok music library, and original music.
Language Feature	Refers to the language used, including mandarin, and other local dialects.
Emphasized theme (Ending)	Refers to the technique of re-emphasizing the theme at the end of the micro-video.
Length	Refers to the length of the micro-video.
Subtitles	Refers to the technique of using subtitles to display the words spoken in the micro-video as written text.

3. Results

Of the 31 provincial level health committees observed, 14 (45.2%) had their own official Tik Tok account, including 6 located in the Central region of China, and 4 in the East and West, respectively. Among them, the health committees in Tianjin and Shanghai had not uploaded any videos, although they had created official accounts. Health committees in Shanxi were the first to release a micro-video on Tik Tok in 2018, while many (64.3%, 9/14) had uploaded their first micro-video in 2019. The total number of followers for all health committees in China was 197,980. The total number of videos uploaded was 962, while the total number of Likes received had reached 1.054 million.

In terms of the 100 most liked micro-videos, none were posted by health committees in Henan, Hunan, Hainan, Guizhou, Inner Mongolia or the NingXia autonomous regions. Instead, health committees from Shanxi, Jilin, Jiangxi, Hubei, Guangdong, and Sichuan provinces had the most popular micro-videos. Table 2 provides further details of the most liked videos.

Table 2. Basic information of Tik Tok accounts run by PHCs.

Province	Region	First Time Video Uploaded	Number of Followers	Number of Uploaded Videos	Number of Updates	Total Number of Likes	Number of Top 100 most liked Micro-Videos
Tianjin	East	Never	26	0	0	0	0
Shanghai	East	Never	4	0	0	0	0
Shanxi	Central	21 June 2018	5145	133	133	31,000	11
Jilin	Central	19 April 2019	13,000	74	75	127,000	14
Jiangxi	Central	12 May 2019	614	19	19	2808	1
Henan	Central	4 April 2019	190	5	5	367	0
Hubei	Central	5 May 2019	8566	121	121	45,000	5
Hunan	Central	10 July 2019	58	5	5	140	0
Guangdong	East	4 September 2018	132,000	478	527	651,000	53
Hainan	East	30 November 2018	274	9	9	580	0
Sichuan	West	23 January 2019	38,000	97	105	196,000	16
Guizhou	West	19 August 2019	54	12	12	51	0
Inner Mongolia	West	25 April 2019	38	6	6	13	0
Ning Xia	West	16 August 2019	11	3	3	27	0
Total			197,980	962	1,015	1,053,986	100

3.1. Distribution of Quantified Impact Dimension

Quantified Impact is defined as the measurement of an official Tik Tok account's influence on the public engagement via Tik Tok. It differs in the top 100 micro-videos in terms of the total number of likes, comments and reposts. Specifically, the total number of likes of the top 100 micro-videos had reached 775,256, ranging from 667 to 177,000. The total number of comments received were 13,579 with zero, being the least, to 6815. Among them, the number of micro-videos that received comments exceeding 1000 was only two, while most micro-videos received less than 100 comments. The total number of reposts amounted to 59,568, with zero being the least and 20,000 being the most. Eleven micro-videos had been reposted at least 1000 times. Table 3 presents further details.

Table 3. The distribution of the Quantified Impact dimension.

Quantified Impact	Min	Max	Median	Sum
Number of Likes	667	177,000	7,752.56	775,256
Number of Comments	0	6815	135.97	13,597
Number of Reposts	0	20,000	595.68	59,568

3.2. Distribution of Video Content Dimension

Video content was divided into four sub-dimensions. In terms of video type, videos involving cartoons took the lead with 27% (27/100), followed by those which involved a documentary (25%, 25/100) or except from TV program (22%, 22/100). For video theme, the topic of health professionals ranked the highest, with 38 out of 100 videos displaying this topic. Videos presenting knowledge about diseases was second, with slightly fewer micro-videos, while the theme of daily diets and health reform was viewed the least number of times with 7% (7/100) and 3% (3/100), respectively. In terms of the emotion involved in the video, over half (58%, 58/100) demonstrated no specific feelings. The feeling of being moved was felt in 19 out 100 micro-videos, followed by the feeling of sense of humor (17%, 17/100), and being excited (6%, 6/100). In terms of characters, 55 out of 100 videos featured healthcare professionals, 12% (12/100) focused on public figures, and 11% (11/100) on the general public, with patients included. The remaining 22% presented no characters.

3.3. Distribution of Video Form Dimension

The format of uploaded micro-videos was divided into five sub-dimensions. For background music used, it was split into three categories: no background music, default music selected from Tik Tok, and original music made by the uploader. 82 out of 100 micro-videos were accompanied by various types of music. Among them, 63.4% (52/82) included original music, produced by the PHC. For the language features, we looked at the local dialects used. Only 3% (3/100) of the micro-videos used local dialects. Mandarin was used in the majority micro-videos for the avoidance of language barriers caused by regional dialects. However, the use of dialects may attract locals in some way.

In terms of length of time of the micro-video, an overwhelming number of videos (98, 98/100) were presented within 60 s. Among them, 11 lasted 0–15 s, 16 from 15–30 s, 28 from 30–45 s, and 43 from 45–60 s. Regarding subtitles, 73 out of 100 showed subtitles. For emphasized theme in the ending scene, only 20% (20/100) of the micro-videos had included this.

4. Discussion

4.1. Principal Findings

This study has provided an overview of the official Tik Tok accounts managed by provincial health committees across mainland China. According to the results, 45.2% (14/31) of the provincial health committees in mainland China have created a Tik Tok account, at the time of data collection.

12 of them had already uploaded their first micro-video, except for those in Tianjin and Shanghai, while many (n = 9) PHCs had uploaded their first micro-video in 2019. It is interesting to note that the adoption of Tik Tok by health departments in provinces with economic prosperity (e.g., Tianjin and Shanghai) lagged behind others. This may be due to the overall health literacy rates in these regions, and effective health education through earlier-adopted social media channels (e.g., Weibo and Wechat). In the case of provinces with economic prosperity, citizens are likely to have a higher level of health literacy, with local health departments delivering better health education. Earlier forms of social media have well-established reputations in communicating health information, which mean the marginal benefit of Tik Tok remains subtle. The diffusion patterns of Tik Tok may not simply apply to economic prosperity and openness, and other factors such as the seriousness of Tik Tok and urgency of adoption, should be taken into consideration. This is consistent with a recent study revealing the complexity of Tik Tok adoption in China, which highlighted the unique function, orientation, production procedures and communicational features compared with pre-existing social media [36]. In our study, we focused on the top 100 most popular micro-videos of all PHCs. Over half of the micro-videos were produced by the Guangdong health committee. For the Quantified Impact, although the PHCs had gained some popularity, a sharp difference was observed between the top 100 most liked micro-videos, in terms of the number of Likes, Comments and Reposts. Many accounts were still in their infancy stage. In terms of video content, many videos showed cartoons or were a documentary produced by the PHC. Themes relating to the promotion of healthy professional images and disease knowledge were most frequently seen in the observed micro-videos. In terms of video format, videos incorporating original music, using formal mandarin language, lasting less than 60 s, and using subtitles, were most commonly followed.

4.2. Followers Are Fundamental to Health Communication on Tik Tok

The effective communication of healthcare information via social media requires considerable followers. Our study revealed that the top 100 most liked micro-videos were mainly from six PHCs, who each had a large following. For example, the Guangdong health committee contributed 53 of the most liked micro-videos and has 130,000 followers, uploading more than 478 micro-videos with over 650,000 likes. Among all accounts, the impact of *Healthy Guangdong* has contributed to more than half of the total number of followers and Likes. At present, *Healthy Guangdong* is the most valuable Tik Tok account from the perspective of quantified impact. This could provide solid evidence that the use of social media by local health departments is often more cautious than that of their counterparts in other government agencies. Since Tik Tok adoption by PHCs is still novel in China, many may be hesitant in its use. In addition, they may have also not mastered the strategies for health communication via the emerging social media channel. Their investment in account promotion and creation of more attractive micro-videos needs strengthening. PHCs are advised to integrate the current impact of other online platforms and establish their reputation on Tik Tok. To achieve this, PHCs can use a social media management tool e.g., Hootsuite, to manage cross-posting of videos across social media channels and schedule content, enabling more consistent posting of content at times which maximize engagement. Furthermore, an introduction or weblink to the official Tik Tok account could be displayed on each PHC official website, Weibo or Wechat account to migrate audiences and build a larger community on Tik Tok.

To attract followers in future, PHCs could create micro-videos related to or engaging with popular topics i.e., reflecting on subjects that concern the general public. By using these as headlines or cover pages, it is likely to gain more public attention. Although popular topics may not be health-related, the micro-video can still be created with the popular topic in-mind. However, the determinants for continued attention still largely depend on the quality of each micro-video. Tik Tok users may be more engaged with a micro-video connected with a popular topic at first but will often become disinterested if the video is not entertaining. To overcome this, PHCs could engage with regionally-admired influencers from e.g., sport or film in China to grow the number of followers and increase public engagement. Since the majority of Tik Tok users are drawn to the platform by entertaining content, better efforts are encouraged to design health-education oriented videos that incorporate comedic elements. PHCs should further consider the creation of docuseries surrounding interesting topics, creating messaging strategies that feature consistent characters e.g., "A Day in the Life of Doctor Z". Meanwhile, they could make greater use of external resources related to public health education, collaborating more frequently with local medical institutes, media and health non-governmental organizations (NGOs), to amplify their influence. For example, in the popular micro-video titled '*I Am A Doctor Not A God*', a rap is created by the Sichuan health committee and Luzhou Renmin Hospital to celebrate the Chinese doctor's day. The rap was adapted from a recent blockbuster film '*Dying to Survive*' or '*I Am Not A God Of Medicine*' and has been popularized since it's upload to Tik Tok.

4.3. Easily Understood Content and Light Format Are Critical

Our study revealed that Tik Tok users prefer the presentation and format of micro-videos to be correlated to their understanding of difficult medical terms or jargons. With regards to content type, animated cartoons and documentary were seen to be popular for content relating to demonstration and for creating a sense of being 'in the moment', to stimulate shared emotion, compared to oral presentations and plain text which were preferred for the sharing of disease knowledge and information on specific drugs. This is consistent with the notion that the narrative story-telling approach has been increasingly adopted to disseminate health-related content in health communication [37]. Meanwhile, the promotion of a health professional's image and disease knowledge were major themes currently viewed. This could be attributed to citizens wanting to get to know their healthcare professionals to obtain different perspectives. For example, a situation-based comedy on overloaded workloads of doctors at New Year Eve brings the public closer to doctors' daily lives, while a micro-video on hypertension management attracts the attention of patients and their care-takers. In addition, the dominant role in micro-videos were that of healthcare professionals. This may be due to medicine being a highly specialized topic where years of training and practice are required before developing informed knowledge. Also, health professionals, including physicians, doctors, and public servants are often easily trusted by the public when sharing health information. The strategy of using public figures for health communication may also be worth applauding. For example, actress Yang Zi and actor Zhang Yishan, favored by young citizens in China, played roles in a scene representing and discussing depression prevention issues.

In terms of format used, a light style in terms of background music, language, length, and subtitles is preferred by content viewers. Although these peripheral factors are not deciding issues when determining video quality, the format could serve as a motivating factor for increasing viewing time [38]. For the creation of health-related micro-videos, PHCs are expected to follow regular patterns in health communication. For example, videos which contain complicated music or too many visual effects can easily distract the audience. The use of vivid cartoons can demonstrate disease knowledge, however, this format could undermine key health information; if one can only remember the cartoon figures, but nothing about the health knowledge, the communication is ineffective. The key health education message should be essential for all micro-video formats. Further efforts are also required to facilitate training and management of Tik Tok account operations for PHCs. To manage Tik Tok accounts more efficiently, PHCs are expected to learn from their peers, as well as other government departments, and allocate more resources to support the development of content and operation of the account.

4.4. Audience-Centered Interactions Are Encouraged

Compared to the total number of Likes and Reposts per micro-video, the total number of Comments was far lower. This may indicate that the public treat health communication via Tik Tok as one-way communication rather than two-way communication. The Tik Tok accounts currently managed by PHCs had few interactions with their audiences; video co-creation can be a means for extending communication between creators and recipients. This is a commonly mentioned problem in previous literature when new information technologies are introduced into public sectors [10,39]. Tik Tok is a valuable co-creation community where the health department can promote healthy lifestyles and impart health-related knowledge, while the users can also generate health related information to impact others, marketers and policy makers. Further interactions require the creators to activate a pro-interaction environment, engage audiences in the content-creation and promotion process, and thus realize the multi-dimensional exchanges and interactions between audiences, service platform and micro-videos.

It could be speculated that micro-videos uploaded by PHCs do not provide enough features for the public to participate in conversation. Meanwhile, in the case of China, where video-based social media has long been regarded as an entertainment platform for amusement, health or science related communication has largely been neglected; a nudge approach by the health department may gradually change the perception hindering effective health communication. In future, PHCs are expected to partner with the Tik Tok platform to improve the image of Tik Tok as a health communication channel. In addition, the audience profile of PHCs is worthy of attention. The analysis of audience characters, i.e., age and locality, will contribute to making targeted health communication strategies more applicable to citizens. If audiences are dominated by young citizens, the most common youth health-related problems should be addressed in the content. Additionally, the video created should consider their preference, daily routine and lifestyle. To initiate conversations, PHCs should find common health concerns, and encourage public participation in the process of creating the micro-video. For example, PHCs could create a micro-video based on popular user discussions, using buzzwords to gain public attention, thus engaging the public in health-related communication.

4.5. Limitations

This study has certain limitations. First, it was a descriptive study exploring PHC use of the Tik Tok platform, a newly introduced micro-video sharing platform. We selected the top 100 most liked micro-videos produced by PHCs, however, number of Likes may not sufficiently measure the popularity of each video, as lots of accounts had been newly created. We did not consider the number of Reposts and Comments. Longer duration is also required to see more dynamics of this new social media platform. Meanwhile, although content analysis is widely used in video analysis, it may still have limitations when demonstrating the special features of micro-videos studied for short duration. Future research can enlarge the study sample, using machine learning or other automatic techniques e.g., using transcriptions, shoot analysis, sentiment analysis or narrative analysis to reveal a more comprehensive picture of Tik Tok accounts run by PHCs.

Second, the reasons for social media adoption and their usage strategies were understudied. As our study centered on the use of Tik Tok accounts, it is possible that other important characteristics may be neglected. For example, the specific conditions of each PHC including administration, level of resources, and public engagement. Meanwhile, our study did not examine the health-related changes resulted from Tik Tok, and additional comparison of the health effect via different social media channels could be of great value to understand the social media use in healthcare.

Third, in our research, we did not investigate the operators of Tik Tok accounts, regarding their selection of content, abiding by the rules, and internal rewards for managing the account. This could lead to variations in Tik Tok adoption. Future study could employ qualitative methods to reveal the 'behind the scenes' story and compare their strategic use across different social media platforms. In addition, the exploration of the recipients of health communication videos via Tik Tok is also worth further attention. For instance, qualitative work that looks into their attitude of watching Tik Tok run by PHCs and their expectations on the content.

5. Conclusions

Less than half of all PHCs in mainland China have established an official Tik Tok account. The value of the Guangdong PHC account is the highest in terms of total number of followers, Likes and Reposts. Content analysis of the top 100 most liked health-related micro-videos revealed that many PHCs are new to operating Tik Tok accounts and struggle to leverage this emerging social media platform. Animated cartoons and documentary-style content, featuring healthcare professionals' and disease knowledge are popular among viewers of health-related micro-videos. More than half of the selected micro-videos focused on health professionals with no specific emotions involved. In addition, original music and subtitles are also easily observed from selected micro-videos. Considering that Tik Tok is a micro-video based social media platform, patient-centered interactions are highly desired for PHCs to create more diverse content with engaging strategies. With many social media users, especially younger generations, now preferring to receive information via video content over written content, PHCs should use Tik Tok to grow engagement levels with citizens, creating content that is unique and personable, and which extends the core values of the PHC. Tik Tok should be viewed as an official means for communicating health information with citizens and not purely an entertainment channel; instead, it should be become an integral part of PHCs social media ecosystems, allowing agencies to interact with citizens on a more personal level, extending communication away from merely written form.

Author Contributions: Conceptualization, C.Z., W.Z., X.X.; methodology, C.Z., W.Z., X.X., J.C.; data curation, C.Z., W.Z., J.C.; data analysis, C.Z., X.X., W.Z., J.C., R.E.; writing—original draft preparation, C.Z., W.Z., X.X., J.C., R.E.; writing—review and editing, C.Z., W.Z., X.X., R.E., J.C.; funding acquisition, X.X. All authors have read and agreed to the published version of the manuscript.

Funding: This paper is supported by National Science Foundation of China, grant number 71734002.

Conflicts of Interest: The authors declare no conflict of interest.

References

1. Wearesocial. Global Social Media Users Pass 3.5 Billion. Available online: http://wearesocial.cn/blog/2019/07/22/global-social-media-users-pass-3-5-billion/ (accessed on 10 October 2019).
2. Agostino, D.; Arnaboldi, M. A Measurement Framework for Assessing the Contribution of Social Media to Public Engagement: An empirical analysis on Facebook. *Public Manag. Rev.* **2016**, *18*, 1289–1307. [CrossRef]
3. Hong, H. Government websites and social media's influence on government-public relationships. *Public Relat. Rev.* **2013**, *39*, 346–356. [CrossRef]
4. Im, T.; Cho, W.; Porumbescu, G.; Park, J. Internet, trust in government, and citizen compliance. *J. Public Adm. Res. Theory* **2012**, *24*, 741–763. [CrossRef]
5. Song, C.; Lee, J. Citizens' Use of Social Media in Government, Perceived Transparency, and Trust in Government. *Public Perform. Manag. Rev.* **2016**, *39*, 430–453. [CrossRef]
6. Zhang, W.; Xu, X.; Zhang, H.; Chen, Q. Online participation chaos: A case study of Chinese government-initiated e-polity square. *Int. J. Public Adm.* **2016**, *39*, 1195–1202. [CrossRef]
7. Wearesocial. Digital 2019 Q2 Global Digital Statshot. Available online: http://wearesocial.cn/blog/2019/04/28/digital-2019-q2-global-digital-statshot/ (accessed on 10 October 2019).
8. Chen, Z.; He, Q.; Mao, Z.; Chung, H.-M.; Maharjan, S. A Study on the Characteristics of Douyin Short Videos and Implications for Edge Caching. Available online: http://arxiv.org/abs/1903.12399 (accessed on 22 October 2019).
9. Yang, S.; Zhao, Y.; Ma, Y. Analysis of the Reasons and Development of Short Video Application—Taking Tik Tok as an Example. In Proceedings of the 2019 9th International Conference on Information and Social Science (ICISS 2019), Manila, Philippines, 12–14 July 2019.
10. Heldman, A.B.; Schindelar, J.; Weaver, J.B. Social Media Engagement and Public Health Communication: Implications for Public Health Organizations Being Truly "Social". *Public Health Rev.* **2013**, *35*. [CrossRef]
11. Deng, Z.; Hong, Z.; Zhang, W.; Evans, R.; Chen, Y. The Effect of Online Effort and Reputation of Physicians on Patients' Choice: 3-Wave Data Analysis of China's Good Doctor Website. *J. Med. Internet Res.* **2019**, *21*, e10170. [CrossRef]
12. Ranney, M.L.; Genes, N. Social media and healthcare quality improvement: A nascent field. *BMJ Qual. Saf.* **2016**, *25*, 389–391. [CrossRef]

13. Tengilimoglu, D.; Sarp, N.; Yar, C.E.; Bektaş, M.; Hidir, M.N.; Korkmaz, E. The consumers' social media use in choosing physicians and hospitals: The case study of the province of Izmir: Choosing Physicians and Hospitals. *Int. J. Health Plan. Manag.* **2017**, *32*, 19–35. [CrossRef]
14. Richter, J.P.; Muhlestein, D.B.; Wilks, C.E. Social media: How hospitals use it, and opportunities for future use. *J. Healthc. Manag.* **2014**, *59*, 447–460. [CrossRef]
15. Zhang, W.; Deng, Z.; Evans, R.; Xiang, F.; Ye, Q.; Zeng, R. Social Media Landscape of the Tertiary Referral Hospitals in China: Observational Descriptive Study. *J. Med. Internet Res.* **2018**, *20*, e249. [CrossRef] [PubMed]
16. Zhang, W.; Deng, Z.; Hong, Z.; Evans, R.; Ma, J.; Zhang, H. Unhappy Patients Are Not Alike: Content Analysis of the Negative Comments from China's Good Doctor Website. *J. Med. Internet Res.* **2018**, *20*, e35. [CrossRef] [PubMed]
17. Zhu, C.; Zeng, R.; Zhang, W.; Evans, R.; He, R. Pregnancy-Related Information Seeking and Sharing in the Social Media Era Among Expectant Mothers: Qualitative Study. *J. Med. Internet Res.* **2019**, *21*, e13694. [CrossRef] [PubMed]
18. Syed-Abdul, S.; Fernandez-Luque, L.; Jian, W.-S.; Li, Y.-C.; Crain, S.; Hsu, M.-H.; Wang, Y.-C.; Khandregzen, D.; Chuluunbaatar, E.; Nguyen, P.A.; et al. Misleading Health-Related Information Promoted Through Video-Based Social Media: Anorexia on YouTube. *J. Med. Internet Res.* **2013**, *15*, e30. [CrossRef] [PubMed]
19. Smailhodzic, E.; Hooijsma, W.; Boonstra, A.; Langley, D.J. Social media use in healthcare: A systematic review of effects on patients and on their relationship with healthcare professionals. *BMC Health Serv. Res.* **2016**, *16*. [CrossRef]
20. Baron, R.J.; Berinsky, A.J. Mistrust in Science—A Threat to the Patient–Physician Relationship. *N. Engl. J. Med.* **2019**, *381*, 182–185. [CrossRef]
21. Househ, M.; Borycki, E.; Kushniruk, A. Empowering patients through social media: The benefits and challenges. *Health Inform. J.* **2014**, *20*, 50–58. [CrossRef] [PubMed]
22. Thackeray, R.; Neiger, B.L.; Smith, A.K.; Van Wagenen, S.B. Adoption and use of social media among public health departments. *BMC Public Health* **2012**, *12*. [CrossRef] [PubMed]
23. Jha, A.; Lin, L.; Savoia, E. The Use of Social Media by State Health Departments in the US: Analyzing Health Communication through Facebook. *J. Community Health* **2016**, *41*, 174–179. [CrossRef]
24. China Network Internet Information Center. *The 44th China Statistical Report on Internet Development*; China Network Internet Information Center: Beijing, China, 2019.
25. Onion Lab and Caasdata. A Report on the Analysis of Government Tik Tok Accounts in 2018. Available online: https://www.useit.com.cn/thread-20984-1-1.html (accessed on 25 October 2019).
26. Chengwei, W.; Liang, M. How do government micro-videos make a difference: A content analysis of government Tik Tok accounts. *E Gov.* **2019**, *7*, 31–40.
27. Yang, P.-C.; Lee, W.-C.; Liu, H.-Y.; Shih, M.-J.; Chen, T.-J.; Chou, L.-F.; Hwang, S.-J. Use of Facebook by Hospitals in Taiwan: A Nationwide Survey. *Int. J. Environ. Res. Public Health* **2018**, *15*, 1188. [CrossRef] [PubMed]
28. Frohlich, D.O.; Zmyslinski-Seelig, A. The Presence of Social Support Messages on YouTube Videos about Inflammatory Bowel Disease and Ostomies. *Health Commun.* **2012**, *27*, 421–428. [CrossRef] [PubMed]
29. Gabarron, E.; Fernandez-Luque, L.; Armayones, M.; Lau, A.Y. Identifying Measures Used for Assessing Quality of YouTube Videos with Patient Health Information: A Review of Current Literature. *Interact. J. Med. Res.* **2013**, *2*, e6. [CrossRef] [PubMed]
30. Tian, Y. Organ Donation on Web 2.0: Content and Audience Analysis of Organ Donation Videos on YouTube. *Health Commun.* **2010**, *25*, 238–246. [CrossRef]
31. Wen, N.; Chia, S.C.; Hao, X. What Do Social Media Say About Makeovers? A Content Analysis of Cosmetic Surgery Videos and Viewers' Responses on YouTube. *Health Commun.* **2015**, *30*, 933–942. [CrossRef]
32. Yoo, J.H.; Kim, J. Obesity in the New Media: A Content Analysis of Obesity Videos on YouTube. *Health Commun.* **2012**, *27*, 86–97. [CrossRef]
33. Paek, H.-J.; Kim, S.; Hove, T.; Huh, J.Y. Reduced Harm or Another Gateway to Smoking? Source, Message, and Information Characteristics of E-Cigarette Videos on YouTube. *J. Health Commun.* **2014**, *19*, 545–560. [CrossRef]
34. Ma, J.; Zhang, W.; Harris, K.; Chen, Q.; Xu, X. Dying online: Live broadcasts of Chinese emerging adult suicides and crisis response behaviors. *BMC Public Health* **2016**, *16*, 774. [CrossRef]

35. Brennan, R.L.; Prediger, D.J. Coefficient Kappa: Some Uses, Misuses, and Alternatives. *Educ. Psychol. Meas.* **1981**, *41*, 687–699. [CrossRef]
36. Liang, M. Government Micro-video: Status quo, challenges and future directions. *E Gov.* **2019**, *7*, 2–10.
37. Frank, L.B.; Murphy, S.T.; Chatterjee, J.S.; Moran, M.B.; Baezconde-Garbanati, L. Telling Stories, Saving Lives: Creating Narrative Health Messages. *Health Commun.* **2014**, *30*, 154–163. [CrossRef] [PubMed]
38. Connelly, B.L.; Certo, S.T.; Ireland, R.D.; Reutzel, C.R. Signaling Theory: A Review and Assessment. *J. Manag.* **2010**, *37*, 39–67. [CrossRef]
39. Hsu, Y.-C.; Chen, T.-J.; Chu, F.-Y.; Liu, H.-Y.; Chou, L.-F.; Hwang, S.-J. Official Websites of Local Health Centers in Taiwan: A Nationwide Study. *Int. J. Environ. Res. Public Health* **2019**, *16*, 399. [CrossRef] [PubMed]

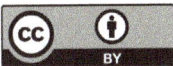

© 2019 by the authors. Licensee MDPI, Basel, Switzerland. This article is an open access article distributed under the terms and conditions of the Creative Commons Attribution (CC BY) license (http://creativecommons.org/licenses/by/4.0/).

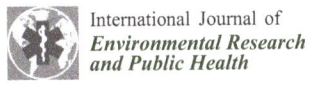

Article

The Perceived Availability of Online Social Support: Exploring the Contributions of Illness and Rural Identities in Adults with Chronic Respiratory Illness

Samantha R. Paige [1,*], Rachel E. Damiani [1], Elizabeth Flood-Grady [1,2], Janice L. Krieger [1] and Michael Stellefson [3]

1. STEM Translational Communication Center, University of Florida, Gainesville, FL 32611, USA; rdamiani@ufl.edu (R.E.D.); efloodgrady@ufl.edu (E.F.-G.); janicekrieger@ufl.edu (J.L.K.)
2. Clinical and Translational Sciences Institute, University of Florida, Gainesville, FL 32610, USA
3. Department of Health Education and Promotion, East Carolina University, Greenville, NC 27858, USA; stellefsonm17@ecu.edu
* Correspondence: paigesr190@ufl.edu

Received: 11 December 2019; Accepted: 27 December 2019; Published: 29 December 2019

Abstract: Joining an online social support group may increase perceived membership to a community, but it does not guarantee that the community will be available when it is needed. This is especially relevant for adults with Chronic Obstructive Pulmonary Disease (COPD), many of whom reside in rural regions and continually negotiate their illness identity. Drawing from social support literature and communication theory of identity, this cross-sectional study explored how COPD illness and geographic identities interact to influence patients' perceived availability of online social support. In April 2018, 575 adults with a history of respiratory symptoms completed an online survey. Patients with a COPD diagnosis reported greater availability of online support. This was partially mediated by a positive degree of COPD illness identity (i.e., being diagnosed with COPD, a history of tobacco use, severe respiratory symptoms, high disease knowledge, and low income but high education). The relationship between COPD illness identity and the availability of online support was strongest among those with low rural identity; however, at lower levels of COPD illness identity, participants with high rural identity reported the greatest degree of available online support. Results have important implications for tailored education approaches across the COPD care continuum by illness and geographic identities.

Keywords: online social support; social identity; communication theory of identity; rural health; chronic obstructive pulmonary disease

1. Introduction

The perceived availability of social support has a positive effect on health behaviors and associated outcomes [1–3], including stress reduction and improved quality of life [4]. Social support is an interpersonal communication process characterized by the exchange of informational and emotional resources among and across networks [5,6]. Identifying and engaging social networks is a prerequisite to achieve associated benefits of social support; however, a significant value of social support lies within the perception that others will be available, should the need for support arise [7].

The Internet transcends lifespan and geographic boundaries to increase users' access to social support. Social support groups exist online and through social media to help patients cope with a particular health condition or risk behavior. These programs, which are intended to supplement traditional offline support, provide patients with emotional and informational resources [8]. Unlike face-to-face support transactions, however, these technology mediated programs reduce the social and contextual cues used to reduce uncertainty and thereby better address informational and communicative needs [9]. The rising number of online support programs and their increased following is a testament for their growing interest among individuals affected by chronic disease [8,10]. A remaining concern is the degree to which patients believe the illness management support will be available when they need it.

Membership in online disease-specific social support programs constitute a "rite of passage" for patients who are diagnosed with a chronic condition [11]. However, there is a degree of social belonging that needs to occur for an individual to sufficiently benefit from online support. In general, people begin to identify as a member of an online social network by learning, negotiating, and adopting the values and attitudes of others [12]. These shared values and beliefs increase the likelihood of engaging in behaviors consistent with group norms [12]. As described by the Communication Theory of Identity (CTI) [13,14], a disconnect between group membership and identity often results in adverse health behaviors and poor communicative outcomes, which can reduce the availability of social support. As such, receiving a diagnosis and joining an online support program may increase perceived membership to a social network (i.e., social identity), but it does not guarantee that the network will be available for support when it is needed.

A unique disease context to study the theoretical intersection between perceived availability of online social support and social identity is Chronic Obstructive Pulmonary Disease (COPD), which is a progressive lower respiratory condition that predominantly affects rural adults over the age of 45 with a history of smoking tobacco [15]. Because COPD is a progressive condition, patients must engage in timely, on-going self-management of symptoms [16]. The self-management of COPD is considered a communal- rather than intrapersonal-level endeavor [17], as it is optimized through care coordination with multiple stakeholders in COPD decision-making. Physical, psychosocial, and social support are noted as critical for patients with COPD to thrive with their condition. Social and psychosocial support include (but are not limited to) emotional regulation, developing relationships and supplementing offline support, as well as navigating services and information about maintaining independence [18]. Although there has been a recent call for expanding access to online social support in COPD [19], these patients are generally older and report challenges when navigating online communities [20]. Therefore, there is a need to understand the social identities that may contribute to the perceived availability of online social support [21], especially among patients who live in isolated rural regions where health disparities persist yet access to the Internet increases.

1.1. Perceived Online Social Support

Social support is broadly conceptualized as "verbal and nonverbal communication between recipients and providers that reduces uncertainty about the situation, the self, the other, or the relationship and functions to enhance a perception of personal control in one's experience" [5] (p. 19). Social support can be perceived (i.e., belief that social support will be available) or received (i.e., exchanged or provided) [22]. An abundance of literature highlights the value of perceived social support in enhancing health promotion and reducing mortality in diverse patient populations [23,24]. For instance, there is evidence supporting the importance of perceptions of an available social network among patients with COPD. The presence of a supportive person or network (e.g., simply residing with a supportive person) is associated with positive health behaviors, including smoking cessation and participation in pulmonary rehabilitation [25]. As such, the perceived availability of social support can generally have a positive effect on patients to enhance their quality of life [26].

There is growing interest in how Internet and social media use impacts patients with COPD [27]. Social media, particularly platforms that provide support for chronic illnesses (e.g., COPD), extend patients' access to informational and emotional resources enabling them to better cope with their illness [8]. This is likely why patients with chronic disease more often participate in online social support than those without a chronic condition [28]. Research exploring the potential of online support groups for COPD patient education has focused on the quality and modality of various self-management topics communicated by diverse sources, including peers and professional organizations [29,30]. Patients with COPD also actively use social media to disclose symptoms (e.g., cough, mucus and sputum, shortness of breath) and seek patient education resources [31]. Martinez and colleagues [32] support this finding, indicating that patients with COPD more frequently (at least weekly) use the Internet if they experience severe symptoms and complications. Nevertheless, these patients generally reside in a rural region and have limited access to health care insurance. As such, the Internet is used as a health care supplement to obtain new information and seek second opinions about a health status or recommendation.

Online social support groups are "any virtual social space where people come together to get and give information or support, to learn, or to find company" [33] (p. 348). The primary focus of research examining the potential of the Internet to facilitate social support among COPD patients has been geared toward its receipt rather than its provision. Giving and receiving social support represents two different acts to achieve communication and behavior-oriented goals. Reblin and Uchino [22] systematically reviewed literature on social support and health-related implications, reporting the need to better understand the mechanisms by which people are motivated to both give and receive social support. These authors posit that that people who give social support may be motivated not only by informational needs, but also to "feel good" about themselves or feel valued by giving back to the community. And while there is evidence that people who receive social support are likely to reciprocate it, there is limited evidence to demonstrate whether or not a diagnosis of COPD contributes to how the availability of online social support is perceived among these patients. Accordingly, this study tested the following hypothesis:

Hypothesis 1: *A positive relationship exists between a diagnosis of COPD and perceived availability of online sources to (a) give and (b) receive social support.*

1.2. Social Identities: Illness and Geographic

Much like social support, the social identities of people are continuously constructed and validated, through interactions with others who may be within and outside of a particular social network. As such, communication is a core element of social identity formation and adaptation [13]. Social identities are cultivated when cultural underpinnings of a particular illness or region are integrated into a person's self-concept to explain the beliefs, values, and behaviors of its members [34]. One type of social identity is illness identity, comprising a set of roles and attitudes that a person develops in relation to their understanding of having a disease or disorder [35]. Simply being diagnosed with a condition does not guarantee that an individual relates with others diagnosed or living with the condition. This phenomenon is extremely relevant to the context of COPD, where smoking tobacco is a primary and stigmatized behavioral risk factor for most people living with the condition, yet there is also a predisposing genetic variant that causes the disease for some who have never smoked tobacco in their lifetime [15]. Knowledge about COPD is suboptimal and considerably conflicted [26], which may affect the degree to which a patient identifies with the condition and others who have been diagnosed. Mass media campaigns (e.g., Tips from Former Smokers© [36]) advertise the "face of COPD" as an older adult, typically a male with a history of heavy smoking tobacco who exhibits respiratory distress that necessitates use of supplemental oxygen [37]. On the contrary, pharmaceutical companies advertise treatments for COPD by highlighting symptoms (e.g., the metaphorical elephant on chest) experienced by middle-to-older age adults who value enjoying time with family. These ads rarely mention risk behaviors (e.g., tobacco use) or equipment (e.g., oxygen tanks) that elicit public stigma. Although these campaigns raise awareness of COPD, they evoke differential emotions (e.g., fear, disgust, hope) to consequently shape the public's view of COPD. To date, however, limited empirical attention has examined—from the perspective of patients diagnosed with COPD—which experiences, symptoms, and demographic characteristics are most influential in shaping this illness identity. Therefore, this study aims to answer the following research question:

RQ 1: *What factors are reported as comprising the chronic respiratory illness identity?*

Those with a strong social identity hold beliefs and engage in behaviors that enhance the image of their group membership to make them distinct from other competing groups [12]. Likewise, people who belong to a particular community, or network, but do not strongly identify with their membership are likely to deviate from established group norms [12]. Because social support is a communicative, coping phenomenon that promotes the health and well-being of its recipients, social identities should, theoretically, function in a manner that is conducive to enhancing the availability of social support. Given widespread adoption of the Internet and its variety of social support forums for COPD [29,31,38,39], it is expected that patients with a strong illness identity will report positive perceptions about available online social support. This study tested the following hypothesis:

Hypothesis 2: *COPD illness identity will positively mediate the relationship between receiving a diagnosis of COPD and perceived availability of online social support.*

Another type of social identity is geographic identity, defined as the aspects of one's self that are derived from the culture and natural environment of a physical location [40]. One salient facet of geographic identity includes the traits, values, and behaviors that emerge from residing in either a rural or urban location. Rural adults, for example, engage in riskier health behaviors (e.g., heavy tobacco use, fewer preventive efforts) and report less trust in government safety and regulatory bodies [41]. Although there are sub-cultures that are apparent in rural areas, the rural culture is generally associated with prioritizing relationships with family [42], and satisfaction with living in the same community for long periods of time without any desire to leave [43]. Consequently, rural adults are more likely to value strongly rooted social networks, particularly those comprised of familiar others (e.g., neighbors) who hold similar cultural beliefs. Given this cultural profile, individuals with a high degree of rural identity may be more likely to receive informational support in online groups comprised of users with similar characteristics. This is unlike those who have a low rural identity, who may be more likely to become immersed in the online experience to exchange support with the intention of building new relationships with others who have dissimilar values. Because rural adults are disproportionately affected by COPD [44] and hold unique cultural values about health and social networks, empirical attention is needed to examine how illness and rural identities interact to affect the perceived availability of online social support. Therefore, this study aims to answer the following research question:

RQ 2: *Does rural identity moderate the mediating effect of COPD illness identity on the perceived availability of online social support?*

2. Materials and Methods

In April 2018, 575 adults participated in a 20-min web-based survey. Patients from a university research registry with chronic lower respiratory conditions (ICD-10 Codes J40-J47), minus J45 "asthma"), were enrolled in the study through a combination of United States Postal Service (USPS) mailer and email notifications (n = 283). Participants were also invited to participate through a publicly accessible university-based research listing website, where a survey description and link were advertised as a "lung health study" (n = 292).

2.1. Measures

Socio-demographics. Items from the Behavioral Risk Factor Surveillance System [45] were used to capture socio-demographic features of the sample. This included age (in years), gender, race, ethnicity, as well as income and education.

COPD diagnosis and identity. Participants were asked whether they have been diagnosed with COPD (1 = Yes; 0 = No). To assess COPD illness identity, participants were asked the degree to which they identified with other patients who live with COPD (1 = fully disagree; 7 = fully agree). This item captured communal identity related to COPD, which differs from existing illness identity measures that assess the degree to which an illness is integrated into an individual's self-identity [46].

COPD knowledge. COPD knowledge was measured with Maples and colleagues' [47] 13-item COPD-Questionnaire (COPD-Q), including items about etiology, pathophysiology, management, and symptoms. Each literacy-sensitive item included three nominal response options (True, False, Not Sure). Correct responses were coded as 1, whereas items answered incorrectly or uncertain by the participant were coded as 0. A summative score was computed for analysis (0 = low knowledge; 13 = high knowledge).

COPD symptom severity. Hallmark COPD symptoms include dyspnea, persistent cough, chest congestion, and fatigue [15]. Reflecting these symptoms, four items were created to assess the degree that these symptoms were present in the participant's life. Each item was anchored on a 5-point Likert-type scale (1 = strongly disagree; 5 = strongly agree). Responses were aggregated and averaged ($\alpha = 0.70$). A score of 0 indicated the absence of symptoms, whereas a 5 indicated a strong symptom presence.

Tobacco use. An item from the Behavioral Risk Factor Surveillance System [45] measured tobacco use. First, participants were asked how long it had been since they last smoked a cigarette. Respondents who selected "15 years or more" or "I have never smoked regularly" were categorized as not recent/current smokers. This cutoff was selected because 15 years after quitting smoking puts an individual at an equal risk of cardiovascular disease as someone who has never smoked [48]. Also, a former 30 pack-year smoker is no longer eligible for lung cancer screening, a common tobacco-associated lung condition, if they quit smoking 15 years ago or more [49]. All other responses were coded as current or recent tobacco users.

Rural location and identity. Perceived rural residence was measured by asking, "to what extent would you describe your current location (where you live)?" Perceived rural identity was measured by asking, "to what extent do you identify as being from a small town/rural or urban/city? Both items were scored based on a 5-point Likert-type scale (1 = city/urban; 5 = small town/rural).

Perceived availability of online social support. The Shakespeare-Finch and Obst [4] 2-Way Social Support Scale was adapted to assess how people reciprocate health-related online social support using a 5-point Likert-type scale (1 = not at all; 5 = always). The original instrument used to measure reciprocal social support was comprised of four scales, which distinguished between emotional and instrumental support. We added language to reflect online social support for the purposes of adaptation. Preliminary analyses found that data produced by these two support styles were highly correlated for the perceived availability of online sources to receive and give support ($r = 0.86$; $p < 0.001$). For the purposes of parsimony, the four scales were collapsed to measure two constructs: perceived availability of sources to (a) give (10 items; $\alpha = 0.93$) and (b) receive (10 items; $\alpha = 0.94$) online social support. Each scale's average score was computed for analyses.

2.2. Data Analysis

SPSS v25 (IBM, Armonk, NY, USA) was used to conduct all statistical analyses, which handled missing data by applying list-wise deletion procedures. Frequency statistics were computed to describe the sample. To answer RQ1, a hierarchical linear regression analysis, with attention to R^2 change, was conducted to examine how socio-demographics, COPD diagnosis and risk factors, and COPD knowledge contributed to COPD illness identity scores. Hayes' PROCESS v3.1 macro was used to test Hypotheses 1–3. Data were fit to Model 15 to carry out two conditional process analyses. Model 15 tests a moderated mediation with two moderations occurring between (a) the independent variable and dependent variable and (b) the mediated variable and dependent variable. This model examines the indirect effect of a COPD diagnosis (independent variable; IV) on the perceived availability of online social support (to give and to receive; dependent variables; DVs) via COPD illness identity differences (Mediator), conditional on level of rural identity (Moderator). For the first interaction effect, the product of COPD status and rural identity was produced to determine the moderation effect on perceived availability of online support (DV 1 = give; DV 2 = receive). For the second interaction, the product of COPD illness identity and rural identity was mean-centered. The Johnson-Neyman technique was used to probe for interactions at different levels of the moderator. Data were normally distributed; therefore, the moderator was collapsed into three levels: $-1SD, M, +1SD$ [50]. PROCESS v3.1 macro uses boot strapping was conducted to generate 95% confidence intervals.

3. Results

Table 1 shows the socio-demographic, COPD-related, and online activities of participants. Participants were, on average, 55 years old and predominantly white, although nearly 20% identified as Hispanic. Over half earned more than $50,000 annually and nearly 80% reported at least some college education.

Perceived residence and rural identity were moderately rural. The Mdn for each item was 3, which is similar to the M (SD) values reported in Table 1. About 10% of participants perceived their residence as extremely (value = 1 on the 5-point Likert-type scaled item) urban/metropolitan (n = 66; 11.7%) and reported the lowest possible degree of rural identity (n = 53 or 9.3%). Conversely, nearly 20% perceived their residence as extremely (value = 5 on the 5-point Likert-type scaled item) small/town rural (n = 103; 18.3%) and reported the highest degree of rural identity (n = 100; 17.5%). A Pearson's r correlation demonstrates that perceived residence and geographic identity has a positive, but not perfect correlation (r = 0.74; $p < 0.001$).

Despite nearly 71% of participants reporting a COPD diagnosis and moderately severe symptoms, participants' COPD illness identity was average (M = 3.16; SD = 1.77), on a 7-point Likert-type scale. Less than half (42.1%) reported as a current smoker or a smoker who quit within the past 15 years. A greater proportion of participants reported never smoking (n = 208; 36.3%), as compared to those who had smoked in the past but quit more than 15 years ago (n = 123; 21.5%). Participants also reported an average degree of COPD knowledge (M = 6.45; SD = 2.74).

Participants perceived a moderate degree of online source availability to give and receive support. Although approximately 20% of the sample reported not having any available online support to receive (n = 110, 19.5%) or give (n = 132; 23.5%) health information, over 60% of participants reported using social media at least five hours each week.

Table 1. Characteristics of the sample ($n = 575$).

Predictor	Descriptive Statistics
Socio-Demographics	
Age, M (SD)	55.14 (12.62)
Gender, n (%)	
Female	256 (44.50)
Male	298 (51.80)
Missing	21 (3.70)
Race, n (%)	
White	474 (82.4)
Black/African American	54 (9.4)
Asian American	12 (2.1)
Native American	13 (2.3)
Other/Multi-Racial	19 (3.3)
Missing	1 (0.7)
Ethnicity, n (%)	
Hispanic	108 (18.8)
Non-Hispanic	433 (75.3)
Missing	34 (5.9)
Income, n (%)	
$24,999 or less	70 (12.2)
$25K–$34,999	60 (10.4)
$35K–$49,999	124 (21.6)
$50K–$74,999	147 (25.6)
$75K or more	156 (27.1)
Missing	18 (3.1)
Education, n (%)	
Less than High School	37 (12.7)
High School or Equivalent	66 (11.5)
College 1–3 Years	180 (31.3)
College 4 or More Years	288 (50.1)
Missing	4 (0.7)
Chronic Obstructive Pulmonary Disease (COPD)-Specific Factors	
COPD Illness Identity, M (SD)	3.16 (1.77)
Respiratory Symptom Severity, M (SD)	2.81 (0.96)
Disease Knowledge, M (SD)	6.45 (2.74)
Smoker (Current, Quit within 15 years), n (%)	242 (42.2)
Reported COPD Diagnosis, n (%)	407 (70.8)
Rural-Specific Factors	
Rural Identity, M (SD)	3.01 (1.22)
Perceived Rural Residence, M (SD)	2.98 (1.29)
Online Activity and Support Behaviors	
Give Online Health Support, M (SD)	2.57 (1.15)
Receive Online Health Support, M (SD)	2.58 (1.16)
Weekly Social Media Use, n (%)	
0–1 h	119 (20.7)
2–4 h	99 (17.2)
5–9 h	63 (11)
10+ h	289 (50.3)
Missing	5 (0.9)

3.1. Research Question 1

Table 2 shows that socio-demographics, COPD diagnosis and risk factors, and COPD knowledge contribute to COPD illness identity. In regard to socio-demographics, only lower income and higher education was associated with a greater COPD illness identity, $F (8, 467) = 3.86, p < 0.001$ ($R^2 = 0.06$, $R^2_{adj} = 0.05$). While controlling for socio-demographics, having a self-reported COPD diagnosis, reporting more severe respiratory symptoms, and identifying as a current/recent smoker were all positively associated with COPD illness identity, $F (11, 464) = 13.17, p < 0.001$ ($R^2 = 0.24, R^2_{adj} = 0.22$). Finally, COPD knowledge was positively associated with COPD illness identity, $F (12, 463) = 16.40$, $p < 0.001$ ($R^2 = 0.30, R^2_{adj} = 0.28$).

Table 2. Hierarchical linear regression of factors contributing to COPD illness identity.

Regression Steps	R^2 Change	b	SE b	95% CI Lower Bound	95% CI Upper Bound
Step 1: Socio-Demographics	0.05 **				
Age		−0.01	0.01	−0.02	0.01
Gender [a]		−0.25	0.15	−0.56	0.05
Race [b]		0.31	0.23	−0.15	0.77
Ethnicity [c]		0.37	0.22	−0.05	0.79
Income [d]		−0.60 **	0.16	−0.91	−0.29
Education [e]		0.57 *	0.23	0.12	1.03
Rural Identity		0.06	0.10	−0.13	0.25
Perceived Rural Residence		−0.02	0.10	−0.21	0.16
Step 2: COPD Experiences	0.22 **				
COPD Diagnosis		0.79 **	0.19	0.42	1.15
Respiratory Symptoms		0.54 **	0.09	0.37	0.71
Smoker [f]		0.32 *	0.15	0.01	0.62
Step 3: COPD Awareness	0.28 **				
COPD Knowledge		0.18 **	0.03	0.12	0.23

Note. CI = Confidence Interval; [a] Gender (1 = Female; 0 = Male); [b] Race (1 = White; 0 = Non-White); [c] Ethnicity (1 = Hispanic; 0 = Non-Hispanic); [d] Income (1 = $50K or more/year; 0 = $49,999 or less/year); [e] Education (1 = At least some college; 0 = High school or less); [f] Smoker (Current or quit within the past 15 years). * $p < 0.05$; ** $p < 0.01$.

3.2. Hypotheses 1–2

Table 3 presents results of conditional process analyses, supporting both H1 and H2. Both models show that factors contributing to COPD illness identity were statistically significant for opportunities to give, $F (501, 8) = 20.15, p < 0.001$ ($R^2 = 0.24$), and receive online support, $F (504, 8) = 21.05, p < 0.001$ ($R^2 = 0.25$). As expected, a COPD diagnosis had a positive, statistically significant association with COPD illness identity in both models ($p < 0.001$). When factors from Table 2 were entered into the same regression step, socioeconomic status and identifying as a current/former tobacco smoker were no longer statistically significant predictors of COPD illness identity.

Table 3 also demonstrates the cumulative models examining COPD status, COPD illness and rural identities while controlling for covariates of perceived availability of online sources to give, $F (497, 12) = 39.57, p < 0.001$ ($R^2 = 0.49$), and receive support, $F (500, 12) = 37.50, p < 0.001$ ($R^2 = 0.47$). Figure 1 shows that COPD diagnosis ($b = 0.76$ and 0.72, respectively) and COPD illness identity ($b = 0.16$ and 0.13, respectively) had a positive, statistically significant association with perceived availability of online sources for which they could give and receive support. In regard to covariates, being younger, residing in a less rural area, and reporting lower COPD knowledge was associated with greater perceived availability of these support sources.

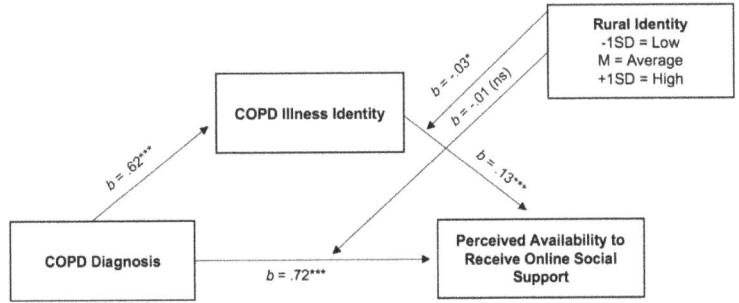

Figure 1a. Perceived availability of online sources to receive health-related social support

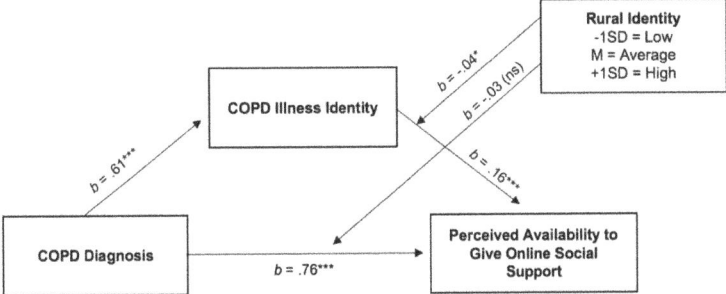

Figure 1b. Perceived availability of online sources to give health-related social support

Figure 1. Conceptual models depicting moderated indirect effects. (**a**) Perceived availability of online sources to receive health-related social support; (**b**) Perceived availability of online sources to give health-related social support. Note. * $p < 0.05$; *** $p < 0.001$; ns = not statistically significant ($p > 0.05$).

3.3. Research Question 2

Table 3 further demonstrates that rural identity moderates the relationship between COPD illness identity and the perceived availability of online sources to give ($b = -0.04$) and receive ($b = -0.03$) support ($p < 0.05$). Figure 2 depicts the moderation effect. Johnson-Neyman analyses indicated that the interaction strength was strongest for low rural identity (effect = 0.24; standard error = 0.04) and weaker for high rural identity (effect = 0.07; standard error = 0.04). Rural identity did not moderate the direct relationship between COPD diagnosis and perceived availability of online social support.

Table 4 demonstrates the direct effect of a COPD diagnosis on the perceived availability of online social support and the indirect effect through COPD illness identity at three levels of rural identity (−1SD, M, +1SD). A partial mediation exists. The non-statistically significant index of moderated mediation indicated that this indirect relationship is independent of rural identity as a moderator.

Table 3. Conditional process analyses of identity on online health-related engagement.

	Regression Models, b (SE) [95% CI]	
Regression Steps	Outcome 1: Perceived Availability to Give Online Support	Outcome 2: Perceived Availability to Receive Online Support
Step 1: COPD Illness Identity		
n(df)	501(8)	504(8)
F Statistic	20.15 ***	21.05 ***
R^2 Value	0.24	0.25
COPD Status	0.61 (0.17) [0.28, 0.95] ***	0.62 (0.17) [0.29, 0.96] ***
Symptom Severity	0.55 (0.08) [0.39, 0.71] ***	0.54 (0.08) [0.38, 0.69] ***
COPD Knowledge	0.17 (0.03) [0.11, 0.22] ***	0.17 (0.03) [0.12, 0.22] ***
Smoker	0.12 (0.15) [−0.16, 0.41]	0.11 (0.15) [−0.18, 0.40]
Perceived Rural Residence	−0.05 (0.06) [−0.02, 0.01]	−0.05 (0.05) [−0.15, 0.06]
Age	−0.01 (0.01) [−0.02, 0.01]	−0.01 (0.01) [−0.02, 0.01]
Income	−0.24 (0.14) [−0.52, 0.03]	−0.24 (0.14) [−0.51, 0.03]
Education	0.40 (0.19) [0.04, 0.77] *	0.35 (0.19) [−0.02, 0.71]
Step 2: Online Support Outcome		
n(df)	497(12)	500(12)
F Statistic	39.57 ***	37.50 ***
R^2 Value	0.49	0.47
COPD Status	0.76 (0.09) [0.57, 0.94] ***	0.72 (0.10) [0.52, 0.91] ***
COPD Illness Identity	0.16 (0.02) [0.11, 0.21] ***	0.13 (0.02) [0.08, 0.18] ***
Rural Identity	−0.01 (0.04) [−0.10, 0.07]	0.01 (0.05) [−0.09, 0.09]
COPD Status * Rural Identity	−0.03 (0.07) [−0.16, 0.11]	−0.01 (0.07) [−0.15, 0.12]
COPD Identity * Rural Identity	−0.04 (0.02) [−0.07, −0.01] *	−0.03 (0.02) [−0.07, 0.00] *
Symptom Severity	−0.05 (0.04) [−0.14, 0.04]	−0.03 (0.04) [−0.12, 0.06]
COPD Knowledge	−0.04 (0.02) [−0.07, −0.01] **	−0.06 (0.02) [−0.09, −0.03] ***
Smoker [a]	0.07 (0.08) [−0.08, 0.23]	0.04 (0.08) [−0.12, 0.20]
Perceived Rural Residence	−0.22 (0.04) [−0.30, −0.13] ***	−0.19 (0.04) [−0.27, −0.10] ***
Age	−0.03 (0.01) [−0.04, −0.03] ***	−0.04 (0.01) [−0.04, −0.03] ***
Income	−0.07 (0.08) [−0.21, 0.08]	−0.14 (0.07) [−0.29, 0.01]
Education	0.16 (0.10) [−0.04, 0.37]	0.19 (0.10) [−0.01, 0.40]

Note. CI = Confidence Interval; [a] Smoker (Current/quit within the past 15 years); * $p < 0.05$; ** $p < 0.01$; *** $p < 0.001$.

Table 4. Direct and indirect effects by geographic identity (−1SD, M, +1SD).

		95% Confidence Interval	
Direct/Indirect Pathway	Effect (Std. Error)	Lower Level	Upper Level
Direct Effect			
COPD Diagnosis -> Give Online Support			
Low Rural Identity	0.79 (0.13)	0.54	1.05
Average Rural Identity	0.76 (0.09)	0.57	0.94
High Rural Identity	0.72 (0.12)	0.49	0.96
COPD Diagnosis -> Receive Online Support			
Low Rural Identity	0.74 (0.13)	0.48	1.00
Average Rural Identity	0.72 (0.10)	0.53	0.91
High Rural Identity	0.71 (0.12)	0.47	0.94
Indirect Effect			
COPD Diagnosis -> COPD Illness Identity -> Give Online Support			
Low Rural Identity	0.13 (0.05)	0.04	0.24
Average Rural Identity	0.10 (0.04)	0.03	0.18
High Rural Identity	0.07 (0.03)	0.02	0.13
COPD Diagnosis -> COPD Illness Identity -> Receive Online Support			
Low Rural Identity	0.10 (0.04)	0.03	0.20
Average Rural Identity	0.08 (0.03)	0.02	0.15
High Rural Identity	0.05 (0.03)	0.01	0.12

Note. Low rural identity (−1SD) = −1.20; Average rural identity (M) = 0.0; High rural identity (+1SD) = 1.20.

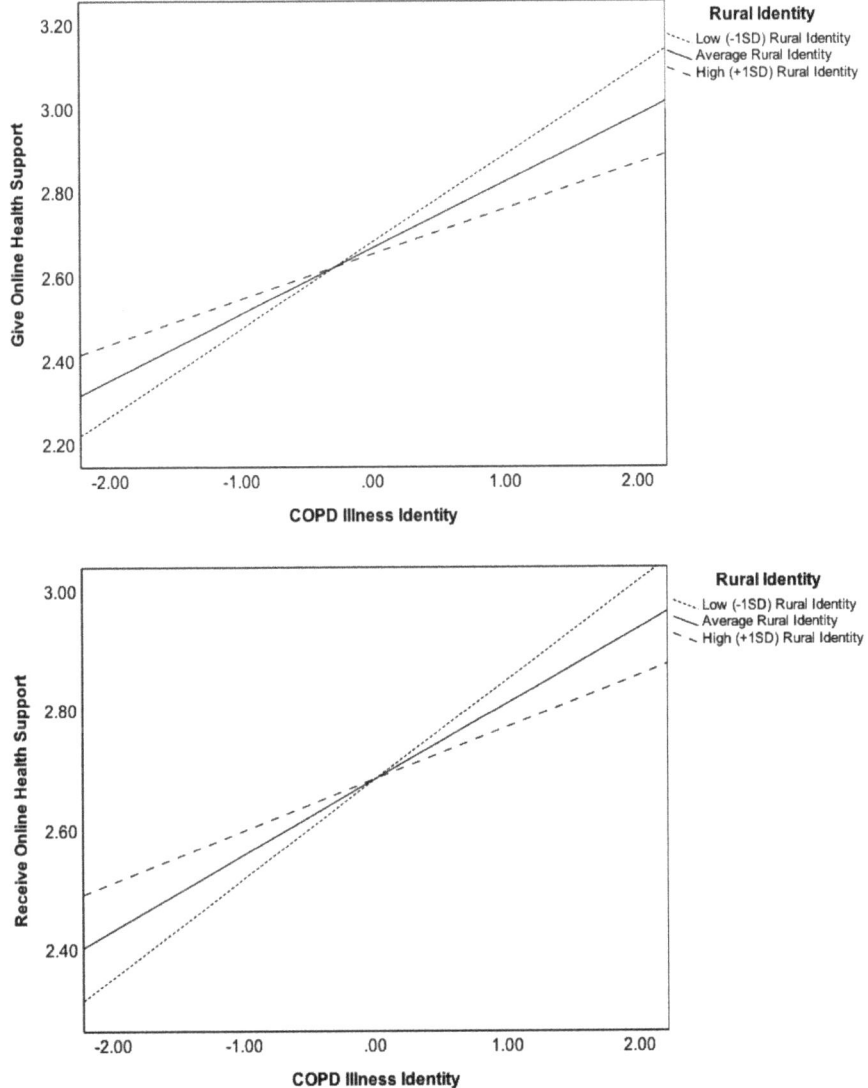

Figure 2. Moderating effect of rural identity on illness identity and reciprocating online support.

4. Discussion

Principal Findings

This study explored how social identities, including illness and rurality, contributed to perceptions of available online sources for giving and receiving social support among patients with a history of respiratory health conditions. Reporting a COPD diagnosis was positively associated with COPD illness identity, as well as perceived availability of online sources for social support. Consistent with social identity and communication literature [13], respondents with a strong COPD illness identity also reported having online sources available for social support. Results also demonstrate that the relationship between COPD illness identity and perceived availability of online social support was strongest among participants with low rural identity. Findings have important implications for considering the interplay of multiple layers of social identity in understanding online social support in COPD.

Socio-demographics, specifically low income and high education, were attributed to COPD illness identity; however, COPD experiences (i.e., having a physician COPD diagnosis, identifying as a current/recent smoker) and symptoms (i.e., reporting more severe respiratory symptoms) explained the greatest amount of variance in identity. Unexpectedly, results demonstrated that neither geographic region, gender, race/ethnicity, nor age was associated with COPD illness identity. These findings underscore the outdated stereotype of COPD as an older white man's disease [37].

Consistent with research that chronic disease populations are more likely than their non-diagnosed counterparts to engage in online media activities [28], self-reporting a COPD diagnosis was positively associated with perceived availability of being able to give and receive online social support. This relationship was partially mediated by COPD illness identity. Interestingly, a greater perception of online social support existed among participants with COPD, who were younger and had low COPD knowledge. Although there is evidence that greater respiratory symptom severity predicts patients' Internet use [27,32], research has demonstrated that high COPD knowledge and less severe symptoms are associated with a higher degree of eHealth literacy (i.e., ability to access, understand, and evaluate online information) [27]. Patients who are at a critical point of illness identity negotiation may not be able to maximize the potential of online social support, because they do not have the optimal skills to do so. Future research is needed to understand how patients navigate these online experiences with varying degrees of knowledge and symptoms.

Rural identity did not moderate the relationship between having a COPD diagnosis and reporting available online support; however, it did interact with COPD illness identity, a partial mediator that explained the relationship between COPD diagnosis and perceived available online support. Results demonstrated that the positive relationship between COPD illness identity and perceived available online social support was strongest among individuals who reported low rural identity. Despite these results, there is evidence that online chronic disease interventions are both effective and accepted in rural regions to promote disease-specific knowledge and psychosocial adaptations [51]. We further examined this relationship and found that patients with a high rural identity reported a greater degree of online social support than their counterparts with low rural identity, but only when COPD illness identity was low. This provides a unique opportunity to promote the early detection of COPD among high-risk rural adults by targeting patients with health education that helps build their communal identity with COPD. Conversely, for urban adults with high COPD illness identity, online interventions that integrate social support may be more effective later in the COPD care continuum, or immediately after a diagnosis when the adoption of new self-management behaviors becomes imperative. Future research is needed to understand the timing and amount of online support interventions across the geographic and care continuums in COPD. This will provide support in culturally adapted respiratory health communication interventions that consider the intersection of illness and geographic identities.

This study examines how two communal identities (i.e., COPD illness and rural) interact to explain how patients with COPD reciprocate online support to cultivate community ties. Although geographic region and culture may not function as part of an individual's COPD illness identity, these social identities have a synergistic effect on perceptions of available online social support. Central to theoretical underpinnings of the CTI [13], identity "gaps" or discrepancies between actual and perceived group membership can lead to poor communicative outcomes. Consistent with this theory, the relationship between COPD risk factors and perceptions of illness identity were more favorable to the perceived availability of online social support for health-related purposes. Reporting an urban residence was positively associated with greater availability of online social support; however, low rural (or urban) identity did not significantly moderate the relationship between COPD status and perceived availability of online social support. The only instance where rural identity moderated the relationship between diagnosis and perceived availability of online social support was in conjunction with a positive COPD illness identity. In future social support research conducted through the theoretical lens of social identity and CTI, identity should be examined as a dynamic and multi-faceted construct that influences perceptions of online social support. Rather than isolate one component of identity (e.g., illness identity), findings emphasize the need to adopt a holistic perspective to understand health behaviors by considering multiple components of communal identity simultaneously.

The perceived availability to give and receive online social support was highly correlated in this study, indicating that this sample comprising predominantly of patients with COPD believe they have support systems on the Internet with whom they can exchange or reciprocate health information. This provides support for the theoretical argument that a person who receives support is likely to reciprocate it [22]. These scales are expected to correlate to some degree [4]; however, we did not expect the association to be so strong in this patient population, which is why we separated the two scales to examine predictors of perceived availability to give and to receive online support. Empirical evidence supports that patients with COPD face challenges navigating online platforms simply to access and evaluate health content from informational websites, and only about 30% of patients with COPD use social media (e.g., Facebook) [27]. In the current study, however, about 60% of participants were active on social media more than 5 h a week, equivalent to nearly one hour each day. It is unclear from this study whether frequent use of social media resulted in a greater degree of perceived availability of online support, or whether being directed to online support forums by a family member, peer, or health care provider resulted in greater use of these media. Regardless, this finding justifies national efforts to increase COPD patients' access and use to online communities [19], which are shown to improve self-management behaviors and health-related outcomes [25,26].

This study does not exist without limitations. A single item measured illness and geographic identities, as valid and reliable measures of these constructs either do not exist or are limited in their theoretical scope. Finally, this was a cross-sectional study, meaning associations are correlative not causative. This presents a potential limitation but highlights an important direction for future research. For example, we aimed to understand what factors are associated with COPD illness identity in this study, and one of those factors was COPD knowledge. It is possible that a person with a high COPD illness identity may be naturally more inclined to seek more information about COPD, thus being more knowledgeable. The potential for reverse causality in the relationship between COPD illness identity and COPD knowledge brings attention to the importance of more experimental and longitudinal research in understanding how illness identities manifest across the care continuum (e.g., screening, diagnosis, and across treatment). Likewise, research is needed to examine the interaction of geographic and illness identities in other health-related contexts, particularly those that are acute and not progressive.

5. Conclusions

This study examines elements of social identity through a communication lens to understand how patients perceive the availability of online health-related social support. Results provide evidence that illness and geographic identities contribute to the perceived availability of online sources of social support in the context of COPD. Further, results facilitate an understanding for the point on the COPD care continuum that rural/urban patients may be most receptive to online social support. Receptivity will be likely in these two contexts: (1) high rural identity coupled with low COPD illness identity, and (2) low rural identity coupled with high COPD illness identity. For rural communities, in particular, social media facilitates opportunities for instrumental and emotional social support that can help adults with respiratory distress recognize the burden of their disease and prompt early detection of exacerbated symptoms.

Author Contributions: Conceptualization, S.R.P., R.E.D., E.F.-G., J.L.K., and M.S.; methodology, S.R.P. and E.F.-G.; software, S.R.P.; validation, S.R.P., R.E.D., E.F.-G., J.L.K., and M.S.; formal analysis, S.R.P. and E.F.-G.; investigation, S.R.P.; resources, S.R.P.; data curation, S.R.P., J.L.K., and M.S.; writing—original draft preparation, S.R.P., R.E.D., and E.F.-G.; writing—review and editing, S.R.P., R.E.D., E.F.-G., J.L.K., and M.S.; visualization, S.R.P., R.E.D., and E.F.-G.; supervision, S.R.P.; project administration, S.R.P.; funding acquisition, S.R.P. All authors have read and agreed to the published version of the manuscript.

Funding: Research reported in this publication was supported by the National Heart, Lung, and Blood Institute of the National Institutes of Health under Award Numbers F31HL132463 and F32HL143938. The content is solely the responsibility of the authors and does not necessarily represent the official views of the National Institutes of Health.

Acknowledgments: Thank you to the University of Florida's Recruitment Center and Integrated Data Repository for assisting in identifying eligible participants for this study. As always, a special thank you to those participants who took their time to complete the survey.

Conflicts of Interest: The authors declare no conflict of interest.

References

1. Lyyra, T.M.; Heikkinen, R.L. Perceived Social Support and Mortality in Older People. *J. Gerontol. B Psychol. Sci. Soc. Sci.* **2006**, *61*, S147–S152. [CrossRef] [PubMed]
2. Steinfield, C.; Ellison, N.B.; Lampe, C. Social Capital, Self-Esteem, and Use of Online Social Network Sites: A Longitudinal Analysis. *J. Appl. Dev. Psychol.* **2008**, *29*, 434–445. [CrossRef]
3. Wright, K.B. Communication in Health-Related Online Social Support Groups/Communities: A Review of Research and Predictors of Participation, Applications of Social Support Theory, and Health Outcomes. *Rev. Commun. Res.* **2016**, *4*, 65–87.
4. Shakespeare-Finch, J.; Obst, P.L. The Development of the 2-Way Social Support Scale: A Measure of Giving and Receiving Emotional and Instrumental Support. *J. Pers. Assess.* **2011**, *93*, 483–490. [CrossRef] [PubMed]
5. Albrecht, T.L.; Adelman, M.B. *Communicating Social Support*; Sage Publications, Inc.: Thousand Oaks, CA, USA, 1987.
6. Cutrona, C.E.; Suhr, J.A. Controllability of Stressful Events and Satisfaction with Spouse Support Behaviors. *Commun. Res.* **1992**, *19*, 154–174. [CrossRef]
7. Uchino, B.N. Understanding the Links Between Social Support and Physical Health: A Life-Span Perspective with Emphasis on the Separability of Perceived and Received Support. *Perspect. Psychol. Sci. J. Assoc. Psychol. Sci.* **2009**, *4*, 236–255. [CrossRef]
8. Rains, S.A.; Peterson, E.B.; Wright, K.B. Communicating Social Support in Computer-Mediated Contexts: A Meta-Analytic Review of Content Analyses Examining Support Messages Shared Online among Individuals Coping with Illness. *Commun. Monogr.* **2015**, *82*, 403–430. [CrossRef]
9. Walther, J.B.; Loh, T.; Granka, L. Let Me Count the Ways: The Interchange of Verbal and Nonverbal Cues in Computer-Mediated and Face-to-Face Affinity. *J. Lang. Soc. Psychol.* **2005**, *24*, 36–65. [CrossRef]
10. Patel, R.; Chang, T.; Greysen, S.R.; Chopra, V. Social Media Use in Chronic Disease: A Systematic Review and Novel Taxonomy. *Am. J. Med.* **2015**, *128*, 1335–1350. [CrossRef]
11. Allen, C.; Vassilev, I.; Kennedy, A.; Rogers, A. Long-Term Condition Self-Management Support in Online Communities: A Meta-Synthesis of Qualitative Papers. *J. Med. Internet Res.* **2016**, *18*, 61. [CrossRef]
12. Hogg, M.A. Social Identity. In *Handbook of Self and Identity*; The Guilford Press: New York, NY, USA, 2003; pp. 462–479.
13. Hecht, M.L.; Lu, Y. Communication Theory of Identity. In *Encyclopedia of Health Communication*; SAGE Publications, Inc.: Thousand Oaks, CA, USA, 2014; pp. 226–227. [CrossRef]
14. Jung, E.; Hecht, M.L. Elaborating the Communication Theory of Identity: Identity Gaps and Communication Outcomes. *Commun. Q.* **2004**, *52*, 265–283. [CrossRef]
15. Centers for Disease Control & Prevention. CDC–COPD Home Page–Chronic Obstructive Pulmonary Disease (COPD). Available online: https://www.cdc.gov/copd/index.html (accessed on 14 November 2017).
16. Han, M.L.K.; Martinez, C.H.; Au, D.H.; Bourbeau, J.; Boyd, C.M.; Branson, R.; Criner, G.J.; Kalhan, R.; Kallstrom, T.J.; King, A.; et al. Meeting the Challenge of COPD Care Delivery in the USA: A Multiprovider Perspective. *Lancet Respir. Med.* **2016**, *4*, 473–526. [CrossRef]

17. Pleasants, R.A.; Riley, I.L.; Mannino, D.M. Defining and Targeting Health Disparities in Chronic Obstructive Pulmonary Disease. *Int. J. Chronic Obstr. Pulm. Dis.* **2016**, *11*, 2475–2496. [CrossRef] [PubMed]
18. Gardener, A.C.; Ewing, G.; Kuhn, I.; Farquhar, M. Support Needs of Patients with COPD: A Systematic Literature Search and Narrative Review. *Int. J. Chronic Obstr. Pulm. Dis.* **2018**, *13*, 1021–1035. [CrossRef]
19. Kiley, J.P.; Gibbons, G.H. COPD National Action Plan: Addressing a Public Health Need Together. *Chest* **2017**, *152*, 698–699. [CrossRef] [PubMed]
20. Paige, S.R.; Stellefson, M.; Krieger, J.L.; Alber, J.M. Computer-Mediated Experiences of Patients with Chronic Obstructive Pulmonary Disease. *Am. J. Health Educ.* **2019**, *50*, 127–134. [CrossRef]
21. Barton, C.; Effing, T.W.; Cafarella, P. Social Support and Social Networks in COPD: A Scoping Review. *J. Chronic Obstr. Pulm. Dis.* **2015**, *12*, 690–702. [CrossRef]
22. Reblin, M.; Uchino, B.N. Social and Emotional Support and Its Implication for Health. *Curr. Opin. Psychiatry* **2008**, *21*, 201–205. [CrossRef]
23. Göz, F.; Karaoz, S.; Goz, M.; Ekiz, S.; Cetin, I. Effects of the Diabetic Patients' Perceived Social Support on Their Quality-of-Life. *J. Clin. Nurs.* **2007**, *16*, 1353–1360. [CrossRef]
24. Prati, G.; Pietrantoni, L. Optimism, Social Support, and Coping Strategies As Factors Contributing to Posttraumatic Growth: A Meta-Analysis. *J. Loss Trauma* **2009**, *14*, 364–388. [CrossRef]
25. Chen, Z.; Fan, V.S.; Belza, B.; Pike, K.; Nguyen, H.Q. Association between Social Support and Self-Care Behaviors in Adults with Chronic Obstructive Pulmonary Disease. *Ann. Am. Thorac. Soc.* **2017**, *14*, 1419–1427. [CrossRef] [PubMed]
26. Lenferink, A.; van der Palen, J.; Effing, T. The Role of Social Support in Improving Chronic Obstructive Pulmonary Disease Self-Management. *Expert Rev. Respir. Med.* **2018**, *12*, 623–626. [CrossRef] [PubMed]
27. Stellefson, M.L.; Shuster, J.J.; Chaney, B.H.; Paige, S.R.; Alber, J.M.; Chaney, J.D.; Sriram, P.S. Web-Based Health Information Seeking and EHealth Literacy among Patients Living with Chronic Obstructive Pulmonary Disease (COPD). *Health Commun.* **2018**, *33*, 1410–1424. [CrossRef]
28. Fox, S. *The Social Life of Health Information*; Pew Res. Center: Washington, DC, USA, 2014; Available online: https://www.pewresearch.org/fact-tank/2014/01/15/the-social-life-of-health-information/ (accessed on 28 December 2019).
29. Paige, S.R.; Stellefson, M.; Chaney, B.H.; Alber, J.M. Pinterest as a Resource for Health Information on Chronic Obstructive Pulmonary Disease (COPD): A Social Media Content Analysis. *Am. J. Health Educ.* **2015**, *46*, 241–251. [CrossRef]
30. Stellefson, M.; Chaney, B.; Ochipa, K.; Chaney, D.; Haider, Z.; Hanik, B.; Chavarria, E.; Bernhardt, J.M. YouTube as a Source of COPD Patient Education: A Social Media Content Analysis. *Chron. Respir. Dis.* **2014**, *11*, 61–71. [CrossRef]
31. Cook, N.S.; Kostikas, K.; Gruenberger, J.B.; Shah, B.; Pathak, P.; Kaur, V.P.; Mudumby, A.; Sharma, R.; Gutzwiller, F.S. Patients' Perspectives on COPD: Findings from a Social Media Listening Study. *ERJ Open Res.* **2019**, *5*, 00128–02018. [CrossRef]
32. Martinez, C.H.; St. Jean, B.L.; Plauschinat, C.A.; Rogers, B.; Beresford, J.; Martinez, F.J.; Richardson, C.; Han, M.K. Internet Access and Use by COPD Patients in the National Emphysema/COPD Association Survey. *BMC Pulm. Med.* **2014**, *14*, 66. [CrossRef]
33. Preece, J. Sociability and Usability in Online Communities: Determining and Measuring Success. *Behav. Inf. Technol.* **2001**, *20*, 347–356. [CrossRef]
34. Charmaz, K. Stories of Suffering: Subjective Tales and Research Narratives. *Qual. Health Res.* **1999**, *9*, 362–382. [CrossRef]
35. Yanos, P.T.; Roe, D.; Lysaker, P.H. The Impact of Illness Identity on Recovery from Severe Mental Illness. *Am. J. Psychiatr. Rehabil.* **2010**, *13*, 73–93. [CrossRef]
36. Centers for Disease Control and Prevention. Tips From Former Smokers® Campaign. Available online: https://www.cdc.gov/tobacco/campaign/tips/index.html (accessed on 6 April 2019).
37. Pederson, A.P.; Hoyak, K.A.K.; Mills, S.; Camp, P.G. Reflecting the Changing Face of Chronic Obstructive Pulmonary Disease: Sex and Gender in Public Education Materials on COPD. *Proc. Am. Thorac. Soc.* **2007**, *4*, 683–685. [CrossRef] [PubMed]
38. Stellefson, M.; Paige, S.R.; Alber, J.M.; Stewart, M. COPD360social Online Community: A Social Media Review. *Health Promot. Pract.* **2018**, *19*, 489–491. [CrossRef] [PubMed]

39. Apperson, A.; Stellefson, M.; Paige, S.R.; Chaney, B.H.; Chaney, J.D.; Wang, M.Q.; Mohan, A. Facebook Groups on Chronic Obstructive Pulmonary Disease: Social Media Content Analysis. *Int. J. Environ. Res. Public Health* **2019**, *16*, 3789. [CrossRef] [PubMed]
40. Proshansky, H.M.; Fabian, A.K.; Kaminoff, R. Place-Identity: Physical World Socialization of the Self. *J. Environ. Psychol.* **1983**, *3*, 57–83. [CrossRef]
41. Rakauskas, M.E.; Ward, N.J.; Gerberich, S.G. Identification of Differences between Rural and Urban Safety Cultures. *Accid. Anal. Prev.* **2009**, *41*, 931–937. [CrossRef]
42. Slama, K. Rural Culture Is a Diversity Issue. *Minn. Psychol.* **2004**, *53*, 9–12.
43. Parker, K.; Horowitz, J.M.; Brown, A.; Fry, R.; Cohn, D.; Igielnik, R. *Similarities and Differences between Urban, Suburban and Rural Communities in America*; Pew Research Center: Washington, DC, USA, 2018; Available online: https://www.pewsocialtrends.org/2018/05/22/what-unites-and-divides-urban-suburban-and-rural-communities/ (accessed on 28 December 2019).
44. Raju, S.; Keet, C.A.; Matsui, E.C.; Drummond, M.B.; Hansel, N.N.; Wise, R.A.; Peng, R.D.; McCormack, M.C. The Impact of Poverty and Rural Residence on Chronic Obstructive Pulmonary Disease (COPD) Prevalence: A Nationwide Analysis. In *C15. Novel Epidemiology of Asthma and Copd (American Thoracic Society International Conference Abstracts)*; American Thoracic Society: Denver, CO, USA, 2015; p. A3904. [CrossRef]
45. Centers for Disease Control and Prevention. BRFSS Survey Data and Documentation. Available online: https://www.cdc.gov/brfss/annual_data/annual_2017.html (accessed on 11 March 2019).
46. Oris, L.; Luyckx, K.; Rassart, J.; Goubert, L.; Goossens, E.; Apers, S.; Arat, S.; Vandenberghe, J.; Westhovens, R.; Moons, P. Illness Identity in Adults with a Chronic Illness. *J. Clin. Psychol. Med. Settings* **2018**, *25*, 429–440. [CrossRef]
47. Maples, P.; Franks, A.; Ray, S.; Stevens, A.B.; Wallace, L.S. Development and Validation of a Low-Literacy Chronic Obstructive Pulmonary Disease Knowledge Questionnaire (COPD-Q). *Patient Educ. Couns.* **2010**, *81*, 19–22. [CrossRef]
48. *The Benefits of Quitting Smoking Over Time*; American Cancer Society: New York, NY, USA, 2018; Available online: https://www.cancer.org/healthy/stay-away-from-tobacco/benefits-of-quitting-smoking-over-time.html (accessed on 22 December 2019).
49. *Final Recommendation Statement: Lung Cancer Screening*; US Preventive Services Task Force: Rockville, MD, USA, 2013; Available online: https://www.uspreventiveservicestaskforce.org/Page/Document/RecommendationStatementFinal/lung-cancer-screening (accessed on 22 December 2019).
50. Cohen, J.; Cohen, P.; West, S.; Aiken, L. *Applied Multiple Regression/Correlation Analysis for Behavioral Sciences*, 3rd ed.; Routledge; Taylor & Francis Group: New York, NY, USA, 2003.
51. Sinclair, C. Effectiveness and User Acceptance of Online Chronic Disease Management Interventions in Rural and Remote Settings: Systematic Review and Narrative Synthesis. *Clin. Med. Insights Ther.* **2015**, *7*. [CrossRef]

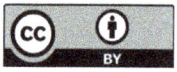

© 2019 by the authors. Licensee MDPI, Basel, Switzerland. This article is an open access article distributed under the terms and conditions of the Creative Commons Attribution (CC BY) license (http://creativecommons.org/licenses/by/4.0/).

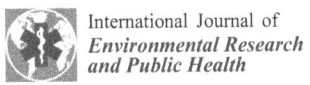

Article

Cultural Differences in Tweeting about Drinking Across the US

Salvatore Giorgi [1,2], David B. Yaden [3], Johannes C. Eichstaedt [4], Robert D. Ashford [5], Anneke E.K. Buffone [3], H. Andrew Schwartz [6], Lyle H. Ungar [1] and Brenda Curtis [2,*]

1. Computer and Information Science Department, University of Pennsylvania, Philadelphia, PA 19104, USA; sgiorgi@sas.upenn.edu (S.G.); ungar@cis.upenn.edu (L.H.U.)
2. National Institutes of Health, National Institute on Drug Abuse, Bethesda, MD 20892, USA
3. Department of Psychology, University of Pennsylvania, Philadelphia, PA 19104, USA; dyaden@sas.upenn.edu (D.B.Y.); buffone.anneke@gmail.com (A.E.K.B.)
4. Department of Psychology & Institute for Human-Centered Artificial Intelligence, Stanford University, Stanford, CA 94305, USA; johannes@jeichstaedt.com
5. Substance Use Disorders Institute, University of the Sciences, Philadelphia, PA 19104, USA; rashford@mail.usciences.edu
6. Department of Computer Science, Stony Brook University, Stony Brook, NY 11794, USA; has@cs.stonybrook.edu
* Correspondence: brenda.curtis@nih.gov

Received: 1 January 2020; Accepted: 8 February 2020; Published: 11 February 2020

Abstract: Excessive alcohol use in the US contributes to over 88,000 deaths per year and costs over $250 billion annually. While previous studies have shown that excessive alcohol use can be detected from general patterns of social media engagement, we characterized how drinking-specific language varies across regions and cultures in the US. From a database of 38 billion public tweets, we selected those mentioning "drunk", found the words and phrases distinctive of drinking posts, and then clustered these into topics and sets of semantically related words. We identified geolocated "drunk" tweets and correlated their language with the prevalence of self-reported excessive alcohol consumption (Behavioral Risk Factor Surveillance System; BRFSS). We then identified linguistic markers associated with excessive drinking in different regions and cultural communities as identified by the American Community Project. "Drunk" tweet frequency (of the 3.3 million geolocated "drunk" tweets) correlated with excessive alcohol consumption at both the county and state levels ($r = 0.26$ and 0.45, respectively, $p < 0.01$). Topic analyses revealed that excessive alcohol consumption was most correlated with references to drinking with friends ($r = 0.20$), family ($r = 0.15$), and driving under the influence ($r = 0.14$). Using the American Community Project classification, we found a number of cultural markers of drinking: religious communities had a high frequency of anti-drunk driving tweets, Hispanic centers discussed family members drinking, and college towns discussed sexual behavior. This study shows that Twitter can be used to explore the specific sociocultural contexts in which excessive alcohol use occurs within particular regions and communities. These findings can inform more targeted public health messaging and help to better understand cultural determinants of substance abuse.

Keywords: excessive drinking; social media; Twitter; natural language processing; American Communities Project

---

1. Introduction

Excessive alcohol consumption, including binge and heavy drinking, is responsible for approximately 88,000 deaths per year in the US, making it the third leading preventable cause of death and a major public health concern [1–3]. Binge drinking, generally defined as having five or more drinks for males and having four or more drinks for females in about 2 hours [4], was reported by 26.4% of people ages 18 or older in 2017 [5]. Binge drinking is associated with adverse health effects such as unintentional injuries (e.g., falls, motor vehicle crashes), alcohol poisoning, interpersonal violence (e.g., homicide, assaults, domestic violence), risky sexual behaviors, and suicide [6]. Additionally, excessive alcohol consumption in the US costs over $250 billion annually, due to the loss in workplace productivity, health care expenses, law enforcement expenses, and motor vehicle crashes [1]. The individual, societal, and economic costs associated with binge drinking has led to repeated calls to monitor alcohol use and its associated adverse health effects as well as to implement public health interventions that reduce alcohol-attributed risks.

A key element of public health alcohol interventions is the monitoring of binge and heavy drinking [7,8]. Traditionally, monitoring involves large surveys (such as the Centers for Disease Control and Prevention's Behavioral Risk Factor Surveillance System; BRFSS) which track trends over time and across specific populations such as metropolitan statistical areas. However, such expensive survey efforts with a limited number of questions cannot shed light on the different cultural practices that lead to excessive drinking, even though such information is necessary to target public health media campaigns [9–11]. Specifically, given the variability in alcohol consumption and associated risks across the United States, it is important to have a granular appreciation for the ways in which different populations within the US engage in excessive alcohol use. Effectively targeted public health communication involves delivering different messages based on predetermined segmentations (e.g., demographic and socioeconomic characteristics), yielding tailored communication which is more likely to persuade individuals [12].

Social media analysis provides an untapped resource for monitoring alcohol consumption at the population level. Social media provides autobiographical language expressing thoughts, emotions, and behaviors, and with the application of machine learning models to such language data, individual psychometric assessments (such as estimates of personality [13]) can be derived. Social media data provide real-time and cost-efficient monitoring of large fractions of populations which in principle can extend across a rich variety of psychological characteristics [14–16]. This data source could provide prevention program planners with the ability to gather information that can be used to tailor public health messaging.

Popular social media platforms in the United States include Facebook, Twitter, Instagram, and Snapchat. Twitter is a free social media platform that allows users to send and receive "tweets" (i.e., short messages limited to 280 characters). As of the last quarter in 2017, Twitter averaged 330 million monthly active users, creating an estimated 500 million tweets per day [17]. Given the widespread use and activity on Twitter as well as the availability of public content at the user level, it has been used in multiple health surveillance studies. For example, Twitter data have been used to track influenza symptoms, estimate alcohol sales volume, and measure depression, HIV prevalence, and heart disease mortality [18–23].

Twitter language data have been used to predict alcohol consumption rates at the county level [24]. Curtis et al. [24] used natural language analysis to associate Twitter language content to rates of alcohol consumption at the county level. Findings revealed that Twitter language data captured cross-sectional patterns of excessive alcohol consumption beyond that of sociodemographic factors (e.g., age, gender, race, income, education). Twitter data have also been used to examine drinking themes and sentiment, showing that drinking tweets contained positive sentiment and as well as themes of wanting, needing, and planning [25]. Social media platforms are also sources of information about substance use patterns in particular sub-populations. For example, the results of a meta-analysis that examined the relationship between young adults' alcohol-related social media engagement and their drinking behavior revealed a relationship between alcohol-related social media engagement and alcohol-related problems [14].

In this study, we examined the feasibility of using Twitter to monitor binge drinking with a focus on regional and cultural differences. Specifically, we addressed the following questions: (1) Do Twitter messages expressing language indicative of excessive alcohol use correlate with county-level alcohol consumption rates? (2) What are the contents of these binge drinking-related tweets? (3) What insights can we gain from examining the regional and cultural variations in the language of these tweets? Finally, (4) can linguistic features, such as pronoun use and valence, help to characterize drunk content within communities? Our aim was to examine the efficacy of social media language analysis as an emerging tool for public health monitoring and intervention.

2. Materials and Methods

2.1. Data

2.1.1. Excessive Alcohol Consumption Data

The BRFSS is a population-based cross-sectional phone health survey of US adults aged ≥ 18 years conducted by state health departments with funding and technical assistance provided by the Centers for Disease Control and Prevention. From the BRFSS (2006–2012), we obtained the prevalence of self-reported binge drinking and heavy drinking (for which county-level estimates had previously been derived; $N = 2192$; [7]). Excessive alcohol consumption was defined as having more than two drinks per day on average (for men) or more than one drink per day on average (for women) or having five or more drinks during a single occasion (for men) or four or more drinks during a single occasion (for women).

2.1.2. Drinking Keyword Filtering

In order to identify tweets related to excessive drinking, we started with 46 drinking-related, unambiguous keywords, such as "hangover", "tailgate", "vodka", and "wasted", introduced in Cavazos-Rehg et al. [25] in addition to our initial keyword "drunk" for a total of 47 keywords (see the full list of keywords in Appendix A, Table A1). These keywords were introduced by Cavazos-Rehg et al. [25] in order to study general drinking-related discussions on Twitter, in terms of sentiment, theme, and source. Since the keywords were used to identify general patterns of drinking, we also used them to identify drinking-related tweets in order to build our "drunk tweet" data set. From our larger Twitter data set (described below), we collected a random sample of roughly 153,000 tweets containing at least one least one of the 47 keywords. Next, for each tweet we created 47 binary indicators for each of our keywords (1 if the tweet contained the keyword, 0 otherwise) and correlated all pairs of binary indicators to identify keyword patterns in the drunk tweets. The results showed that most drinking keywords were relatively rare and did not correlate with other keywords, including "drunk". The three most common words "sober" ($N = 4120$), "bar" ($N = 2218$), and "ale" ($N = 2124$). Additionally, most keywords did not co-occur within the same tweet. Therefore, we chose to limit our data set to tweets which contained the word "drunk", to focus on tweets describing the act of drinking itself, rather than its effects (e.g., "hungover" and "hangover").

2.1.3. Twitter Data

A random 10% of Twitter data were collected between June 23, 2009 to April 17, 2014, augmented with a 1% sample from April 17, 2014 to February 5, 2015 [26,27]. This resulted in approximately 37.6 billion tweets. The Tweets were then filtered so that the word "drunk" appeared in the tweet (we removed any tweets that contained the phrase "drunk in love" due to the popular song title). This resulted in a set of roughly 24.9 million tweets. All non-English tweets were removed using the Python package langid [28]. After language filtering, 19.3 million tweets remained which were then mapped to US counties. Using the geolocation methods described in Reference [29], we used self-reported location information in user profiles and latitude/longitude coordinates attached to tweets to map tweets to US counties and county equivalents (henceforth "counties"). This resulted in 3.3 million "drunk tweets" spread over 3095 counties. Finally, we limited our analysis to counties with at least 1000 words within the drunk tweets, for a total of $N = 1573$ counties in our final data set. Summary results are given in Figure 1a and a US map of drunk tweet frequency in Figure 1b.

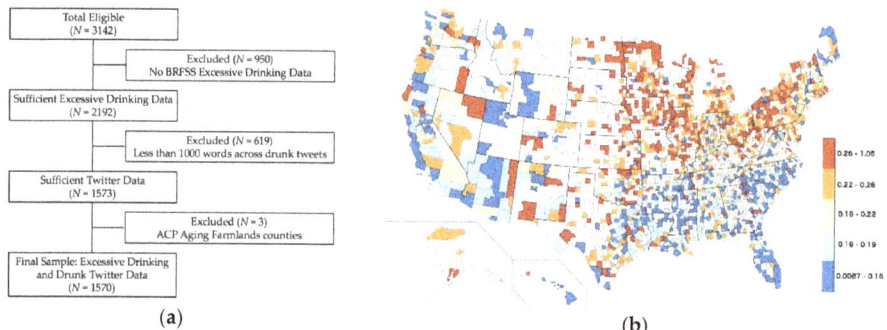

Figure 1. Data description: (**a**) inclusion criteria for this study; (**b**) map of drunk tweet frequency (quintiles, red = high; blue = low).

2.1.4. American Communities Project

In addition to county- and state-level analyses, we also looked at 15 community types identified by the American Communities Project (ACP) [30]. The ACP is a county-level clustering based on 36 demographic, socio-economic, and cultural indicators including population density, income, race, and religious affiliation and developed by George Washington University's School of Media and Public Affairs. Sample communities include Big Cities, College Towns, Hispanic Centers, and Rural Middle America. Note that this county clustering does not depend on spatial proximity, for example, the Big Cities cluster contains counties across the US which contain large metropolitan areas such as Los Angeles and Philadelphia. We argue that this clustering scheme gives more culturally coherent interpretation to expressions of drinking on social media than either counties or states. Additionally, restricting the analysis to a small number of distinct community types allows for the possibility of public health officials developing more culturally tailored messaging and interventions than if our analyses were restricted to states (which are often socio-demographically heterogeneous) or counties (for which there are over 3000 units). We limited our analysis to ACP communities for which at least 25% of the counties met our 1000 "drunk" word threshold. This resulted in 14 ACP communities across $N = 1570$ counties (with Aging Farmlands dropped due to the fact insufficient data).

2.2. Topic Modeling

The set of English-filtered "drunk" tweets (19.3 million) were used to create a set of 100 "drunk" topics using latent Dirichlet allocation (LDA) [31]. To create the drunk topics, we (1) tokenized each tweet (i.e., broke up each tweet into words and word phrases), (2) identified those words and phrases most associated with drunk tweets, (3) filtered the tweets to only contain the most discriminative words (i.e., removed words not significantly associated with drunk tweets), and (4) ran the LDA algorithm over the full set of filtered drunk tweets. Each step is described in detail below.

In their natural form, tweets exist as strings of text which need to be broken up into words whose frequency can be recorded. Early versions of this process ("tokenizing") used white spaces to split a sentence into words, but we used a more modern version designed to handle social media language data (which may include, for example, ":)!" to be broken up into ":)" and "!") [32]. This allowed us to describe the frequency of every word in a tweet as the fraction of the total number of words ("tokens") in that tweet (i.e., Step 1 in the preceding paragraph). We also encoded if a word was used at all in a given tweet (as a "binary" feature: 1 if a token is present in the message, 0 if otherwise). We further recorded the relative frequency of phrases (such as "happy birthday") which we detected by observing them to be more frequently co-occurring words than chance would suggest based on the frequency of "happy" and "birthday".

In Step 2, we found the words and word phrases associated with "drunk" tweets. We randomly sampled 1 million random tweets from our "drunk" set and gathered 1 million random "non-drunk" messages (i.e., messages without the word "drunk") from roughly the same time span. We then calculated a weighted log odds ratio, using an informative Dirichlet prior to estimate the difference in frequency of a word across two corpora (i.e., drunk tweets and non-drunk tweets) [33,34]. This method uses the z score of the log odds ratio in order to control the variance of a given word's frequency, while the prior shrinks the word frequency towards known frequencies from a large background corpus.

In the third step, we filtered each of the 19.3 million drunk messages to only contain 5000 tokens most associated with "drunk" tweets (i.e., any word *not* within the top 5000 significantly correlated tokens was removed from the tweet). Using these 19.3 million filtered messages, we created 100 topics using LDA. The LDA topics were estimated using Gibbs sampling [35] with the MALLET software package [36]. For an extended description of this process, see Schwartz et al. [13].

Finally, in Step 4, we calculated county-level topic loadings for each of the 100 drunk topics using:

$$P(topic|county) = \sum_{\{token \in topic\}} P(topic|token) \times P(token|county). \tag{1}$$

Here $P(topic|token)$, the probability of a topic given a token, was derived via the LDA process and $P(token|county)$ was estimated using the relative frequency of the token in the county. These topic frequencies were then used as independent variables in the statistical analysis.

2.3. Statistical Methods

2.3.1. Drunk Tweeting and Excessive Drinking

We first explored the relationship between Twitter language data identified as "drunk tweets" and excessive drinking by correlating the frequency of drunk tweets (i.e., the number of drunk tweets divided by the total number of tweets within a county) with the BRFSS measure of excessive drinking. We did this at the county, state, and ACP levels (both the state and ACP level variables were calculated as county-level averages).

2.3.2. Differential Language Analysis

We use differential language analysis (DLA) to identify (1) language characterizing counties higher and lower in excessive drinking and (2) drunk language most associated with individual ACP communities [13]. For the former (1), we individually regressed (via a least squares linear regression) each language feature (i.e., county-level topic frequencies for each of the 100 drunk topics) against the BRFSS excessive drinking measure. For the latter (2), we attempted to identify regional trends in drunk tweets by identifying topics most associated with each ACP community. To do this, we created a county-level dummy outcome for each of the 14 ACP communities in our sample (1 if the county is in the ACP community, 0 if otherwise). We considered the association of all 100 drunk topics with all 14 ACP communities using Cohen's d which quantifies the differences in means among subsamples of counties in units of pooled standard deviations. Additionally, for each topic we computed the *p*-value associated with its coefficient in a logistic regression. For both (1) and (2), we applied a Benjamini–Hochberg correction to the significance threshold ($p < 0.05$) of the false discovery rate for multiple comparisons [37].

2.3.3. Self versus Other Drinking

We looked at references to self and other drinking in our drunk tweets. For each county, we calculated the relative frequency of the word "I" (self) in our drunk tweets as well the frequency of "he", "she", and "they" (other). We then standardized (i.e., mean centered and normalized) both the "self" and "other" scores.

2.3.4. Sentiment

Finally, we examined the relationship between sentiment and personal pronouns. To measure personal pronoun use, we used the "personal pronoun" dictionary in the Linguistic Inquiry Word Count (LIWC) which contains 93 distinct pronouns [38]. This method simply counts the number of occurrences of each pronoun within each ACP community. To measure positive sentiment, we used the National Resource Council (NRC) Hashtag Sentiment Lexicon which is designed to estimate tweet sentiment in a robust fashion [39]. This lexicon differs from LIWC, in that each word in the lexica contains a weight and thus gives us a weighted sum of all positive sentiment words occurring in each ACP community.

3. Results

3.1. Community Correlations with Excessive Drinking

The frequency with which people tweet the word "drunk" (as a percentage of all tweets) is moderately correlated with excess drinking at both the county (Pearson's $r = 0.26$) and state (Pearson's $r = 0.45$) level as shown in Table 1. Across the 14 categories of counties determined by the American Communities Project (ACP), we observed a relationship between excessive drinking rates and drunk tweet frequency with trending significance (Pearson's $r = 0.55$, $p = 0.053$), seen in the linear relationship in Figure 2. Based on the ACP classification, on the one hand, we observed that areas with stronger religious identification (LDS Enclaves (Latter-Day Saints; Mormon) and Evangelical Hubs) as well as the African American South were both lowest in excessive drinking and drunk tweeting.

Table 1. Correlations between drunk tweet frequency and excess drinking at the county, state, and American Communities Project levels. Reported Pearson's r with 95% confidence intervals in square brackets.

Spatial Unit	N	Correlation with Excessive Drinking
County	1573	0.26 [0.21, 0.31] ($p < 0.001$)
State	46	0.45 [0.18, 0.72] ($p = 0.002$)
American Communities Project (ACP)	14	0.55 [−0.007, 1.103] ($p = 0.053$)

On the other hand, we observed that College Towns were near the top in excessive drinking and were distinguished from all other categories of communities by the extent to which they tweet about drinking. After College Towns, Rural Middle America and Middle Suburbs tweeted the most about drinking. These two communities are predominantly white (91% in Rural Middle America and 85% in Middle Suburbs) and low income.

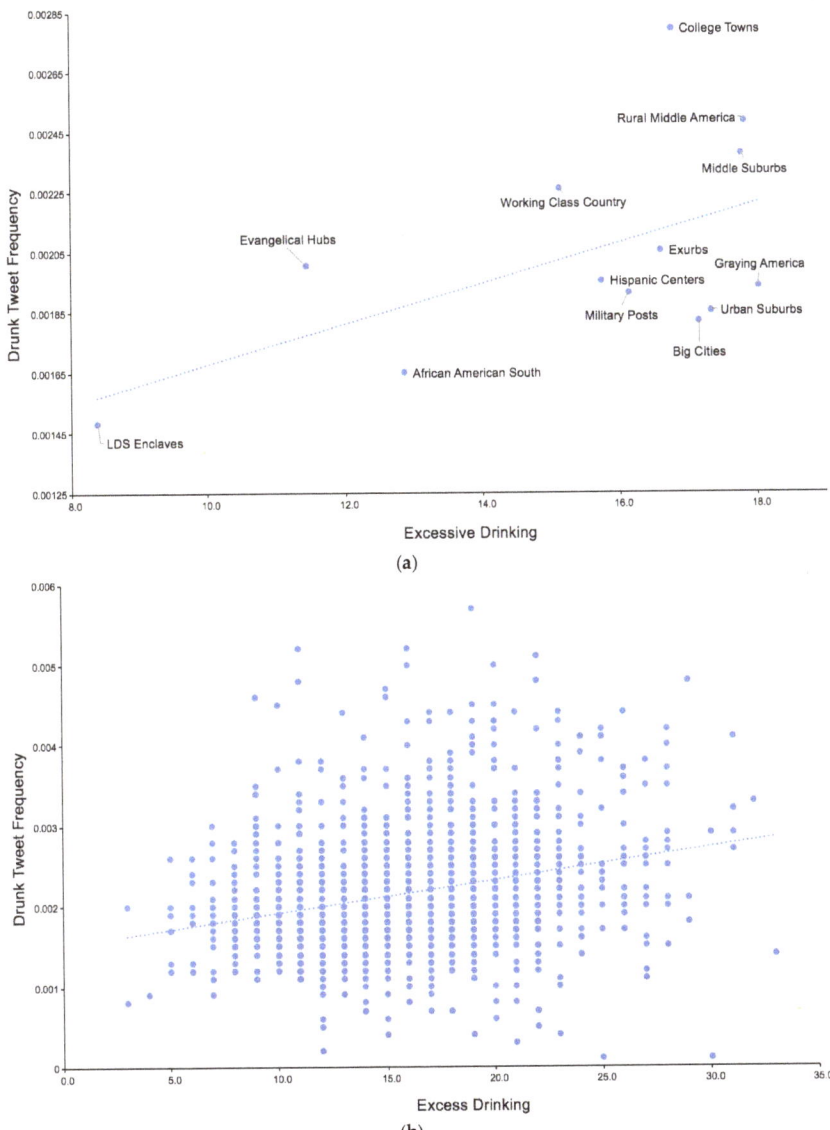

Figure 2. Frequency of drinking tweets versus excessive drinking levels: (**a**) ACP classification (county averages) and (**b**) county level.

3.2. Differential Language Analysis

Figure 3 shows the drunk topics most associated with high levels of excessive drinking at the county level. These topics include a number of hashtags related to drinking and partying with friends ("#fun", "#shots", "#lastnight", "#drunksanta"), two topics related to drinking with family ("my cousins", "my mom", "my aunts", "with my dad", "my brother") as well as a DUI-related topic ("got pulled" arrested", "pleads") and a topic mentioning falling both asleep and down the stairs.

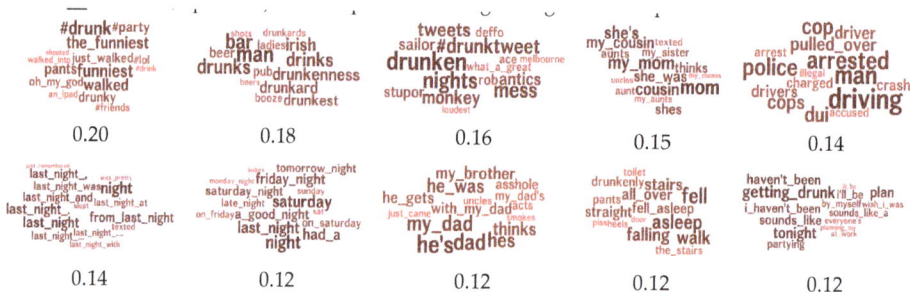

Figure 3. Drunk topics most positively correlated with county-level excess drinking. Reported Pearson's r, $p < 0.05$ after Benjamini–Hochberg correction.

In terms of the ACP, Figure 4 presents the topics associated with four ACP communities: (a) African American South, (b) College Towns, (c) Hispanic Centers, and (d) Evangelical Hubs. These particular communities and topics were selected from the top five most correlated topics (i.e., highest Cohen's d). These communities and topics provide insight into the kind of social contexts in which drinking is discussed.

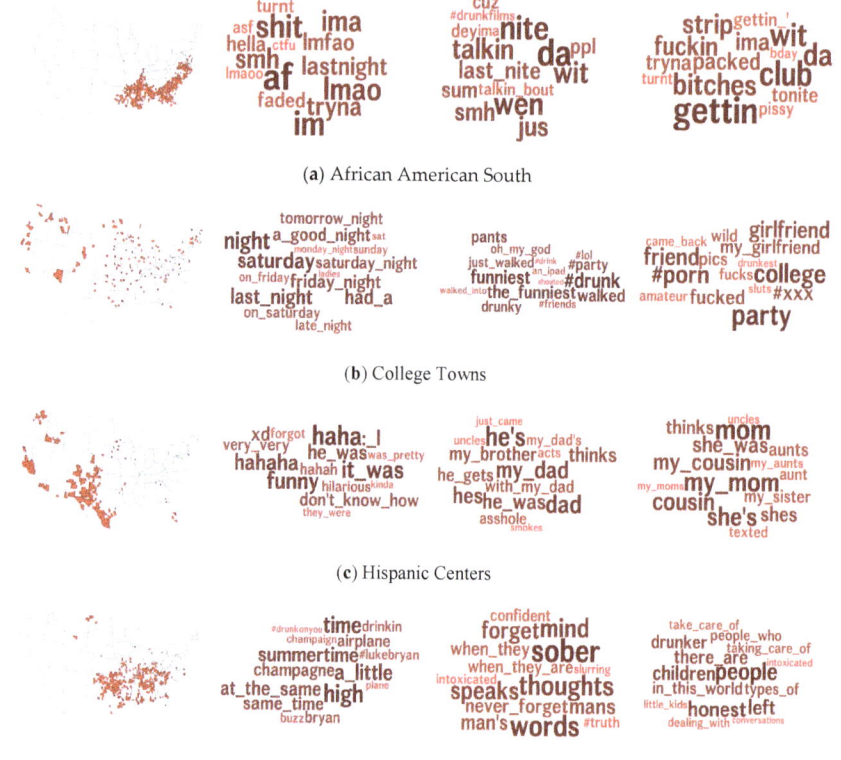

Figure 4. Maps and drunk topics most associated with four ACP communities: (a) African American South, (b) College Towns, (c) Hispanic Centers, and (d) Evangelical Hubs. Left most plots indicate the counties (red) within each ACP community.

African American communities, besides showing higher use of African American English ("tryna", "da", "ima"), also mentioned (night) clubs [40]. College Towns discussed drinking on the weekends ("friday night", "Saturday", "a good night") and drinking humor ("the funniest", "drunky", "oh my god") as well as sex-related topics ("pics", "#porn", "party", "fucks"). In Hispanic centers, the social context of drinking was often foregrounded ("my dad", "my mom", "my cousin"). Evangelical Hubs used particular terms to reference drinking ("buzz", "drinkin", "high") but also to reference sobriety ("sober", "intoxicated", "never forget") and responsibility ("take care of", "dealing with", "little kids").

3.3. Self versus Other Drinking

Tweeting about drinking may both reference one's own behaviors ("I am drunk and fell asleep") as opposed to references to others' behaviors ("He was drunk and fell down the stairs"). To differentiate these kinds of references, we compared mentions of the word "I" (self; first person) against mentions of "he", "she" and "they" (other; third person) among drinking-related tweets in Table 2. LDS Enclaves, Rural Middle America, and College Towns all have an overall pattern of impersonal tweeting about drinking (using fewer pronouns both about the self and others). The African American South marks the contrary case, where tweeting about drinking was personal with higher reference to both self and other drinking.

Table 2. Standardized (z scored) relative frequency of "I" and "he/she/they" within drunk tweets.

	Self	Other
Hispanic Centers	1.90	0.18
African American South	1.53	2.55
Middle Suburbs	1.00	0.18
Military Posts	0.97	0.38
Urban Suburbs	0.73	0.18
Big Cities	0.31	0.77
Native American Lands	−0.59	0.38
LDS Enclaves	−0.61	−1.20
Graying America	−0.69	0.58
Rural Middle America	−0.74	−1.59
College Towns	−0.75	−1.20
Exurbs	−0.81	−0.41
Evangelical Hubs	−0.97	−0.01
Working Class Country	−1.26	−0.80

3.4. Sentiment

How does the personal/impersonal nature about tweeting relate to the way drinking is perceived across types of communities? Figure 5 shows how the personal nature of tweeting about drinking (measured as the relative frequency of personal pronouns) relates to the sentiment of the tweets. We generally observed that positive tweets about drinking tend to be more impersonal and thus may reference general practices or cultural norms more so than experiences of oneself or others; this was particularly true in College Towns. Inversely, tweets containing personal pronouns tended to be more negative in valence with Hispanic Centers sharing by far the most personal content.

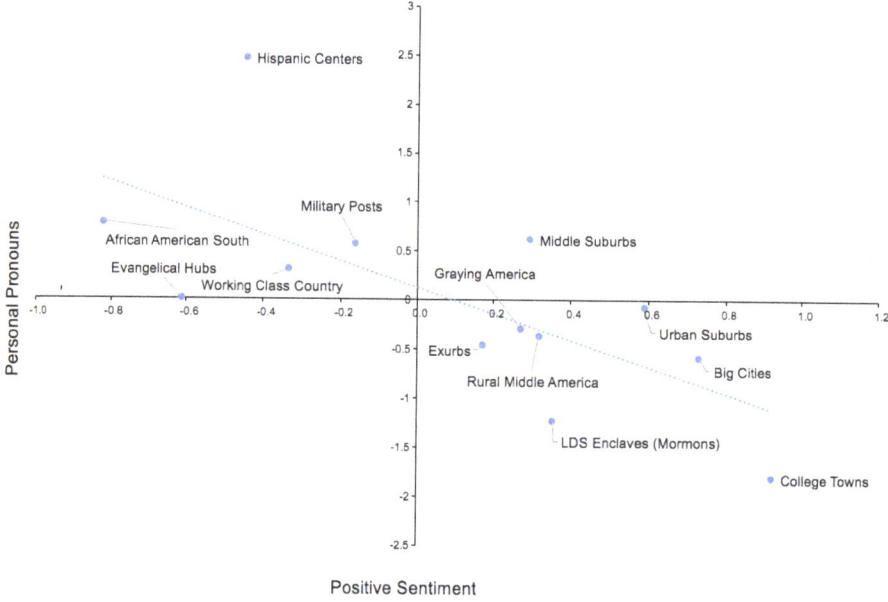

Figure 5. Scatter plot of personal (versus impersonal) tweeting against positive sentiment across the 14 ACP community types. Sentiment is based on the NRC positive sentiment model. Both dimensions were standardized.

4. Discussion

In this study, we found that Twitter can be used as a lens into regional and community context around excessive alcohol use. Communities differed both in *how much* they tweet about drinking and *how* they tweet about drinking. This suggests that Twitter can be used to estimate trends in health behaviors across counties and that a similar methodology can be applied to comorbid conditions such as substance use, depression, and anxiety. In light of our research questions, *how much* addresses our first question: do Twitter messages expressing language indicative of excessive alcohol use correlate with county-level alcohol consumption rates. The *how* addresses the remaining three questions: What are the contents of binge drinking-related tweets? Can pronoun use and valence help characterize drunk tweet content? Finally, what insights can we gain from examining the regional and cultural variations in the language of these tweets?

First, we answer our initial research question in the affirmative: we found that the frequency of "drunk tweeting" accurately captured the trend in the rates of excessive drinking captured by phone surveys administered by the CDC. This finding dovetails with previous studies that showed that simple keyword searches on Twitter predict county-level outcomes (i.e., flu keywords predict influenza-like illness statistics and "drunk" predicts alcohol sales) [18]. This finding underscores the promise for social media platforms to be used as a public health tool for monitoring health-related behaviors. Additionally, the results suggest that religious communities are both the least likely to drink excessively and Tweet about drinking, while university and white, low-income communities see the most tweeting about drinking. The LDS Enclaves finding in particular provides a methods check, as the Mormon religion does not permit drinking, so it should be—and is—at the bottom of this ranking.

Second, in regard to *how* communities Tweet about drinking, we found two main dimensions of distinction addressing our research questions on the content of drunk-related tweets and how this content varies regionally and culturally. Topic analyses revealed that drinking may get discussed either in the form of celebratory endorsements of the cultural practice of drinking (e.g., in College Towns) or in a cautionary manner (e.g., by Mormon communities). Communities also differed in how much discussions around drinking take the form of *personal* behaviors (of both oneself and others) versus how much they are referenced *impersonally* as cultural practices. Between these two dimensions, we found a trend suggesting that disclosures with personal pronouns tended to be more negative, and more impersonal references to cultural norms and practices tended to be more positive. This was mostly the case in College Towns. This suggests that drinking may be perceived positively as a shared practice and negatively "when it happened to me last night". While the interpretation of these differences of language use around drinking requires additional research to confirm, they represent interesting and potentially important avenues to explore the relevance to public health intervention and messaging to these communities. For example, changing the view of drinking as a social practice towards the negative may prove fruitful, perhaps akin to the successful messaging around smoking which made a "cool" practice a distasteful one.

There are also suggestions of strong regional differences in mentions of family (e.g., aunts, cousins, and parents) with Hispanic Centers having a number of significant family-related topics. We note that Hispanic Centers were highest in self-drinking and, therefore, these communities were talking about both family drinking and self-drinking.

A notable standout in terms of communities was College Towns, which tweeted about drinking at a much higher frequency than the excessive drinking rate would suggest. We suspect this reflects a younger and more social media friendly population than most of the other ACP communities. Sexual themes were also associated with College Towns. We note that both porn (#xxx, #porn, sluts) and significant others (my girlfriend, friend) were contained within the same topic. Previous studies have found both substance abuse and pornography consumption as risk factors for male sexual aggression on college campuses [41].

Using publicly available Twitter data as a surveillance system has been used across a number of health-related outcomes including excessive drinking [24]. A similar surveillance study examined hashtags co-occurring in tweets mentioning e-cigarettes while also looking at rates of tobacco-related tweets across the US. [42]. This study contextualized e-cigarette tweets in terms of both co-occurring hashtags and across *spatially* connected regions (i.e., Mid-Atlantic, Southwest, and the West Coast). The present study differs in that drunk tweets were contextualized across *culturally* connected regions, namely, the American Communities Project classification—counties grouped via socio-demographic measures as opposed to groups of adjacent counties.

This study was limited in several ways. These analyses were conducted using aggregated Twitter data and regional drinking figures drawn from large-scale surveys conducted by the CDC. These findings should be replicated using individual-level data with linked self-reports and language. Similar studies have shown associations between self-reported behavior and tweet content. In particular, Unger et al. [43] showed that posting positive tweets about tobacco had a significant association with tobacco use within the past month.

There is also the potential for a selection bias. It may be that only certain types of people tweet about being drunk. However, people do tweet a lot about smoking marijuana, even when and where it is illegal [44]. It may be that there are fewer social taboos on Twitter in regard to discussing substance use than in "polite conversation" thus allowing users a relative sense of freedom to post what they wish. Here again, individual-level data with self-reported drinking behavior and personal language will help to determine whether this is an issue.

Twitter bots can be a source of noise as well as false behaviors and attitudes. Previous studies on social media and e-cigarettes have shown that bots are more likely to reference new e-cigarette products than human Twitter users [40]. One can imagine similar patterns in drinking-related tweets—bots might be more likely to tweet about a new alcoholic beverage or drinking-related social event. Thus, future studies should examine similar relationships between social media bots and mentions of alcohol consumption.

The words, phrases, and linguistic themes that emerge from natural language processing are predictive of outcomes of interest, yet care must be taken when interpreting the results, and for final validity, they should be tested in confirmatory studies that test the identified associations as hypotheses.

5. Conclusions

Excessive alcohol use was reflected and detectable in patterns of social media language. Regions and communities differed both in terms of the quantity and content of social media posts about drinking. We found that tweets about being drunk were predictive of different "styles" of excessive drinking behavior across types of communities derived from demographic and socio-economic indicators in the American Communities Project. The particular words, phrases, and linguistic themes most associated with particular regions and communities can provide insight into sociocultural alcohol use contexts and may help to shape more personalized public health messages and interventions to these populations.

Author Contributions: Conceptualization, B.C., J.C.E. and L.H.U.; methodology, B.C., S.G., H.A.S. and L.H.U.; software, S.G and H.A.S.; formal analysis, S.G.; data curation, S.G.; writing—original draft preparation, R.D.A., B.C., J.C.E., S.G. and D.B.Y.; writing—review and editing, A.E.K.B., J.C.E., S.G., H.A.S., L.H.U. and D.B.Y.; visualization, J.C.E. and S.G.; supervision, B.C., H.A.S., and L.H.U.; funding acquisition, B.C. and L.H.U. All authors have read and agreed to the published version of the manuscript.

Funding: This research was supported in part by the Intramural Research Program of the NIH, National Institute on Drug Abuse (NIDA), NIDA grant R01DA039457, and the Templeton Research Trust.

Conflicts of Interest: The authors declare no conflict of interest.

Appendix A

In Table A1 we list all of our drinking keywords.

Table A1. Full list of drinking keywords.

alcohol	bottle	hangover	pub
alcoholics	bottles	happy hour	shot(s)
alcoholism	brewery	hungover	sober
ale	champagne	lager	tailgate
bar	ciroc	liquor	tailgating
beer	cocktail	lounge	tequila
beer goggles	cocktails	margarita(s)	tipsy
beers	drank	pint	vodka
booze	drink	pints	wasted
boozey	drinking	pregame	whiskey
boozy	gin	pregaming	wine

References

1. Centers for Disease Control and Prevention (CDC). *Alcohol-Related Disease Impact (ARDI)*; CDC: Atlanta, GA, USA, 2008.
2. Mokdad, A.H.; Marks, J.S.; Stroup, D.F.; Gerberding, J.L. Actual causes of death in the United States, 2000. *JAMA* **2004**, *291*, 1238–1245. [CrossRef] [PubMed]
3. Stahre, M.; Roeber, J.; Kanny, D.; Brewer, R.D.; Zhang, X. Contribution of excessive alcohol consumption to deaths and years of potential life lost in the United States. *Prev. Chronic Dis.* **2014**, *11*, E109. [CrossRef] [PubMed]
4. Drinking Levels Defined. Available online: https://www.niaaa.nih.gov/alcohol-health/overview-alcohol-consumption/moderate-binge-drinking (accessed on 20 December 2019).
5. Alcohol Facts and Statistics. Available online: https://www.niaaa.nih.gov/publications/brochures-and-fact-sheets/alcohol-facts-and-statistics (accessed on 20 December 2019).
6. White, A.; Hingson, R. The burden of alcohol use: Excessive alcohol consumption and related consequences among college students. *Alcohol Res. Curr. Rev.* **2013**, *35*. [CrossRef]

7. Xu, F.; Mawokomatanda, T.; Flegel, D.; Pierannunzi, C.; Garvin, W.; Chowdhury, P.; Salandy, S.; Crawford, C.; Town, M. Surveillance for certain health behaviors among states and selected local areas—Behavioral Risk Factor Surveillance System, United States, 2011. *Morb. Mortal. Wkly. Rep. Surveill. Summ.* **2014**, *63*, 1–149.
8. Lyerla, R.; Stroup, D.F. Toward a Public Health Surveillance System for Behavioral Health. *Public Health Rep.* **2018**, *133*, 360–365. [CrossRef] [PubMed]
9. Lynn, P.; Japec, L.; Lyberg, L. What's so special about cross-national surveys? In Proceedings of the International Workshop on Comparative Survey Design and Implementation (CSDI), Madrid, Spain, 10–12 March 2005; GESIS: Mannheim, Germany, 2006; Volume 12, pp. 7–20.
10. Dillman, D.A. Mail and other self-administered surveys in the 21st century: The beginning of a new era. *Retrieved May* **1998**, *30*, 2005.
11. Diener, E.; Oishi, S.; Lucas, R.E. National accounts of subjective well-being. *Am. Psychol.* **2015**, *70*, 234. [CrossRef]
12. Matz, S.C.; Gladstone, J.J.; Stillwell, D. Money buys happiness when spending fits our personality. *Psychol. Sci.* **2016**, *27*, 715–725. [CrossRef]
13. Schwartz, H.A.; Eichstaedt, J.C.; Kern, M.L.; Dziurzynski, L.; Ramones, S.M.; Agrawal, M.; Shah, A.; Kosinski, M.; Stillwell, D.; Seligman, M.E.; et al. Personality, gender, and age in the language of social media: The open-vocabulary approach. *PLoS ONE* **2013**, *8*, e73791. [CrossRef]
14. Curtis, B.L.; Lookatch, S.J.; Ramo, D.E.; McKay, J.R.; Feinn, R.S.; Kranzler, H.R. Meta-Analysis of the Association of Alcohol-Related Social Media Use with Alcohol Consumption and Alcohol-Related Problems in Adolescents and Young Adults. *Alcohol. Clin. Exp. Res.* **2018**, *42*, 978–986. [CrossRef]
15. Stavrakantonakis, I.; Gagiu, A.E.; Kasper, H.; Toma, I.; Thalhammer, A. An approach for evaluation of social media monitoring tools. *Common Value Manag.* **2012**, *52*, 52–64.
16. Nguyen, Q.C.; McCullough, M.; Meng, H.W.; Paul, D.; Li, D.; Kath, S.; Loomis, G.; Nsoesie, E.O.; Wen, M.; Smith, K.R.; et al. Geotagged US tweets as predictors of county-level health outcomes, 2015–2016. *Am. J. Public Health* **2017**, *107*, 1776–1782. [CrossRef] [PubMed]
17. Kursuncu, U.; Gaur, M.; Lokala, U.; Thirunarayan, K.; Sheth, A.; Arpinar, I.B. Predictive analysis on Twitter: Techniques and applications. In *Emerging Research Challenges and Opportunities in Computational Social Network Analysis and Mining*; Springer International Publishing: Cham, Switzerland, 2019; pp. 67–104.
18. Culotta, A. Lightweight methods to estimate influenza rates and alcohol sales volume from Twitter messages. *Lang. Resour. Eval.* **2013**, *47*, 217–238. [CrossRef]
19. Culotta, A. Estimating county health statistics with twitter. In Proceedings of the 32nd Annual ACM Conference on Human Factors in Computing Systems, Toronto, ON, Canada, 26 April–1 May 2014; ACM: New York, NY, USA; pp. 1335–1344.
20. Eichstaedt, J.C.; Schwartz, H.A.; Kern, M.L.; Park, G.; Labarthe, D.R.; Merchant, R.M.; Jha, S.; Agrawal, M.; Dziurzynski, L.A.; Sap, M.; et al. Psychological language on Twitter predicts county-level heart disease mortality. *Psychol. Sci.* **2015**, *26*, 159–169. [CrossRef]
21. Ginsberg, J.; Mohebbi, M.H.; Patel, R.S.; Brammer, L.; Smolinski, M.S.; Brilliant, L. Detecting influenza epidemics using search engine query data. *Nature* **2009**, *457*, 1012. [CrossRef]
22. Jena, A.B.; Karaca-Mandic, P.; Weaver, L.; Seabury, S.A. Predicting new diagnoses of HIV infection using internet search engine data. *Clin. Infect. Dis.* **2013**, *56*, 1352–1353. [CrossRef]
23. Paul, M.J.; Dredze, M. You are what you tweet: Analyzing twitter for public health. In Proceedings of the Fifth International AAAI Conference on Weblogs and Social Media, Barcelona, Spain, 17–21 July 2011.
24. Curtis, B.; Giorgi, S.; Buffone, A.E.; Ungar, L.H.; Ashford, R.D.; Hemmons, J.; Summers, D.; Hamilton, C.; Schwartz, H.A. Can Twitter be used to predict county excessive alcohol consumption rates? *PLoS ONE* **2018**, *13*, e0194290. [CrossRef]
25. Cavazos-Rehg, P.A.; Krauss, M.J.; Sowles, S.J.; Bierut, L.J. "Hey everyone, I'm drunk." An evaluation of drinking-related Twitter chatter. *J. Stud. Alcohol Drugs* **2015**, *76*, 635–643. [CrossRef]
26. Preotiuc-Pietro, D.; Samangooei, S.; Cohn, T.; Gibbins, N.; Niranjan, M. Trendminer: An architecture for real time analysis of social media text. In Proceedings of the Sixth International AAAI Conference on Weblogs and Social Media, Dublin, Ireland, 4–7 June 2012.

27. Giorgi, S.; Preotiuc-Pietro, D.; Buffone, A.; Rieman, D.; Ungar, L.H.; Schwartz, H.A. The remarkable benefit of user-level aggregation for lexical-based population-level predictions. In Proceedings of the 2014 Conference on Empirical Methods in Natural Language Processing (EMNLP), Brussels, Belgium, 31 October–4 November 2018; pp. 1167–1172.
28. Lui, M.; Baldwin, T. langid. py: An off-the-shelf language identification tool. In Proceedings of the Association for Computational Linguistics 2012 System Demonstrations, Jeju Island, Korea, 8–14 July 2012; pp. 25–30.
29. Schwartz, H.A.; Eichstaedt, J.C.; Kern, M.L.; Dziurzynski, L.; Lucas, R.E.; Agrawal, M.; Park, G.J.; Lakshmikanth, S.K.; Jha, S.; Seligman, M.E.; et al. Characterizing geographic variation in well-being using tweets. In Proceedings of the Seventh International AAAI Conference on Weblogs and Social Media, Boston, MA, USA, 8–11 July 2013.
30. Chinni, D.; Gimpel, J. *Our Patchwork Nation: The Surprising Truth about the" Real" America*; Penguin: New York, NY, USA, 2011.
31. Blei, D.M.; Ng, A.Y.; Jordan, M.I. Latent dirichlet allocation. *J. Mach. Learn. Res.* **2003**, *3*, 993–1022.
32. Schwartz, H.A.; Giorgi, S.; Sap, M.; Crutchley, P.; Ungar, L.; Eichstaedt, J. DLATK: Differential language analysis toolkit. In Proceedings of the 2017 Conference on Empirical Methods in Natural Language Processing: System Demonstrations, Copenhagen, Denmark, 9–11 September 2017; pp. 55–60.
33. Monroe, B.L.; Colaresi, M.P.; Quinn, K.M. Fightin' words: Lexical feature selection and evaluation for identifying the content of political conflict. *Political Anal.* **2008**, *16*, 372–403. [CrossRef]
34. Jurafsky, D.; Chahuneau, V.; Routledge, B.R.; Smith, N.A. Narrative framing of consumer sentiment in online restaurant reviews. *First Monday* **2014**, *19*, 4. [CrossRef]
35. Gelfand, A.E.; Smith, A.F. Sampling-based approaches to calculating marginal densities. *J. Am. Stat. Assoc.* **1990**, *85*, 398–409. [CrossRef]
36. McCallum, A.K. Mallet: A machine Learning for Language Toolkit. 2002. Available online: http://mallet.cs.umass.edu (accessed on 22 July 2015).
37. Benjamini, Y.; Hochberg, Y. Controlling the false discovery rate: A practical and powerful approach to multiple testing. *J. R. Stat. Soc. Ser. B (Methodol.)* **1995**, *57*, 289–300. [CrossRef]
38. Pennebaker, J.W.; Boyd, R.L.; Jordan, K.; Blackburn, K. *The Development and Psychometric Properties of LIWC2015*; The University of Texas at Austin: Austin, TX, USA, 2015.
39. Mohammad, S.M.; Kiritchenko, S.; Zhu, X. NRC-Canada: Building the state-of-the-art in sentiment analysis of tweets. *arXiv* **2013**, arXiv:1308.6242.
40. Green, L.J. *African American English: A Linguistic Introduction*; Cambridge University Press: Cambridge, UK, 2002.
41. Carr, J.L.; VanDeusen, K.M. Risk factors for male sexual aggression on college campuses. *J. Fam. Violence* **2004**, *19*, 279–289. [CrossRef]
42. Allem, J.P.; Ferrara, E.; Uppu, S.P.; Cruz, T.B.; Unger, J.B. E-cigarette surveillance with social media data: Social bots, emerging topics, and trends. *JMIR Public Health Surveill.* **2017**, *3*, e98. [CrossRef]
43. Unger, J.B.; Urman, R.; Cruz, T.B.; Majmundar, A.; Barrington-Trimis, J.; Pentz, M.A.; McConnell, R. Talking about tobacco on Twitter is associated with tobacco product use. *Prev. Med.* **2018**, *114*, 54–56. [CrossRef]
44. Nguyen, A.; Hoang, Q.; Nguyen, H.; Nguyen, D.; Tran, T. Evaluating marijuana-related tweets on Twitter. In Proceedings of the 2017 IEEE 7th Annual Computing and Communication Workshop and Conference (CCWC), Las Vegas, NV, USA, 9–11 January 2017; pp. 1–7.

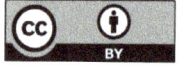

© 2020 by the authors. Licensee MDPI, Basel, Switzerland. This article is an open access article distributed under the terms and conditions of the Creative Commons Attribution (CC BY) license (http://creativecommons.org/licenses/by/4.0/).

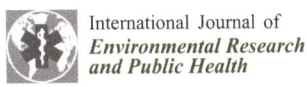

Commentary

Practical and Ethical Considerations for Schools Using Social Media to Promote Physical Literacy in Youth

Trevor Bopp [1,*] and Michael Stellefson [2]

1. Department of Sport Management, University of Florida, Gainesville, FL 32611, USA
2. Department of Health Education and Promotion, East Carolina University, Greenville, NC 27858, USA; stellefsonm17@ecu.edu
* Correspondence: tbopp@ufl.edu; Tel.: +1-352-294-1663

Received: 31 December 2019; Accepted: 12 February 2020; Published: 14 February 2020

Abstract: The rapid development of social media has led to its increased use by children and adolescents for health and well-being purposes. Accordingly, social interactions resulting from social media use can be further integrated into physical and health education pedagogy. Given the relationship between increased physical literacy and positive health outcomes, best practices and lessons learned from social media use in the healthcare industry should be adopted by health and physical educators practicing in schools. Thus, the purpose of this paper is to comment on several practical and ethical challenges and opportunities associated with using social media to improve physical literacy among youth. Specifically, two of the most prominent issues are discussed in depth: (1) integration of social media in physical education settings that educate children and adolescents about the biopsychosocial effects of physical activity, and (2) use of wearable technologies among youth to accrue experiences that enhance physical literacy competencies. In our opinion, health and physical educators who utilize the ALL-ENGAGE Playbook described in this commentary will successfully reach, engage, and impact students with popular social media that adequately promotes physical literacy, including through experiential use of wearable technologies.

Keywords: physical literacy; social media; ethics; health education; wearable technology

1. Introduction

The rapid development of social media has led to its increased use by children and adolescents for health and well-being purposes [1]. Six types of social media platforms are commonly used in health education/promotion: (1) social networking (e.g., Facebook); (2) blog comments and forums; (3) microblogging (e.g., Twitter); (4) media sharing (e.g., Instagram); (5) book marketing; and (6) social news [2]. Such platforms, along with the Internet and other mobile technologies, are now being widely utilized to share health information [3]. Social media thus affords new opportunities for peer-to-peer health information exchange and self-management support, as well as digital disease detection and monitoring [4]. One in five United States (U.S.) children and adolescents are affected by obesity [5], which subsequently hinders motor skill development and physical activity levels [6,7], so it is imperative that educational systems begin to carefully consider how innovative technologies, such as social media, can help youth become more physically literate and active. Although YouTube is one of the most utilized and popular social media sites for all users, particularly for video content [8], younger populations are more likely to use Instagram and Snapchat, with 72% and 69%, respectively, of U.S. teens frequently on these social media platforms [1]. These popular social media websites are particularly useful for delivering targeted persuasive messages that can easily be acted on and shared with online social network members [2]. Furthermore, the integration of social media, technology, and consumer-driven online health information has very strong potential to revolutionize youth health and wellness education programs [9,10].

The education industry continues to transform and progress with the advancement of technology. Recently, there has been a marked increase in the number of virtual schools that capitalize on the low-cost and accessible use of web-based and mobile pedagogical tools [11]. Physical education, in particular, is currently experiencing tremendous growth in the number of classes offered through distance education platforms. Over half ($n = 31$) of U.S. states allow academic credit to be earned through participation in virtual physical education (VPE) courses [12]. Delivery of VPE courses can serve as a viable alternative for students who may travel regularly due to extracurricular activities (e.g., for the arts, music, or sports), reside in remote geographical locations, and/or have special needs or disabilities. Other ideal candidates for VPE include students who may be insecure about their physical skills or abilities, or who may want to take classes that are not offered at their own school due to a lack of certified instructors or insufficient facilities and/or fitness equipment [12,13].

As a desired outcome of physical education in the U.S. [14], physical literacy should be a primary consideration in the development of both traditional physical education and VPE courses. Physical literacy in the U.S. is defined as "the ability, confidence, and desire to be physically active for life" [15] (p. 3). Being physically literate contributes to a healthy life-course trajectory as it is both the foundation for, and enhanced by, physical activity [16]. As such, high physical literacy can help youth manage their weight and reduce health risks [17,18]. Unfortunately, many U.S. school systems and educators find it difficult to reorient and implement change in physical education to focus on enhancing physical literacy [19–21]. One approach used to overcome current barriers is increasing the scalability of VPE courses and online resources [22]. Programs such as VPE show promise in enhancing physical literacy among youth who are particularly vulnerable to health disparities resulting from a lack of physical activity [13].

Unfortunately, physical educators are not always comfortable with using VPE learning management systems (e.g., Blackboard, WebCT, and Moodle). Most notably, teachers express difficulty initiating and maintaining communication about physical activity with their students. They also encounter challenges monitoring students' actual engagement in physical activity [23]. Vollum [10] put forward social media as a potential remedy for overcoming challenges faced by online instructors. Understanding that physical and health education should be "nurturing, empowering, motivating and engaging for all students" (p. 562), Vollum argues that the social interactions resulting from social media have become integrated into standard physical and health education pedagogy. Given the relationship between increased physical literacy and positive health and academic outcomes [15,16,24], it stands to reason that best practices and lessons learned from social media use in the healthcare industry be adopted by health and physical educators practicing in schools. Thus, the purpose of this paper is to consider and provide commentary on several practical and ethical challenges, as well as opportunities, for using social media to improve physical literacy among youth. Further, we introduce and suggest the use of the ALL-ENGAGE Playbook for school administrators and physical educators to consider when integrating social media and technology as pedagogical tools.

2. Practical and Ethical Issues

The healthcare industry has capitalized on these social media trends and other online health resources to virtually monitor and manage patients, as well as to disseminate and serve as a collaborative online resource for health information [3,4]. However, with these positive gains have come ethical concerns particular to social media applications. Previous work completed to assess online physical literacy resources, such as YouTube, revealed not only a desire for quality physical literacy information and content, but also an online community with high standards that places value on such information [25]. Physical education instructors in school systems should be cognizant of these expected quality standards. As standards evolve over time, they will undoubtedly affect the potential of social media to enhance virtual student-to-student, student-to-teacher, and student-to-industry networking opportunities, as well as the availability, accrual, and dissemination of physical literacy information and resources for students.

McKee [3] has described ethical issues of privacy, anonymity, data collection, and patient surveillance on social media. Issues such as these sparked the need for new progressive ethical standards for using social media in health care [9]. Denecke [4] discussed ethical concerns associated with the increased use of web-based technology and social media in healthcare settings. With these concerns in mind, we now consider the following two critical issues most closely associated with utilizing social media to improve youth physical literacy in schools: (1) the integration of social media in elementary, middle, and high school settings that educate children and adolescents about physical literacy, and (2) the use of wearable technologies among these youth during physical education to learn more about physical literacy competencies.

2.1. Integration of Social Media in Physical Education Settings that Educate Children and Adolescents about Physical Literacy

The inherent practical and ethical challenges associated with youth using these popular social media websites and applications (apps) include problems with obtaining consent from their parents or guardians, as well as the privacy of youth and their level of comfort sharing personal information online [4] about their own physical literacy (e.g., body, motor skills, movement, physical activity and fitness, and value and accountability). Physical literacy can be a very personal and individualized journey [26]. One primary benefit of VPE and social media usage is the provision of a safe and potentially private space for students who may be insecure about their physical skills and abilities [13]. Thus, it is critical that educational protocols and policies be explicit regarding storage and usage of, and access to, student data. Students and parents/guardians should also be fully informed about, and understand clearly, that to which they are consenting [27].

However, administrators should be accountable for and concerned not only about the data and student-created content that is collected and stored. Use of misleading educational physical and health information on social media can be very dangerous for youth and the spread of unverified health claims can also be very harmful. Nevertheless, sharing personal experiences to establish meaningful person-to-person connections is central to the social media experience and has the potential to empower users to become more activated in terms of health information-seeking and health-related decision-making [28,29]. Physical education teachers who elect to incorporate social media into the classroom environment should be conscientious about how social media is used to mitigate barriers to youth physical literacy that may exacerbate existing health disparities.

Regarding this practical and ethical challenge, it is imperative that social media platforms be reconfigured and adapted as an educational tool for communication between students and teachers. A common misunderstanding about social media is that it serves as a podium for delivering a message. Instead, social media enables teachers to talk with their students rather than simply talking at them. Talking with students on social media helps to build a sense of trust and adds a personal touch [2]. However, student–teacher online relationships can be ethically questionable and should be maintained in a safe, trusting, and professional manner [4].

Social media should provide engaging, supportive, applicable, and practical physical literacy information and resources. For example, using images and videos of role model child/adolescent actors taking part in healthy physical activity is more likely to capture students' attention and enhance message comprehension. Posts with visual images also typically receive more clicks, shares, comments, and likes on social media [30,31]. However, the applicability, acceptability, and reach of social media posts is often limited due to the large number of posts constantly being made on popular social media channels. Conversely, if educators do not attentively monitor students' social media conversations, these conversations can quickly become unpredictable and result in confusion and frustration for the students [32]. Likewise, if educators do not consistently add and update physical and health education content, the social media sites they manage are likely to lack robust and informative conversations [33].

Currently, there are few models available to health and physical education specialists that describe guidelines for planning, implementing, and evaluating social media pages for health promotion and disease management. Therefore, a new social media awareness, outreach, and engagement "playbook" was developed to foster meaningful interaction with priority audiences [2]. The ALL-ENGAGE Playbook [34] is a social media framework, inspired by evidence-based social media guidelines, including those provided by the Centers for Disease Control and Prevention (CDC) [35–37], that should be considered by physical education teachers and programs to establish and facilitate worthwhile participation and discussion with students. This would involve: assessing social media channels to best reach student(s); listening to social media conversations to identify trending physical activity and literacy topics; leveraging existing gaps and opportunities for using social media in physical education; editing course posting calendars to manage social media administration; networking with peers who have similar physical activity/education interests; generating new social media content that is search engine optimized (SEO); adapting social media policies to facilitate interactivity and diverse opinions; guiding students to current, accurate, and evidence-based physical activity and health/wellness information; and evaluating social media pages through systematic analysis of performance indicators. Table 1 outlines plays, action steps, and goals associated with each element of the ALL-ENGAGE Playbook.

Table 1. Goal-Directed Plays and Action Steps in the ALL-ENGAGE Social Media Playbook.

Play	Action Steps	Goal(s)
Assess social media channels	• Research active keywords • Identify social media websites regularly accessed (daily or almost daily) by students and youth • Determine capacity to use social media	Understand students' current and potential usage of popular social media for physical literacy, physical activity, and health/wellness information
Listen to social media conversations	• Manage and monitor social media interactions between and among students (e.g., discussions, posted comments, pictures and videos) • Review posted content and feedback left on relevant websites or blogs [38] • Join the conversation	Identify trending physical literacy, physical activity, and health/wellness information, discussion topics, concerns, and questions Describe student interests, knowledge, physical and health literacy, and cultural perspectives on physical activity and education
Leverage existing gaps and opportunities	• Answer student questions on social media • Address discussions that never concluded • Repurpose evidence-based physical education content to start a new conversation on social media	Make social media a valuable space for student-to-teacher interaction and communication Address physical activity and literacy management questions and concerns
Edit course posting calendars	• Create a story board that personalizes and humanizes posted physical education materials and content • Program third-party social media management software • Schedule times for when a message is to be sent out on any day or time of the week	Post to a social media site (e.g., Instagram, YouTube, Facebook) at least three times per week, with 3-5 h per week spent engaging with users Post to Twitter or Snapchat at least once daily, with 3–5 h a week spent managing feeds
Network with students and other social media users	• "Like" status updates and comments • Cross promote content from reputable sources, agencies, and influencers [35] • Offer Q&A social media sessions with physical activity experts	Connect students with industry professionals and other educational social media users who share similar physical activity and health/wellness interests

Table 1. Cont.

Play	Action Steps	Goal(s)
Generate new social media content	<ul><li>Post user-generated content (UGC) that is search engine optimized (SEO)</li><li>Share content in language understood and used by students</li><li>Involve student group work whenever possible</li></ul>	Increase physical activity and literacy information accessibility that reinforces important content for students and other potential stakeholder audiences Increase the frequency of interactions and improve user engagement
Adapt social media policies	<ul><li>Develop social media moderator policies and trainings [39]</li><li>Post a social media code of conduct and grading rubric for students</li><li>Document best practices for posting, moderating, and communicating on social media</li></ul>	Facilitate student-to-student and student-to-teacher interactivity and engagement Maintain healthy and informative participation, with a diversity of opinions related to cultural, spiritual, and political beliefs and opinions
Guide student users	<ul><li>Deliver physical activity and health/wellness resources</li><li>Drive students to useful, interesting, and action-oriented posts</li><li>Train teachers and administrators to remove destructive posts that may personally attack others</li></ul>	Create brand (i.e., course) recognition Engage students and discuss current topics and issues that they find relevant
Evaluate social media pages	<ul><li>Observe social media page activity</li><li>Collect and process evaluation data</li><li>Interpret key performance indicators on social media [38]</li></ul>	Monitor progress toward reaching short-term, intermediate, and long-term physical literacy Learn from mistakes and make program modifications accordingly

Figure 1 demonstrates the cyclical nature of the ALL-ENGAGE Playbook strategy, with a focus on the use of social media to build physical literacy competencies. Systematically planning for social media use in physical education is important given that prior work acknowledges increased risks for negative outcomes such as breaches of student confidentiality and unprofessional student-to-student or student-to-teacher interactions [4]. For example, educators who use social media to improve physical literacy should seek to remove all personally identifying student information from all posted content [2]. It is also important to monitor privacy settings on social media to limit the exposure of content outside of students within the class. Personal and professional social media profiles should be separate, with declared conflicts of interest made clear [2]. Additionally, anyone using social media tools should be required to have specific training. When preparing training for teachers and students, topics should include hashtag use, uploading content, updating profile pictures, and sharing media [40]. Educators should also be trained to remove destructive posts and students who violate stated social media policies [41]. They should additionally encourage youth to avoid potentially harmful material on social media (e.g., misguided instructions on how to exercise); consider the consequences of taking social media actions before posting, commenting, or sharing content with others; report derogatory comments pertaining to a person's gender, race, or religion; and stay cautious of commercially motivated objectives, such as selling unregulated fitness products [42].

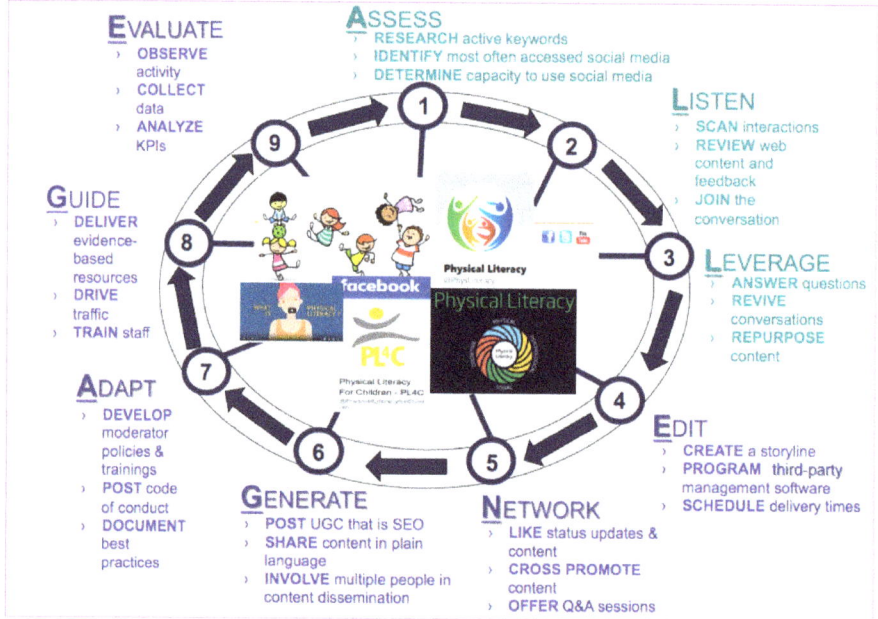

Figure 1. ALL-ENGAGE Playbook for advancing youth physical literacy on social media.

Daum and Buschner [23] found that teachers had a difficult time offering immediate feedback and constructive visual cues on students' movement and physical activity assignments and this hindered both the applicable teaching and in-depth learning of motor skills. Social media apps might not currently be capable of addressing such issues. Thus, social media pedagogy should adapt teaching capabilities to meet the academic needs and learning styles of today's youth, particularly as it pertains to social interactions in modern culture [10]. Required training would need to be developed in accordance with the ALL-ENGAGE social media playbook (Figure 1). Training teachers to become active communicators and disseminators on social media may help address parental perceptions that social media contains mostly inaccurate and biased information. Schools should adopt policies and administer training programs continuously on a semester-by-semester basis to focus on appropriate and ethically responsible use of social media in physical education and VPE.

2.2. The Use of Wearable Technologies among Youth

Young peoples' understanding, use, and need for digital physical activity and health technologies varies and is greatly influenced by schools, physical education, sports, family, and peers [43]. Thus, the use of such digital physical and health technologies in the school system can be very beneficial to students' physical literacy development, in both traditional physical education settings and VPE classes, yet presents similar, previously mentioned, ethical concerns with issues of data security, accountability, and privacy. To this end, the Guide phase of the ALL-ENGAGE playbook encourages the utilization of evidence-based digital activity and health resources and technologies. Further, the Evaluate phase describes means by which such tools can be evaluated to determine their impact on youth physical literacy and related outcomes. Wearable health technologies and trackers are typically designed for the general user to monitor particular health metrics (e.g., heart rate, steps, distance traveled) and connect to a database, via phone or internet, to allow users to manage, learn, and adjust their physical activity accordingly based on their shared data [44]. Such information would be valuable to students and teachers as it would provide them with more opportunities for varied and in-depth charting of their physical literacy journey [16,45]. Other software and technologies, such as augmented and virtual reality, can be utilized by mobile devices to aid in student development of physical literacy. It has been found that augmented reality applications, when integrated into cell phones, had a positive impact on physical education students' learning and advancing their spatial awareness and distance estimation [46]. Taken together, integrating and cross-referencing the data collected from wearable technologies and social media sites allows educators to better understand the impact of social interactions, spatial location and environment, psychological states and affect, and other behaviors on student physical activity levels and engagement [47].

Concerns with privacy, security, and accountability have previously been discussed, but it is important to note other potential issues resulting from the use of social media and mobile technologies. For instance, wearable technologies have been found to be helpful in detecting early indications of youth's mental health, but involved real-time and immediate monitoring of social media, sleep, and activity, which required end-users' trust and active engagement with administrators [48]. Kerner and Goodyear [49] found evidence that wearing such devices negatively impacted physical competence and perceived autonomy due to daily activity targets (e.g., 10,000 steps per day), as well as contributed to amotivation towards physical activity and healthy lifestyles. Lastly, we must remark on the significance of access and equity in the wearing of digital activity trackers among students from marginalized communities. Requiring and/or capitalizing on the use of wearable technologies can have unintended consequences that may exasperate discrepancies in schools' financial and community resources for youth, as well as (a lack of) conducive environments and time for youth to be physically active [50,51]. Parameters should thus be put into place that will afford all students from the same schools or districts the opportunity to participate in VPE and/or the use of wearable and mobile educational technologies, along with a transparent protocol that will monitor students' mental and affective experiences with these devices.

3. Conclusions

While social media may become the way of the future for conveying and disseminating physical education to youth, its use is largely unregulated, with limited oversight provided by trained professionals. As social media becomes more integrated into school-based physical education, teachers will likely play an important role in monitoring information that is being shared. In this capacity, school administrators should engage with the public to address physical activity and health-related misconceptions or misinformation on social media in a manner that is non-confrontational and enlightening. The purpose of this paper was to consider and provide commentary on several practical and ethical challenges and to discuss opportunities for using social media to improve physical literacy among youth. To this end, we summarized two of the major practical and ethical issues surrounding the use of social media in physical education settings where physical literacy is promoted. The use of social media and wearable physical activity and health-related technologies in such settings raises some concerns with respect to privacy, security, trust, and accountability, but should be considered due to unprecedented opportunities for educating youth about the principles that guide physically literate and healthy lifestyles. While there is no one-size-fits-all approach to the use of such web-based applications and mobile devices, we introduce and suggest the use of the ALL-ENGAGE Playbook for consideration by school administrators and physical educators when integrating social media and technology as pedagogical tools. While the ALL-ENGAGE Playbook has yet to be tested in social media research among children and adolescents, we feel that there is great potential in implementing this innovative framework to promote physical literacy in youth populations. Moreover, physical educators who choose to utilize the ALL-ENGAGE Playbook in practice may be more likely to successfully reach, engage, and impact youth with social-media-based programming that enables students to learn about and enhance their physical literacy, especially through use of wearable technologies.

Author Contributions: Conceptualization, T.B. and M.S. formal analysis, T.B. and M.S.; resources, T.B. and M.S.; writing—original draft preparation, T.B. and M.S.; writing—review and editing, T.B. and M.S.; visualization, T.B. and M.S. All authors have read and agreed to the published version of the manuscript.

Funding: This research received no external funding.

Conflicts of Interest: The authors declare no conflict of interest.

References

1. Anderson, M.; Jiang, J. Teens, Social Media & Technology 2018. Available online: https://www.pewresearch.org/internet/2018/05/31/teens-social-media-technology-2018/ (accessed on 5 February 2020).
2. Bensley, R.J.; Thackeray, R.; Stellefson, M. Using social media. In *Community and Public Health Education Methods: A Practical Guide*; Bensley, R.J., Brookins-Fisher, J., Eds.; Jones & Barlette Learning: Burlington, MA, USA, 2019; pp. 149–167.
3. McKee, R. Ethical issues in using social media for health and health care research. *Health Policy* **2013**, *110*, 298–301. [CrossRef]
4. Denecke, K.; Bamidis, P.; Bond, C.; Gabarron, E.; Househ, M.; Lau, A.Y.S.; Mayer, M.A.; Merolli, M.; Hansen, M. Ethical issues of social media usage in healthcare. *Yearb. Med. Inform.* **2015**, *10*, 137–147. [CrossRef] [PubMed]
5. Healthy Schools: Childhood Obesity Facts. Available online: https://www.cdc.gov/healthyschools/obesity/facts.htm (accessed on 27 December 2019).
6. Robinson, L.E.; Stodden, D.F.; Barnett, L.M.; Lopes, V.P.; Logan, S.W.; Rodrigues, L.P.; D'Hondt, E. Motor competence and its effect on positive developmental trajectories of health. *Sports Med.* **2015**, *45*, 1273–1284. [CrossRef] [PubMed]
7. Malina, R.M. Top 10 research questions related to growth and maturation of relevance to physical activity, performance, and fitness. *Res. Q. Exerc. Sport* **2014**, *85*, 157–173. [CrossRef] [PubMed]
8. Maina, A. Small Business Trends 20 Popular Media Sites Right Now. Available online: https://smallbiztrends.com/2016/05/popular-social-media-sites.html (accessed on 5 February 2020).
9. DeCamp, M. Ethical issues when using social media for health outside professional relationships. *Int. Rev. Psychiatr.* **2015**, *27*, 97–105. [CrossRef] [PubMed]
10. Vollum, M.J. The potential for social media use in K-12 physical and health education. *Comput. Hum. Behav.* **2014**, *35*, 560–564. [CrossRef]
11. Molnar, A.; Miron, G.; Elgeberi, N.; Barbour, M.K.; Huerta, L.; Shafer, S.R.; Rice, J.K. *Virtual Schools in the U.S.*; National Education Policy Center: Boulder, CO, USA, 2019; Available online: http://nepc.colorado.edu/publication/virtual-schools-annual-2019 (accessed on 5 February 2020).
12. Society of Health and Physical Educators. *2016 Shape of the Nation: Status of Physical Education in the USA*; SHAPE America: Reston, VA, USA, 2016.
13. Rhea, D.J. Virtual physical education in the K-12 setting. *J. Phys. Educ. Rec. Dance* **2011**, *82*, 5–50. [CrossRef]
14. Society of Health and Physical Educators. *National Standards & Grade-Level Outcomes for K-12 Physical Education*; Human Kinetics: Champaign, IL, USA, 2014.
15. *Physical Literacy in the United States: A Model, Strategic Plan, and Call to Action*; Aspen Institute Sports & Society Program: Washington, DC, USA, 2015; Available online: http://aspenprojectplay.org/sites/default/files/PhysicalLiteracy_AspenInstitute.pdf (accessed on 5 February 2020).
16. Green, N.R.; Roberts, W.M.; Sheehan, D.; Keegan, R.J. Charting physical literacy journeys within physical education settings. *J. Teach. Phys. Educ.* **2018**, *37*, 272–279. [CrossRef]
17. Healthy Places: Physical Activity. Available online: https://www.cdc.gov/healthyplaces/healthtopics/physactivity.htm (accessed on 27 December 2019).
18. *Physical Activity Guidelines for Americans*, 2nd ed.; U.S. Department of Health and Human Services: Washington, DC, USA, 2018.
19. Bopp, T.; Stellefson, M.; Weatherall, B.; Spratt, S. Promoting physical literacy for disadvantaged youth living with chronic disease. *Am. J. Health Educ.* **2019**, *50*, 153–158. [CrossRef]
20. Naylor, P.J.; Nettlefold, L.; Race, D.; Hoy, C.; Ashe, M.C.; Higgins, J.W.; McKay, H.A. Implementation of school based physical activity interventions: A systematic review. *Prev. Med.* **2015**, *72*, 95–115. [CrossRef]
21. Roetert, E.P.; MacDonald, L.C. Unpacking the physical literacy concept for K-12 physical education: What should we expect the learner to master? *J. Sport Health Sci.* **2015**, *4*, 108–112. [CrossRef]

22. Mosier, B. Virtual physical education: A call for action. *J. Phys. Educ. Rec. Dance* **2012**, *83*, 6–10. [CrossRef]
23. Daum, D.N.; Buschner, C. The status of high school online physical education in the United States. *J. Teach. Phys. Educ.* **2012**, *31*, 86–100. [CrossRef]
24. Castelli, D.M.; Centeio, E.E.; Beighle, A.E.; Carson, R.L.; Nicksic, H.M. Physical literacy and comprehensive school physical activity programs. *Prev. Med.* **2014**, *66*, 95–100. [CrossRef]
25. Bopp, T.; Vadeboncoeur, J.D.; Stellefson, M.; Weinsz, M. Moving beyond the gym: A content analysis of YouTube as an information resource for physical literacy. *Int. J. Environ. Res. Public Health* **2019**, *16*, 3335. [CrossRef]
26. Whitehead, M. Definition of physical literacy and clarification of related issues. *J. Sport Sci. Phys. Educ.* **2013**, *65*, 29–34.
27. Wang, Y. Big opportunities and big concerns of big data in education. *Tech Trends* **2016**, *60*, 381–384. [CrossRef]
28. Hacker, J.; Wickramasinghe, N.; Durst, C. Can health 2.0 address critical healthcare challenges? Insights from the case of how online social networks can assist in combatting the obesity epidemic. *Australas. J. Inf. Syst.* **2017**, *21*, 1–7. [CrossRef]
29. Stellefson, M.; Alber, J.M.; Wang, M.Q.; Eddy, J.M.; Chaney, B.H.; Chaney, J.D. Use of health information and communication technologies to promote health and manage behavioral risk factors associated with chronic disease: Applications in the field of health education. *Am. J. Health Educ.* **2015**, *46*, 185–191. [CrossRef]
30. Strekalova, Y.A.; Krieger, J.L. A picture really is worth a thousand words: Public engagement with the national cancer institute on social media. *J. Cancer Educ.* **2017**, *32*, 155–157. [CrossRef]
31. Thesis, S.K.; Burke, R.M.; Cory, J.L.; Fairley, T.L. Getting beyond impressions: An evaluation of engagement with breast cancer-related Facebook content. *Mhealth* **2016**, *2*, 41. [CrossRef] [PubMed]
32. Park, A.; Hartzler, A.L.; Huh, J.; Hsieh, G.; McDonald, D.W.; Pratt, W. "How Did we get here?": Topic drift in online health discussions. *J. Med. Internet Res.* **2016**, *18*, e284. [CrossRef] [PubMed]
33. Cole-Lewis, H.; Perotte, A.; Galica, K.; Dreyer, L.; Griffith, C.; Schwarz, M.; Augustson, E. Social network behavior and engagement within a smoking cessation Facebook page. *J. Med. Internet Res.* **2016**, *18*, e205. [CrossRef] [PubMed]
34. Stellefson, M.; Paige, S.; Alber, J.; Chaney, B.; Chaney, D.; Chappell, C. Development of the ALL-ENGAGE Playbook for Planning, Implementing, and Evaluating Social Media in Health Promotion and Disease Management. In *Poster Presented at the Annual Meeting and Expo of the American Public Health Association*; American Public Health Association: Atlanta, GA, USA, 2017; Available online: https://apha.confex.com/apha/2017/meetingapp.cgi/Paper/388257 (accessed on 5 February 2020).
35. *The Health Communicator's Social Media Toolkit*; Centers for Disease Control and Prevention: Atlanta, GA, USA, 2011. Available online: https://www.cdc.gov/healthcommunication/ToolsTemplates/SocialMediaToolkit_BM.pdf (accessed on 30 December 2019).
36. *Social Media Guidelines and Best Practices*; Centers for Disease Control and Prevention: Atlanta, GA, USA, 2012. Available online: http://www.cdc.gov/SocialMedia/Tools/guidelines/pdf/FacebookGuidelines.pdf (accessed on 5 February 2020).
37. *CDC Enterprise Social Media Policy*; Centers for Disease Control and Prevention: Atlanta, GA, USA, 2015. Available online: www.cdc.gov/socialmedia/tools/guidelines/pdf/social-media-policy.pdf (accessed on 5 February 2020).
38. Neiger, B.L.; Thackeray, R.; Van Wagenen, S.A.; Hanson, C.L.; West, J.H.; Barnes, M.D.; Fagen, M.C. Use of social media in health promotion: Purposes, key performance indicators, and evaluation metrics. *Health Promot. Pract.* **2012**, *13*, 159–164. [CrossRef] [PubMed]
39. Alber, J.M.; Paige, S.; Stellefson, M.; Bernhardt, J.M. Social Media self-efficacy of health education specialists: Training and organizational development implications. *Health Promot. Pract.* **2016**, *17*, 915–921. [CrossRef]
40. Brankley, L.; Davies, J. Environmental Scan of Social Media at Ontario Public Health Units. Available online: www.wdgpublichealth.ca/?q=ldcp (accessed on 9 February 2017).
41. Huh, J.; Marmor, R.; Jiang, X. Lessons learned for online health community moderator roles: A mixed-methods study of moderators resigning from WebMD communities. *J. Med. Internet Res.* **2016**, *18*, e247. [CrossRef]
42. Lau, A.Y.; Gabarron, E.; Fernandez-Luque, L.; Armayones, M. Social media in health—What are the safety concerns for health consumers? *Health Inf. Manag. J.* **2012**, *41*, 30–35. [CrossRef]
43. Goodyear, V.A.; Armour, K.M.; Wood, H. Young people learning about health: The role of apps and wearable devices. *Learn. Media Technol.* **2019**, *4*, 193–210. [CrossRef]

44. Meyer, J.; Boll, S. Digital health devices for everyone! *IEEE Pervasive Comput.* **2014**, *13*, 10–13.
45. Durden-Myers, E.J.; Green, N.R.; Whitehead, M.E. Implications for promoting physical literacy. *J. Teach. Phys. Educ.* **2018**, *37*, 262–271. [CrossRef]
46. Gómez-García, M.; Trujillo-Torres, J.M.; Aznar-Díaz, I.; Cáceres-Reche, M.P. Augment reality and virtual reality for the improvement of spatial competences in physical education. *J. Hum. Sport Exerc.* **2018**, *13*, S189–S198. [CrossRef]
47. Bagot, K.S.; Matthews, S.A.; Mason, M.; Squeglia, L.M.; Fowler, J.; Gray, K.; Herting, M.; May, A.; Colrain, I.; Godino, J.; et al. Current, future and potential use of mobile and wearable technologies and social media data in the ABCD study to increase understanding of contributors to child health. *Dev. Cogn. Neurosci.* **2018**, *32*, 121–129. [CrossRef] [PubMed]
48. Dewa, L.H.; Lavelle, M.; Pickles, K.; Kalorkoti, C.; Jaques, J.; Pappa, S.; Aylin, P. Young adults' perceptions of using wearables, social media and other technologies to detect worsening mental health: A qualitative study. *PLoS ONE* **2019**, *14*, e0222655. [CrossRef] [PubMed]
49. Kerner, C.; Goodyear, V.A. The motivational impact of wearable healthy lifestyle technologies: A self-determination perspective on Fitbits with adolescents. *Am. J. Health Educ.* **2017**, *48*, 287–297. [CrossRef]
50. Esmonde, K.; Jette, S. Assembling the 'Fitbit subject': A Foucauldian-sociomaterialist examination of social class, gender and self-surveillance on Fitbit community message boards. *Health* **2018**. [CrossRef]
51. Schaefer, S.E.; Ching, C.C.; Breen, H.; German, J.B. Wearing, thinking, and moving: Testing the feasibility of fitness tracking with urban youth. *Am. J. Health Educ.* **2016**, *47*, 8–16. [CrossRef]

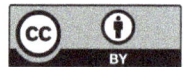

© 2020 by the authors. Licensee MDPI, Basel, Switzerland. This article is an open access article distributed under the terms and conditions of the Creative Commons Attribution (CC BY) license (http://creativecommons.org/licenses/by/4.0/).

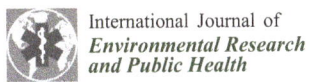

Article

The Direct and Indirect Effects of Online Social Support, Neuroticism, and Web Content Internalization on the Drive for Thinness among Women Visiting Health-Oriented Websites

Nikol Kvardova *, Hana Machackova and David Smahel

Faculty of Social Studies, Masaryk University, 60200 Brno, Czech Republic; hmachack@fss.muni.cz (H.M.); smahel@fss.muni.cz (D.S.)
* Correspondence: nikol.kvardova@fss.muni.cz

Received: 31 December 2019; Accepted: 1 April 2020; Published: 2 April 2020

Abstract: One of the debates about media usage is the potential harmful effect that it has on body image and related eating disturbances because of its representations of the "ideal body". This study focuses on the drive for thinness among the visitors of various health-oriented websites and online platforms because neither has yet been sufficiently studied in this context. Specifically, this study aims to bring more insight to the risk factors which can increase the drive for thinness in the users of these websites. We tested the presumption that web content internalization is a key factor in this process, and we considered the effects of selected individual factors, specifically the perceived online social support and neuroticism. We utilized survey data from 445 Czech women (aged 18–29, M = 23.5, SD = 3.1) who visited nutrition, weight loss, and exercise websites. The results showed a positive indirect link between both perceived online social support and neuroticism to the drive for thinness via web content internalization. The results are discussed with regard to the dual role of online support as both risk and protective factor. Moreover, we consider the practical implications for eating behavior and weight-related problems with regard to prevention and intervention.

Keywords: drive for thinness; health-oriented websites; online social support; neuroticism; web content internalization

1. Introduction

Considering Western culture and its orientation toward appearance, young girls and women are susceptible to the desire to be thin so they would achieve an ideal body shape [1,2]. According to the Tripartite Influence Model [3], women internalize idealized thin body shapes from the media, which includes traditional mass media and the internet, including health-oriented websites. Exposure to thin-ideal content can have a negative impact on women because it is associated with their drive for thinness and eating disturbances [4,5].

In this study, we focus on the drive for thinness, which is motivation for a thin or thinner body and the desire to lose weight [1,6]. It is considered a risk factor for well-being because it is associated with decreased psychological health and the later development of anorexia and bulimia nervosa [7,8]. Because of its potential harm, it is crucial to understand the factors that are associated with the drive for thinness. Although previous studies investigated the role of the media in relation to the drive for thinness [1,5,9], there is a lack of evidence for health-oriented websites and the role they play in promoting weight loss. We intend to contribute to this area by focusing on these types of websites within the theoretical framework of the Tripartite Influence Model [3]. Moreover, our aim is to enrich this model, which posits socio-cultural influences on eating disturbances, by including the role of the individual factors associated with the drive for thinness. Specifically, we examine the role of these websites for the perceived online social support, neuroticism, and internalization, and their direct and indirect effects on the drive for thinness.

As a result, our aim is to extend the knowledge about the role of health-related websites in the development of eating disorders by showing how and for whom these online spaces pose a risk. Based on our conclusions, we propose recommendations for prevention and intervention efforts.

1.1. Drive for Thinness and Health-Oriented Websites

The drive for thinness is a motivational orientation toward having a thin or thinner body and a desire to lose weight [1,6]. It emerges as a motivated behavior in order to reduce body-related discontent [10], which is manifested by eating restraint and a preoccupation with body shape and weight [11]. It is considered a risk factor to women's health because it is associated with decreased psychological well-being, like body dissatisfaction [10], body-related anxiety [12], lower self-esteem [8], or perceived stress [13]. Moreover, the drive for thinness is one of the diagnostic criteria for anorexia and bulimia nervosa, and it is associated with the later development of both [7,8,11]. The ideal of thinness [1], the drive for thinness, and related eating disorders are more prevalent in women than in men [14]. Therefore, we focused the study on women.

Considering the potential detrimental effects, it is important to understand the factors which exacerbate the drive for thinness. According to the Tripartite Influence Model [3], there are three main influences on disordered eating: parents, peers, and the media. The role of the media has been highly debated in relation to disordered eating. In the past two decades, substantial attention has been given to the role of new technologies, such as social networking sites, eating- and exercise-related websites, personal blogs with pro-eating disorder content, and various health-related discussion forums [15]. We focus on websites related to weight loss, nutrition, and exercise. These websites act as important sources for general online information related to nutrition, fitness, weight loss, and a healthy lifestyle. There are plenty of websites that address these topics, including personal blogs, informational websites for particular health-related themes, discussion forums, and social-networking groups [16,17]. Websites can be focused on weight loss, body shaping, healthy lifestyle, eating, dieting, nutrition plans for specific illnesses, recipes, and exercising [15,18,19]. Visitors may go through content, read articles, make and read comments, and obtain advice and inspiration. Moreover, websites can serve as a social environment where people interact with messages, comments, and evaluations, and they are places where people can receive support from other visitors [20–22].

However, these websites can have a negative impact on women because they display content that is associated with the drive for thinness, body dissatisfaction, and eating disturbances [4,5,23,24]. Specifically, some of these websites display pro-ED (pro-eating disorder) content that suggests that maintaining an eating disorder is a positive lifestyle choice [25]. They also contain positive comments about being thin, guilt-inducing messages related to food, stigmatization about weight, and expressions of negativity about being fat or overweight. They include content related to dieting and eating restraint, and the promotion of a thin-ideal appearance [18,26]. This appearance-oriented content can have a negative effect on women through the maintenance of weight- and appearance-related concerns [27].

The current study focuses on young female visitors of health-oriented websites in the Czech Republic. According to the data from Eurostat [28], 54% of Czech women aged 16 to 29 searched for online health-related information in 2016, which is the year when the data for our study was collected. The European average during that time was 60% of young women. Concerning the general usage of the internet, 95% of Czech women aged 16 to 29 stated that they used the internet in the preceding three months in 2016, whereas the European average was 96% [29]. This means that the usage of the internet and the online health seeking behavior among Czech women is similar as in other European countries.

1.2. Internalization

The negative effect of the exposure to the appearance-related online content can be explained with the Tripartite Influence Model, which suggests that the link between exposure to media ideals and eating disorders is not direct. It proposes that internalization of the appearance ideals serves as a mediating factor interfering association between media effect and disordered eating [30]. Media impact on disordered eating via internalization, as proposed by Tripartite Influence Model, was examined and supported by previous studies [31–35]. In the context of developing and maintaining eating disturbances, internalization is the process of adopting socially and culturally defined norms about body shape, which are commonly maintained as body ideals in everyday social interactions and in the media. By internalizing these ideals, one's conception of self could be affected because the ideals can come to represent personal standards against which one could appraise self and others [34]. Since the idealized appearance depicted by the media does not always correspond with one's real body shape, inconsistencies can emerge between the internalized norm and the actual body. Internalized ideals and perceived discrepancies can lead to consideration about how to obtain this ideal body [1]. This in turn results in disordered eating.

Several studies investigated specifically drive for thinness and how it is related to internalized appearance ideals in adolescent girls and young adult women. Internalization is a significant factor associated with the drive for thinness in both categories [1,8,15,35,36]. Moreover, the mediational role of internalization in the association between media exposure and the drive for thinness was supported [15,35]. However, less attention has been given to the individual factors which may be salient in this process and help explain who is susceptible to internalize media content. Therefore, in this study, we focus on two factors: online social support and neuroticism.

1.3. Online Social Support

Research has shown that seeking support from others is a frequent motivation for using health-oriented websites and participating in health-related online groups [37–39]. The online space offers various ways to get in touch with others, so there are also diverse ways to seek help and receive support. Social support, which in this context is mostly provided as emotional support, is expressed through emotions, empathy, and as informational support, like sharing knowledge regarding eating or fitness activities [21,40].

Online social support has been investigated as an important factor among people who struggle with eating disorders. For instance, women who engaged in an internet weight loss community mentioned encouragement, motivation, information, and shared experiences as significant resources. They appreciated the accessibility, the anonymity, and the non-judgmental interactions as unique characteristics of internet-mediated support [21]. Moreover, examinations of ED discussion forums and ED-oriented support groups have revealed that these online sites provide relevant information, emotional support, personal disclosure, help, friendship, peer support, and a safe space to ventilate feelings [20,22,39,41].

Though receiving social support is, in many occasions, a very beneficial process, we also examine its potential for the reinforcement of the drive for thinness via increased internalization. This process can be described with two theories: Social Identity Theory, which refers to an individual's knowledge of belonging and the perceived emotional and value significance of group membership [42]; and the Self-Categorization Theory [43,44], which depicts how membership in social groups affects an individual's behavior. Social identity refers to an individual's knowledge of belonging and perceived emotional and value significance of group membership [42]. Social identity can act as the basis for both giving and receiving social support. Perceived social support can additionally promote the sense of shared identity and the subjective importance of one's group membership [19,42,45,46]. Subsequently, social identity and group membership are associated with the internalization of group norms. The norms and attitudes shared within the group are internalized as personal standards and the individuals act accordingly [47]. On websites related to weight loss, nutrition, and exercise, users share body-appearance standards, which are demonstrated by the website content, and have discussions about ideal appearance and figure [18]. With these shared interests, the goals, the mutual interaction, and the social support that are exchanged among visitors, the websites have a social character. Thus, consistent with the Social Identity Theory approach, the perceived social support from the health-oriented websites can promote a sense of shared social identity and the perception of salience within the website group membership. Consequently, norms and standards regarding body appearance can be internalized even more.

1.4. Neuroticism

Neuroticism is defined in terms of the inclination to emotional reactivity, instability, perceived anxiety, and high vulnerability when coping with stress [33,48,49]. Individuals who are high in neuroticism are excitable, easily upset, and prone to experiences that are unpleasant [50]. They are also more sensitive to criticism; they experience higher levels of rejection; and they have lower self-esteem [51]. In prior research, neuroticism has been connected to the increased drive for thinness in women [52,53], to heightened food and body preoccupation [54], to body dissatisfaction [55], to the self-regulation of eating attitudes (e.g., food temptation) [56], and even to eating disorder diagnosis [48,57] and binge eating [58,59]. According to Fischer, Schreyer, Coughlin, Redgrave, and Guarda [52], the facets of neuroticism, including irritability and difficulty with emotional regulation, are risk factors for developing an ED. Moreover, disordered eating is associated with neuroticism because it can serve as a coping mechanism with which neurotic individuals deal with negative feelings [58,60].

In this study, we examine neuroticism as a risk factor for increased internalization, which can lead to a stronger drive for thinness. The link was proposed by Scoffier-Mériaux et al. [56], who hypothesized internalization as a mediator between neuroticism and unhealthy dieting behavior. This model was subsequently tested by Martin and Racine [49], who examined the mediating roles of thin and athletic-ideal internalization in association between neuroticism, body dissatisfaction, and compulsive exercise. Using the sample of 531 college students (58% women) aged 18–44, they found that thin-ideal internalization mediated the link between neuroticism and body dissatisfaction, and the internalization of athletic ideals mediated the effect of neuroticism on compulsive exercise. Moreover, several prior studies have found that neuroticism is associated with higher internalization [49,50,56,61]. To explain this link, Roberts and Good [50] suggest that women with increased neuroticism compare themselves to attractive people, and this comparison is more likely to result in negativity due to their emotional liability. This negative effect, which arises from the incongruity between the internalized body ideal and the actual body shape, can result in an increased drive for thinness, as has been proposed by previous studies [52,53]. Therefore, we hypothesize that internalization may be a mechanism through which neuroticism is positively linked to the drive for thinness in women.

1.5. Research Goals

This study focuses on the drive for thinness, which is considered a risk for women's well-being. It aims to enhance our understanding of the risk factors that contribute to its development, specifically with regard to the influence of media and the role of individual factors in young women. Previous studies have shown that the media can have a negative effect on women because exposure to its content is associated with their desire to have a thin body shape [1,5,9]. However, these studies mainly investigated traditional media (i.e., TV, magazines) and pro-eating-disorder websites. There is a lack of research in health-oriented websites, which are currently popular. These websites display content that is associated with the drive for thinness, body dissatisfaction, and eating disturbances [4,5,23,24]. Therefore, our aim is to fill this gap and bring more insight into the association between visiting health-related websites and the drive for thinness among women. Furthermore, our study aims to enrich the Tripartite Influence Model [3], which is the theoretical framework that explains eating disturbances with socio-cultural factors, by incorporating neuroticism and perceived social support as individual factors. Specifically, we test whether web content internalization mediates the effect of these factors. We propose that increased neuroticism and perceived online social support positively affects web content internalization, which in turn affects the drive for thinness. Considering that disordered eating can be related to age and Body Mass Index [62–64], we also control for both of these factors.

2. Materials and Methods

2.1. Study Sample

This study uses data from a project which focused on the visitors of websites oriented toward nutrition, weight loss, and exercise. The data were collected through an online survey between May and October 2016. Participants were recruited with an invitation on 65 Czech websites, web magazines, social networking sites, blogs, and discussion forums that focused on weight loss, diet, eating habits, and exercise. The original sample comprised of 1002 respondents (81.6% women, aged 13 to 62, M = 24.8, SD = 6.9). The project was approved by the Research Ethics Committee of the University.

The current study focuses on a subsample of 445 young adult women, aged 18 to 29 (M = 23.5, SD = 3.1). Because the ideal of thinness is aimed mainly at women [1] and the drive for thinness and eating disorders are more prevalent in women [14], we focused on women in our study. Moreover, young adult women were the major part of the health-oriented website visitors in the project, and we did not have a sufficient amount of data from participants of other ages and genders. The original sample of women in the age range from 18 to 29 comprised of 632 participants. We excluded respondents based on their motivation for visiting health-oriented websites and because of missing data. We excluded women who reported that the reason for their website visits was because of the health issues of someone else (as indicated by the question *Do you visit the sites about nutrition or sports not for yourself, but mainly because you want to help with the nutrition or sport of another person (partner, child, parent, etc.)?*) (N = 37). In addition, participants with a substantial number of missing values for the key variables (N = 150) were excluded, and there were no significant age differences between our sample and excluded respondents (t = 0.37, p = 0.71)).

2.2. Measures

2.2.1. Perceived Online Social Support

Perceived online social support was assessed using three items adapted from Graham, Papandonatos, Kang, Moreno, and Abrams [65]: *I get advice and support here that I would not get elsewhere*; *It is encouraging to know that there are other people making similar efforts (with regard to nutrition or sport)*; and *I feel that other visitors (or authors) of sites are giving me support*, with answers that ranged from 1 = Definitely does not apply to 4 = Definitely applies. A higher score indicated higher perceived support. The internal consistency was acceptable (ω = 0.72, M = 2.8, SD = 0.7).

2.2.2. Neuroticism

We measured neuroticism with three items from the short 15-item Big Five Inventory [66]. The items were *I worry a lot*; *I get nervous easily*; and *I remain calm in tense situations* (reverse scored). Participants answered on a six-point scale that ranged from 1 = Does not apply to 6 = Definitely applies. A higher score indicated higher neuroticism. The internal consistency was acceptable (ω = 0.67, M = 3.7, SD = 1.1).

2.2.3. Web Content Internalization

Internalization was measured using the question "To what extent do the following statements apply to you in regards to these sites?" with three items that were adapted from Cusumano and Thompson [67]: *I compare my appearance with people on these sites*; *I try to look like the people on these sites*; and *The content on these sites inspires me in how to look attractive*. Participants answered on a six-point scale that ranged from 1 = Does not apply to 6 = Definitely applies. A higher score indicated higher web content internalization. The internal consistency was satisfactory (ω = 0.81, M = 2.4, SD = 0.8).

2.2.4. Drive for Thinness

The Drive for Thinness subscale from Eating Disorder Inventory-3 [68] was used. The scale consisted of seven items (e.g., *I feel extremely guilty after overeating*; *I am preoccupied with the desire to be thinner*). Participants responded on a six-point scale that ranged from 1 = Never to 6 = Always. A higher score indicated a higher drive for thinness. The internal consistency was satisfactory ($\omega = 0.86$, M = 3.4, SD = 1.2). The latent variable was constructed with the parceling approach; specifically, we made three parcels, combining low-loading and high-loading items [69]. Parcels were computed as a mean of the items.

2.2.5. BMI

Participants provided information about their current weight (in kilograms) and height (in centimeters). BMI was computed as follows: Weight (kg)/Height (m)^2.

3. Results

We examined the correlations among the variables (Table 1): perceived online social support, neuroticism, web content internalization, and the drive for thinness. The results were as expected: the drive for thinness was positively correlated with online social support ($r = 0.11$, $p = 0.03$), web content internalization ($r = 0.51$, $p < 0.001$), and neuroticism ($r = 0.23$, $p < 0.001$). Web content internalization was positively associated with online social support ($r = 0.24$, $p < 0.001$) and neuroticism ($r = 0.16$, $p < 0.001$). Additionally, the drive for thinness was positively associated with BMI ($r = 0.20$, $p < 0.001$), but not with age ($r = 0.02$, $p = 0.67$).

Table 1. Correlations among variables.

Examined Variables	Drive for Thinness	Online Support	Neuroticism	Internalization	BMI	Age
Drive for thinness						
Online support	0.11 *					
Neuroticism	0.23 *	−0.01				
Internalization	0.51 *	0.24 *	0.16 *			
BMI	0.20 *	0.07	0.10 *	0.02		
Age	0.02	0.002	−0.04	−0.05	0.15 *	

Note: * designates $p < 0.05$.

To test our presumptions, Structural Equation Modeling (SEM) was used with a Robust Maximum Likelihood (MLR) estimator. We used R software, and lavaan, semTools, and semPlot packages. We tested a model with indirect effects, predicting drive for thinness. We included neuroticism and online social support as predictors, the web content internalization as a mediator of the effect of neuroticism and social support, and age and BMI as controls. The model had an acceptable fit, CFI = 0.98, TLI = 0.97, RMSEA = 0.04. Results are displayed in Figure 1 and Table 2.

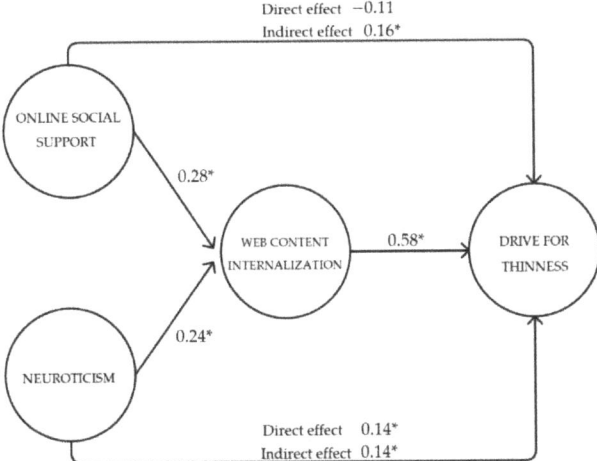

Figure 1. Path diagram with standardized regression coefficients (β). Note: * designates $p < 0.05$.

Perceived online social support from health-oriented websites predicted web content internalization (β = 0.28, $p < 0.001$). Perceived online social support did not have a strong direct effect on the drive for thinness, though the effect was weak and marginally significant (β = −0.11, $p = 0.06$; CI = −0.61; 0.01). Moreover, we found a significant indirect effect for online social support on the drive for thinness via web content internalization (β = 0.16, $p = 0.001$).

Neuroticism predicted web content internalization (β = 0.24, $p < 0.001$), and it had a direct effect on the drive for thinness (β = 0.14, $p = 0.01$). Moreover, we found a significant indirect effect for neuroticism on the drive for thinness through web content internalization (β = 0.14, $p < 0.001$). Therefore, the link between neuroticism and the drive for thinness was partially mediated by the web content internalization. Regarding controls, BMI positively predicted the drive for thinness (β = 0.17, $p = 0.001$), but there was no association between age and the drive for thinness (β = 0.02, $p = 0.60$).

Table 2. Structural Equation Modeling (SEM) predicting the drive for thinness and web content internalization.

Drive for Thinness		b	SE	p	β	CI
BMI		0.05	0.01	0.001	0.17	(0.03; 0.07)
Age		0.008	0.02	0.60	0.02	(−0.03; 0.05)
Web content internalization		0.77	0.09	<0.001	0.58	(0.59; 0.95)
Online social support	Direct effect	−0.30	0.16	0.06	−0.11	(−0.61; 0.01)
	Indirect effect	0.44	0.13	0.001	0.16	(0.19; 0.69)
Neuroticism	Direct effect	0.14	0.06	0.01	0.14	(0.02; 0.26)
	Indirect effect	0.14	0.04	<0.001	0.14	(0.06; 0.22)
Web content internalization		b	SE	p	β	CI
Online social support		0.57	0.16	<0.001	0.28	(0.26; 0.88)
Neuroticism		0.18	0.05	<0.001	0.24	(0.08; 0.28)

4. Discussion

In our study, we examined the factors associated with the drive for thinness in young adult women who visited websites oriented toward weight loss, nutrition, and exercise. Specifically, we investigated the perceived online social support of other website visitors, the neuroticism, and the web content internalization of the body appearance standards, and their direct and indirect effects on the drive for thinness. Our objective was to investigate whether the web content internalization mediates the links among the perceived online social support, the neuroticism, and the drive for thinness. We found support for our presumption: both online support and neuroticism were positively linked with the tendency for internalization, which, in turn, increased the drive for thinness.

In our data, we found a substantial connection between internalization and the drive for thinness. Our findings are in line with the Tripartite Influence Model [3,31–33], which suggests that body image concerns and eating disorders are affected by socio-cultural factors (e.g., media pressure, parental criticism, peer criticism) and indirectly through the internalization of the medialized body ideals. Moreover, we enriched the propositions of the Tripartite Influence Model [3] by including individual factors. This line of research was recently developed in studies that focused on perfectionism, self-esteem, depression, and anxiety [30–34,70]. This focus helps to better understand the risk factors, which strengthen the tendency for internalization.

Specifically, we found that perceived support increased the drive for thinness via its reinforcement of internalization. Our findings correspond to knowledge regarding ED (eating disorders) online groups, in which perceived support was connected to a higher sense of belonging and the acceptance of thin-ideal norms [20,22,39,71]. ED online groups and communities act as an important source of support that can be difficult to obtain elsewhere for individuals who struggle with ED and body image concerns [39,41]. However, support received from these online groups can be detrimental to women's health because it endorses negative attitudes toward their bodies and promotes extremely thin body shapes as attainable standards. Haas et al. [72] examined the social support on pro-anorexia websites and discovered that visitors received support for eating restraint and reinforcement for their negative views of themselves and their bodies. Sowles et al. [73] pointed out that members of the pro-ED online community disseminate images that depict thin body shapes and promote the thin ideal by labeling them as their desired goals. Similar findings emerged from a study by Marcus [40], who found that members of a pro-anorexic community shared photos of extremely thin bodies to motivate users to maintain their diets and to outline the beauty standards of the group. In this manner, women are encouraged to adopt body appearance standards that lead to a desire for a thin body. The findings of our study suggest that these processes apply not only to ED online groups, but to health-related websites as well.

Health-oriented websites, with their opportunities for social interaction (e.g., discussion with other users about specific health-related topics, personal messages, inspiration, sharing experiences, memories, feelings), enable visitors to receive social support. The perceived social support is associated with the acceptance of group norms due to the higher subjective salience of the social group to which the individuals belong [40,44,47]. In line with social identity theory [44], the stronger identification with a group would result in the acceptance of group norms and, in the case of websites focusing on nutrition and fitness—these probably supported the thin and fitness-oriented images of the ideal body. Thus, though the perceived support is often seen as a positive aspect of online interaction, in these instances, it may result in negative outcomes. However, when interpreting these results, the limitations of this study should be taken into consideration. Due to the correlational nature of the data used, it was not possible to draw causal conclusions. Thus, the association between online social support and the drive for thinness may work in the opposite direction, meaning that women with a stronger drive for thinness may more often seek social support for their goals and efforts in the online space and, specifically, via health-oriented websites.

Moreover, this finding should also be compared to the results for the direct effect of support on the drive for thinness. This effect was rather weak and just marginally significant; however, it may indicate that the role of support is diverse. If we disentangle the indirect effect that positively affects the drive for thinness from the direct effect, we find that support negatively affected the drive for thinness. To interpret this finding, we should acknowledge that perceived support helps to increase overall well-being [74–76], which decreases the tendency for unhealthy and disordered eating habits [77,78]. Thus, perceived online social support can actually function as both a risk and a protective factor. On one hand, it may contribute to the development of the drive for thinness via increased internalization. On the other hand, it may also serve as a buffer for this negative effect, probably via the increase of overall well-being, which was not included in this study. This presumption could be pursued in future examinations.

Thus, we still need to consider other factors which underlie the internalization of the web content. Our study focused on neuroticism, which showed to be positively linked to the drive for thinness and also had an indirect effect via internalization. Therefore, the effect of neuroticism on women's drive for thinness was partially mediated by the internalization of the body appearance standards displayed on health-oriented websites. In line with prior studies [49,50,52,53,56,61], our findings showed that people with heightened neuroticism are more prone to accepting the norms, and, probably because of the increased tendency for social comparison, tend more to strive to be thin.

However, besides the mediated effect, we also found a direct positive link to the drive for thinness. This suggests that increased internalization is not the only mechanism through which people with neurotic traits can be more at risk. However, considering that we found support for the tendency for heightened internalization from the websites, and upon the propositions of the Tripartite Influence Model [3], we could expect that the mechanism could be similar in relation to parental and peer norms, which have not been measured in this study. This poses one of the limitations for our study.

Concerning other limitations, it should be stressed that we used cross-sectional correlational data based on a sample that was self-selected through health-oriented websites. Thus, though we examined the proposed model for the mechanisms to increase the drive for thinness, the research design complicates drawing causal conclusions. Future research should implement a longitudinal research design to make more reliable causal conclusions and to capture potential reciprocal associations. Moreover, we were not able to control for the effects of additional variables on the drive for thinness. These are factors (e.g., body dissatisfaction) [79] that are related to the drive for thinness and disordered eating, and it would be appropriate to control for their effects to obtain more accurate results. Furthermore, we do not have information about the specific content that respondents encountered. It would be useful to incorporate objective measures and directly observe the effects of participants' exposure to online content. Finally, although the thin ideal displayed in the media and the related drive for thinness is more prominent in women [1], future research could focus on men, their internalization of the body appearance norms, and their motivations for body change.

In the current study, our aim was to propound a model that comprises of the individual factors that affect women's drive for thinness. Based on our findings, we can formulate several implications. According to the theory and the available data, we propose the following processes: online social support from the visitors of health-oriented websites and neuroticism affect the drive for thinness, and these links are mediated by the internalization of body appearance standards. Thus, alongside previous research in this area [1,8,15,35,36], our study supported the predictive role of internalization in the drive for thinness among women. Specifically, our study provided insight into the internalization of the content of health-oriented websites, which had not been sufficiently investigated and had not been taken into account in relation to women's drive for thinness. Our results imply that it is crucial to acknowledge health-oriented websites and their potential impact on women, especially in the context of the internalization of body appearance norms. Health-oriented websites, which are not generally acknowledged as harmful to women's body image, can be a significant source of body appearance norms and subsequent body image concerns [18]. As was discovered in the current study, women internalize body ideals from health-oriented websites and this, in turn, increases their drive for thinness. This connection should be actively acknowledged by health-care professionals. It is important for professionals to ask their clients who have ED-related problems about their technology usage and to provide them with space to talk about it [80]. Thus, in the context of the current study, health-care professional should discuss with clients who are struggling with EDs their usage of health-oriented websites, specifically with a focus on their exposure to the thin- or fitness-ideal content.

We also showed that both online support and neuroticism present risk factors because they can increase the tendency for internalization and, in turn, increase the drive for thinness. Therefore, it is important to be aware of the possible negative effect that online social support may have on women and to address it when preventing or reducing the drive for thinness. However, the findings of this study showed that online social support can function both as a risk and a protective factor. Thus, when discussing the use of health-oriented websites with ED clients, it is important to disentangle the different forms of social support that women receive from the visitors of these platforms. In addition, neurotic individuals experience higher levels of negative emotions and stress, which makes them more susceptible [52,53]. Based on our results, we suggest that preventive health programs, intervention, individual psychotherapy, counseling, and other health policies can be focused on the reduction of the negative emotions and stress in women. These can also help the reduction of the internalization of the body appearance standards promoted on health-oriented websites.

5. Conclusions

This study focused on the factors associated with the drive for thinness in young adult women who visited weight loss, nutrition, and exercise websites. These platforms are currently of high use, yet they have not been sufficiently studied in relation to eating disturbances. We examined the direct and indirect effects of perceived online social support from fellow website visitors, neuroticism, and the web content internalization of the body appearance standards on the drive for thinness. Our findings supported the predictive role of web content internalization on the drive for thinness in women. Moreover, we showed that the perceived online support from the health-oriented websites and neuroticism can pose risk factors because they are associated with a higher tendency for internalization and, in turn, with a stronger drive for thinness. Our results indicate that it is crucial to acknowledge health-oriented websites and their potential impact on women and their drive for thinness, especially in the context of the internalization of body appearance standards. We also discuss the role of social support, and its double role of risk and protection. Our findings can be used to establish prevention and intervention efforts to help individuals who struggle with body image and eating disturbances.

Author Contributions: Writing—original draft preparation, N.K.; writing—review and editing, N.K., H.M. and D.S..; supervision, H.M. and D.S.; project administration, H.M. and D.S.; formal analysis, N.K. All authors have read and agreed to the published version of the manuscript.

Funding: This research and the APC were funded by Czech Science Foundation, grant number 19-27828X (project FUTURE).

Conflicts of Interest: The authors declare no conflict of interest.

References

1. Pritchard, M.; Cramblitt, B. Media Influence on Drive for Thinness and Drive for Muscularity. *Sex Roles* **2014**, *71*, 208–218. [CrossRef]
2. Warren, C.S.; Gleaves, D.H.; Cepeda-Benito, A.; Fernandez, M.D.C.; Rodriguez-Ruiz, S. Ethnicity as a Protective Factor against Internalization of a Thin Ideal and Body Dissatisfaction. *Int. J. Eat. Disord.* **2005**, *37*, 241–249. [CrossRef] [PubMed]
3. Thompson, J.K.; Heinberg, L.J.; Altabe, M.; Tantleff-Dunn, S. *Exacting Beauty: Theory, Assessment, and Treatment of Body Image Disturbance*; American Psychological Association: Washington, DC, USA, 1999.
4. Harper, K.; Sperry, S.; Thompson, J.K. Viewership of Pro-Eating Disorder Websites: Association with Body Image and Eating Disturbances. *Int. J. Eat. Disord.* **2008**, *41*, 92–95. [CrossRef] [PubMed]
5. Juarez, L.; Soto, E.; Pritchard, M.E. Drive for Muscularity and Drive for Thinness: The Impact of Pro-Anorexia Websites. *Eat. Disord.* **2012**, *20*, 99–112. [CrossRef]
6. Jones, M.E.; Blodgett Salafia, E.H.; Hill, B.D. The Effect of Parental Warmth on Girls' Drive for Thinness: Do Both Parents Matter? *J. Child Fam. Stud.* **2019**, *28*, 182–191. [CrossRef]

7. De Pasquale, C.; Pistorio, M.L.; Tornatore, E.; De Berardis, D.; Fornaro, M. The Relationship between Drive to Thinness, Conscientiousness and Bulimic Traits during Adolescence: A Comparison between Younger and Older Cases in 608 Healthy Volunteers. *Ann. Gen. Psychiatry* **2013**, *12*. [CrossRef]
8. Fernandez, S.; Pritchard, M. Relationships between Self-Esteem, Media Influence and Drive for Thinness. *Eat. Behav.* **2012**, *13*, 321–325. [CrossRef]
9. Tiggemann, M. The Role of Media Exposure in Adolescent Girls' Body Dissatisfaction and Drive for Thinness: Prospective Results. *J. Soc. Clin. Psychol.* **2006**, *25*, 523–541. [CrossRef]
10. Sands, R. Reconceptualization of Body Image and Drive for Thinness. *Int. J. Eat. Disord.* **2000**, *28*, 397–407. [CrossRef]
11. Wiederman, M.W.; Pryor, T.L. Body Dissatisfaction, Bulimia, and Depression among Women: The Mediating Role of Drive for Thinness. *Int. J. Eat. Disord.* **2000**, *27*, 90–95. [CrossRef]
12. Brunet, J.; Sabiston, C.M.; Dorsch, K.D.; McCreary, D.R. Exploring a Model Linking Social Physique Anxiety, Drive for Muscularity, Drive for Thinness and Self-Esteem among Adolescent Boys and Girls. *Body Image* **2010**, *7*, 137–142. [CrossRef] [PubMed]
13. Warren, C.S.; Holland, S.; Billings, H.; Parker, A. The Relationships between Fat Talk, Body Dissatisfaction, and Drive for Thinness: Perceived Stress as a Moderator. *Body Image* **2012**, *9*, 358–364. [CrossRef] [PubMed]
14. Galmiche, M.; Déchelotte, P.; Lambert, G.; Tavolacci, M.P. Prevalence of Eating Disorders over the 2000–2018 Period: A Systematic Literature Review. *Am. J. Clin. Nutr.* **2019**, *109*, 1402–1413. [CrossRef] [PubMed]
15. Tiggemann, M.; Miller, J. The Internet and Adolescent Girls' Weight Satisfaction and Drive for Thinness. *Sex Roles* **2010**, *63*, 79–90. [CrossRef]
16. Bissonnette-Maheux, V.; Provencher, V.; Lapointe, A.; Dugrenier, M.; Dumas, A.A.; Pluye, P.; Straus, S.; Gagnon, M.P.; Desroches, S. Exploring Women's Beliefs and Perceptions About Healthy Eating Blogs: A Qualitative Study. *J. Med. Internet Res.* **2015**, *17*, e87. [CrossRef]
17. Ransom, D.C.; La Guardia, J.G.; Woody, E.Z.; Boyd, J.L. Interpersonal Interactions on Online Forums Addressing Eating Concerns. *Int. J. Eat. Disord.* **2010**, *43*, 161–170. [CrossRef]
18. Boepple, L.; Thompson, J.K. A Content Analysis of Healthy Living Blogs: Evidence of Content Thematically Consistent with Dysfunctional Eating Attitudes and Behaviors. *Int. J. Eat. Disord.* **2014**, *47*, 362–367. [CrossRef]
19. Smahel, D.; Machackova, H.; Smahelova, M.; Cevelicek, M.; Almenara, C.A.; Holubcikova, J. *Digital Technology, Eating Behaviors, and Eating Disorders*; Springer: Cham, Switzerland, 2018.
20. Flynn, M.A.; Stana, A. Social Support in a Men's Online Eating Disorder Forum. *Int. J. Mens. Health* **2012**, *11*, 150–169. [CrossRef]
21. Hwang, K.O.; Ottenbacher, A.J.; Green, A.P.; Cannon-Diehl, M.R.; Richardson, O.; Bernstam, E.V.; Thomas, E.J. Social Support in an Internet Weight Loss Community. *Int. J. Med. Inform.* **2010**, *79*, 5–13. [CrossRef]
22. McCormack, A. Individuals with Eating Disorders and the Use of Online Support Groups as a Form of Social Support. *CIN Comput. Inform. Nurs.* **2010**, *28*, 12–19. [CrossRef]
23. Custers, K.; Van den Bulck, J. Viewership of Pro-Anorexia Websites in Seventh, Ninth and Eleventh Graders. *Eur. Eat. Disord. Rev.* **2009**, *17*, 214–219. [CrossRef] [PubMed]
24. Rouleau, C.R.; Von Ranson, K.M. Potential Risks of Pro-Eating Disorder Websites. *Clin. Psychol. Rev.* **2011**, *31*, 525–531. [CrossRef] [PubMed]
25. Turja, T.; Oksanen, A.; Kaakinen, M.; Sirola, A.; Kaltiala-Heino, R.; Räsänen, P. Proeating Disorder Websites and Subjective Well-Being: A Four-Country Study on Young People. *Int. J. Eat. Disord.* **2017**, *50*, 50–57. [CrossRef] [PubMed]
26. Ging, D.; Garvey, S. 'Written in These Scars Are the Stories I Can't Explain': A Content Analysis of pro-Ana and Thinspiration Image Sharing on Instagram. *New Media Soc.* **2018**, *20*, 1181–1200. [CrossRef]
27. Carrotte, E.R.; Vella, A.M.; Lim, M.S. Predictors of "Liking" Three Types of Health and Fitness-Related Content on Social Media: A Cross-Sectional Study. *J. Med. Internet Res.* **2015**, *17*, e205. [CrossRef] [PubMed]
28. Eurostat. Women Aged 16–29 Using the Internet For Seeking Health-Related Information. Available online: https://appsso.eurostat.ec.europa.eu/nui/show.do?dataset=isoc_ci_ac_i&lang=en (accessed on 28 March 2020).
29. Eurostat. Women Aged 16–29 Using the Internet in Last Three Months. Available online: https://appsso.eurostat.ec.europa.eu/nui/show.do?dataset=isoc_ci_ifp_iu&lang=en (accessed on 28 March 2020).

30. Van Den Berg, P.; Thompson, J.K.; Obremski-Brandon, K.; Coovert, M. The Tripartite Influence Model of Body Image and Eating Disturbance A Covariance Structure Modeling Investigation Testing the Mediational Role of Appearance Comparison. *J. Psychosom. Res.* **2002**, *53*, 1007–1020. [CrossRef]
31. Huxley, C.J.; Halliwell, E.; Clarke, V. An Examination of the Tripartite Influence Model of Body Image: Does Women's Sexual Identity Make a Difference? *Psychol. Women Q.* **2015**, *39*, 337–348. [CrossRef]
32. Keery, H.; van den Berg, P.; Thompson, J.K. An Evaluation of the Tripartite Influence Model of Body Dissatisfaction and Eating Disturbance with Adolescent Girls. *Body Image* **2004**, *1*, 237–251. [CrossRef]
33. Pokrajac-bulian, A. Thin-Ideal Internalization and Comparison Process as Mediators of Social Influence and Psychological Functioning in the Development of Disturbed Eating Habits in Croatian College Females. *Psychol. Top.* **2008**, *17*, 221–245.
34. Jones, D.C.; Vigfusdottir, T.H.; Lee, Y. Body Image and the Appearance Culture among Adolescent Girls and Boys: An Examination of Friend Conversations, Peer Criticism, Appearance Magazines, and the Internalization of Appearance Ideals. *J. Adolesc. Res.* **2004**, *19*, 323–339. [CrossRef]
35. Gilbert, S.C.; Crump, S.; Madhere, S.; Schutz, W. Internalization of the Thin Ideal as a Predictor of Body Dissatisfaction and Disordered Eating in African, African-American, and Afro-Caribbean Female College Students. *J. Coll. Stud. Psychother.* **2009**, *23*, 196–211. [CrossRef]
36. Low, K.G.; Charanasomboon, S.; Brown, C.; Hiltunen, G.; Long, K.; Reinhalter, K.; Jones, H. Internalization of the Thin Ideal, Weight and Body Image Concerns. *Soc. Behav. Pers.* **2003**, *31*, 81–90. [CrossRef]
37. Peebles, R.; Wilson, J.L.; Litt, I.F.; Hardy, K.K.; Lock, J.D.; Mann, J.R.; Borzekowski, D.L.G. Disordered Eating in a Digital Age: Eating Behaviors, Health, and Quality of Life in Users of Websites with pro-Eating Disorder Content. *J. Med. Internet Res.* **2012**, *14*. [CrossRef] [PubMed]
38. Reijo, S. Dietary Blogs as Sites of Informational and Emotional Support. *Inf. Res.* **2010**, *15*, 2.
39. Tong, S.T.; Heinemann-LaFave, D.; Jeon, J.; Kolodziej-Smith, R.; Warshay, N. The Use of Pro-Ana Blogs for Online Social Support. *Eat. Disord.* **2013**, *21*, 408–422. [CrossRef]
40. Marcus, S.R. Thinsperation vs. Thickseperation: Comparing pro-Anorexic and Fat Acceptance Image Posts on a Photo-Sharing Site. *Cyberpsychology* **2016**, *10*. [CrossRef]
41. Kendal, S.; Kirk, S.; Elvey, R.; Catchpole, R.; Pryjmachuk, S. How a Moderated Online Discussion Forum Facilitates Support for Young People with Eating Disorders. *Health Expect.* **2017**, *20*, 98–111. [CrossRef]
42. Chiu, C.M.; Huang, H.Y.; Cheng, H.L.; Sun, P.C. Understanding Online Community Citizenship Behaviors through Social Support and Social Identity. *Int. J. Inf. Manag.* **2015**, *35*, 504–519. [CrossRef]
43. Tajfel, H.; Turner, J.C. An integrative theory of intergroup conflict. In *The Social Psychology of Intergroup Relation*; Brooks-Cole: Monrerey, CA, USA, 1979.
44. Tajfel, H. *Social Identity and Intergroup Relations*; Cambridge University Press: Cambridge, MA, USA, 2010.
45. Deaux, K. Reconstructing Social Identity. *Soc. Personal. Soc. Psychol.* **1993**, *19*, 4–12. [CrossRef]
46. Haslam, S.A.; O'Brien, A.; Jetten, J.; Vormedal, K.; Penna, S. Taking the strain: Social identity, social support, and the experience of stress. *Br. J. Soc. Psychol.* **2005**, *44*, 355–370. [CrossRef]
47. Stets, J.E.; Burke, P.J. Identity Theory and Social Identity Theory. *Soc. Psychol. Q.* **2000**, *63*, 224–237. [CrossRef]
48. Gual, P.; Pérez-Gaspar, M.; Martinez-Gonzalez, M.A.; Lahortiga, F.; de Irala-Estévez, J.; Cervera-Enguix, S. Self-Esteem, Personality, and Eating Disorders: Baseline Assessment of a Prospective Population-Based Cohort. *Int. J. Eat. Disord.* **2002**, *31*, 261–273. [CrossRef] [PubMed]
49. Martin, S.J.; Racine, S.E. Personality Traits and Appearance-Ideal Internalization: Differential Associations with Body Dissatisfaction and Compulsive Exercise. *Eat. Behav.* **2017**, *27*, 39–44. [CrossRef] [PubMed]
50. Roberts, A.; Good, E. Media Images and Female Body Dissatisfaction: The Moderating Effects of the Five-Factor Traits. *Eat. Behav.* **2010**, *11*, 211–216. [CrossRef]
51. Rozgonjuk, D.; Ryan, T.; Kuljus, J.K.; Täht, K.; Scott, G.G. Social Comparison Orientation Mediates the Relationship between Neuroticism and Passive Facebook Use. *Cyberpsychology* **2019**, *13*. [CrossRef]
52. Fischer, L.K.; Schreyer, C.C.; Coughlin, J.W.; Redgrave, G.W.; Guarda, A.S. Neuroticism and Clinical Course of Weight Restoration in a Meal-Based, Rapid-Weight Gain, Inpatient-Partial Hospitalization Program for Eating Disorders. *Eat. Disord.* **2017**, *25*, 52–64. [CrossRef]
53. Kjelsås, E.; Augestad, L.B. Gender, Eating Behavior, and Personality Characteristics in Physically Active Students. *Scand. J. Med. Sci. Sports* **2004**, *14*, 258–268. [CrossRef]

54. Ellickson-Larew, S.; Naragon-Gainey, K.; Watson, D. Pathological Eating Behaviors, BMI, and Facet-Level Traits: The Roles of Conscientiousness, Neuroticism, and Impulsivity. *Eat. Behav.* **2013**, *14*, 428–431. [CrossRef]
55. MacNeill, L.P.; Best, L.A.; Davis, L.L. The Role of Personality in Body Image Dissatisfaction and Disordered Eating: Discrepancies between Men and Women. *J. Eat. Disord.* **2017**, *5*, 44. [CrossRef]
56. Scoffier-Mériaux, S.; Falzon, C.; Lewton-Brain, P.; Filaire, E.; d'arripe-Longueville, F. Big Five Personality Traits and Eating Attitudes in Intensively Training Dancers: The Mediating Role of Internalized Thinness Norms. *J. Sports Sci. Med.* **2015**, *14*, 627–633.
57. Cervera, S.; Lahortiga, F.; Martinez-Gonzalez, M.A.; Gual, P.; de Irala-Estevez, J.; Alonso, Y. Neuroticism and Low Self-Esteem as Risk Factors for Incident Eating Disorders in a Prospective Cohort Study. *Int. J. Eat. Disord.* **2003**, *33*, 271–280. [CrossRef] [PubMed]
58. Izydorczyk, B. Neuroticism and Compulsive Overeating (A Comparative Analysis of the Level of Neuroticism and Anxiety in a Group of Females Suffering from Psychogenic Binge Eating, and in Individuals Exhibiting No Mental or Eating Disorders). *Arch. Psychiatry Psychother.* **2012**, *14*, 5–13.
59. Koren, R.; Munn-Chernoff, M.A.; Duncan, A.E.; Bucholz, K.K.; Madden, P.A.F.; Heath, A.C.; Agrawal, A. Is the Relationship between Binge Eating Episodes and Personality Attributable to Genetic Factors? *Twin Res. Hum. Genet.* **2014**, *17*, 65–71. [CrossRef] [PubMed]
60. Henderson, Z.B.; Fox, J.R.E.; Trayner, P.; Wittkowski, A. Emotional Development in Eating Disorders: A Qualitative Metasynthesis. *Clin. Psychol. Psychother.* **2019**, *26*, 440–457. [CrossRef] [PubMed]
61. Heinberg, L.J.; Coughlin, J.W.; Pinto, A.M.; Haug, N.; Brode, C.; Guarda, A.S. Validation and Predictive Utility of the Sociocultural Attitudes toward Appearance Questionnaire for Eating Disorders (SATAQ-ED): Internalization of Sociocultural Ideals Predicts Weight Gain. *Body Image* **2008**, *5*, 279–290. [CrossRef] [PubMed]
62. Chaudhari, B.; Tewari, A.; Vanka, J.; Kumar, S.; Saldanha, D. The Relationship of Eating Disorders Risk with Body Mass Index, Body Image and Self-Esteem among Medical Students. *Ann. Med Health Sci. Res.* **2017**, *7*, 144–149.
63. Dada, G.; Feixas, G.; Compañ, V.; Montesano, A. Self-Construction, Cognitive Conflicts, and Disordered Eating Attitudes in Young Women. *J. Constr. Psychol.* **2012**, *25*, 70–89. [CrossRef]
64. Rojo-Moreno, L.; Rubio, T.; Plumed, J.; Barberá, M.; Serrano, M.; Gimeno, N.; Conesa, L.; Ruiz, E.; Rojo-Bofill, L.; Beato, L.; et al. Teasing and Disordered Eating Behaviors in Spanish Adolescents. *Eat. Disord.* **2013**, *21*, 53–69. [CrossRef]
65. Graham, A.L.; Papandonatos, G.D.; Kang, H.; Moreno, J.L.; Abrams, D.B. Development and validation of the online social support for smokers scale. *J. Med Internet Res.* **2011**, *13*, e69. [CrossRef]
66. Lang, F.R.; John, D.; Lüdtke, O.; Schupp, J.; Wagner, G.G. Short assessment of the Big Five: Robust across survey methods except telephone interviewing. *Behav. Res. Methods* **2011**, *43*, 548–567. [CrossRef]
67. Cusumano, D.L.; Thompson, J.K. Media influence and body image in 8–11-year-old boys and girls: A preliminary report on the multidimensional media influence scale. *Int. J. Eat. Disord.* **2001**, *29*, 37–44. [CrossRef]
68. Garner, D.M. *Eating Disorder Inventory-3. Professional Manual*; Psychological Assessment Resources: Lutz, FL, USA, 2004.
69. Little, T.D.; Cunningham, W.A.; Shahar, G.; Widaman, K.F. To Parcel or Not to Parcel: Exploring the Question, Weighing the Merits. *Struct. Equ. Model.* **2002**, *9*, 151–173. [CrossRef]
70. Menzel, J.E.; Sperry, S.L.; Small, B.; Thompson, J.K.; Sarwer, D.B.; Cash, T.F. Internalization of Appearance Ideals and Cosmetic Surgery Attitudes: A Test of the Tripartite Influence Model of Body Image. *Sex Roles* **2011**, *65*, 469–477. [CrossRef]
71. McKinley, C.J. Investigating the influence of threat appraisals and social support on healthy eating behavior and drive for thinness. *Health Commun.* **2009**, *24*, 735–745. [CrossRef] [PubMed]
72. Haas, S.M.; Irr, M.E.; Jennings, N.A.; Wagner, L.M. Communicating Thin: A Grounded Model of Online Negative Enabling Support Groups in the pro-Anorexia Movement. *New Media Soc.* **2011**, *13*, 40–57. [CrossRef]
73. Sowles, S.J.; McLeary, M.; Optican, A.; Cahn, E.; Krauss, M.J.; Fitzsimmons-Craft, E.E.; Wilfley, D.E.; Cavazos-Rehg, P.A. A Content Analysis of an Online Pro-Eating Disorder Community on Reddit. *Body Image* **2018**, *24*, 137–144. [CrossRef]

74. Espeleta, H.C.; Beasley, L.; Bohora, S.; Ridings, L.E.; Silovsky, J.F. Depression in Latina mothers: Examining the roles of acculturation, enculturation, social support, and family resources. *Cult. Divers. Ethn. Minority Psychol.* **2019**, *25*, 527–538. [CrossRef]
75. Grieve, R.; Indian, M.; Witteveen, K.; Anne Tolan, G.; Marrington, J. Face-to-face or Facebook: Can social connectedness be derived online? *Comput. Hum. Behav.* **2013**, *29*, 604–609. [CrossRef]
76. Ibrahim, N.; Che Din, N.; Ahmad, M.; Amit, N.; Ghazali, S.E.; Wahab, S.; Abdul Kadir, N.; Halim, F.W.; Halim, M.R.T.A. The role of social support and spiritual wellbeing in predicting suicidal ideation among marginalized adolescents in Malaysia. *BMC Public Health* **2019**, *19*, 553. [CrossRef]
77. Fitzsimmons, E.E.; Bardone-Cone, A.M. Coping and social support as potential moderators of the relation between anxiety and eating disorder symptomatology. *Eat. Behav.* **2011**, *12*, 21–28. [CrossRef]
78. Wonderlich-Tierney, A.L.; Vander Wal, J.S. The effects of social support and coping on the relationship between social anxiety and eating disorders. *Eat. Behav.* **2010**, *11*, 85–91. [CrossRef] [PubMed]
79. Keski-Rahkonen, A.; Bulik, C.M.; Neale, B.M.; Rose, R.J.; Rissanen, A.; Kaprio, J. Body Dissatisfaction and Drive for Thinness in Young Adult Twins. *Int. J. Eat. Disord.* **2005**, *37*, 188–199. [CrossRef] [PubMed]
80. Šmahelová, M.; Čevelíček, M.; Nehybková, E.; Šmahel, D.; Čermák, I. Is It Important to Talk about Technologies with Eating Disorder Clients? The Health-Care Professional Perspective. *Health Commun.* **2019**, *34*, 31–38. [CrossRef] [PubMed]

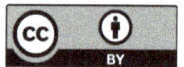

© 2020 by the authors. Licensee MDPI, Basel, Switzerland. This article is an open access article distributed under the terms and conditions of the Creative Commons Attribution (CC BY) license (http://creativecommons.org/licenses/by/4.0/).

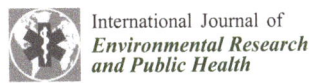

Commentary

Evolving Role of Social Media in Health Promotion: Updated Responsibilities for Health Education Specialists

Michael Stellefson [1,*], Samantha R. Paige [2], Beth H. Chaney [1] and J. Don Chaney [1]

1. Department of Health Education and Promotion, East Carolina University, Greenville, NC 27858, USA; chaneye@ecu.edu (B.H.C.); chaneyj@ecu.edu (J.D.C.)
2. STEM Translational Communication Center, University of Florida, Gainesville, FL 32611, USA; paigesr190@ufl.edu
* Correspondence: stellefsonm17@ecu.edu

Received: 26 December 2019; Accepted: 8 February 2020; Published: 12 February 2020

Abstract: The use of social media in public health education has been increasing due to its ability to remove physical barriers that traditionally impede access to healthcare support and resources. As health promotion becomes more deeply rooted in Internet-based programming, health education specialists are tasked with becoming more competent in computer-mediated contexts that optimize both online and offline consumer health experiences. Generating a better understanding of the benefits and drawbacks to using social media in the field is important, since health education specialists continue to weigh its advantages against potential concerns and barriers to use. Accordingly, this Special Issue aims to explore social media as a translational health promotion tool by bridging principles of health education and health communication that examine (1) the method with which social media users access, negotiate, and create health information that is both actionable and impactful for diverse audiences; (2) strategies for overcoming challenges to using social media in health promotion; and (3) best practices for designing, implementing, and evaluating social media forums in public health. In this commentary, we discuss the updated communication and advocacy roles and responsibilities of health education specialists in the context of social media research and practice.

Keywords: social media; health education; health promotion

1. Introduction

Our understanding of health and the impact of behavioral, sociocultural, and system-level factors on health outcomes has evolved significantly over the past several decades [1]. Advances in technology are central to this evolution, as adoption of mobile devices connected to the Internet continues to grow across sociodemographic groups and geographic regions. One technological advancement accessed regularly is social media, which is used by 2.82 billion people worldwide [2]. Social media is defined as activities, practices, and behaviors among communities of users who gather online to share information, knowledge, and opinions using conversational media [3]. There are tens of thousands of health-promotion-related social media websites that are currently available to the public [1]. In health promotion, social media is commonly accessed for networking and community building purposes, as well as for informing healthcare decision-making between patients and providers [4].

The use of social media in public health education and promotion has been increasing in the United States (U.S.), due, in part, to its ability to remove physical barriers that traditionally impede access to healthcare support and resources. In 2017, Dr. Zsuzsanna Jakab, The World Health Organization (WHO)'s Regional Director of Europe, described the intersection of electronic health (eHealth) in public health as a "beautiful marriage" that celebrates the global commitment and dedication towards reaping the benefits of eHealth for all [5]. Patients, clinicians, mobile health, and social media all play unique roles in health promotion, highlighting the need to for secure data management that can facilitate more personalized medicine and more equitable public health policies [5]. Today, it is difficult to imagine public health without social media. Although social media is viewed as acceptable and usable among multiple audiences and shows much promise in promoting health equity among disadvantaged populations (e.g., low income, rural, and older adults) [6], there remains inconsistent empirical evidence on the effectiveness of social media to improve public health outcomes and trends [7,8]. In order to optimize the potential of social media to improve public health, there is a need to effectively leverage these technological tools to create scalable, culturally adapted health promotion programs and campaigns. Unfortunately, evidence remains limited on how to do this within the field of health promotion [6,9]. Generating a better understanding regarding the benefits and drawbacks to using social media in health promotion is important, since health education specialists weigh its advantages against potential concerns over misinformation being shared to the public at large [10].

Central to social media is interactivity. Social media facilitates greater information sharing and opportunities for community building through an Internet-mediated dialogue that allows users to create their own content (e.g., blogs, online discussion boards). This content, in turn, can become invaluable for health education specialists who are seeking formative research to design, adapt, and evaluate programs and campaigns with priority audiences. Consistently, social media hosts opportunities for consumers to exchange strategic health messages on popular social media channels, including Facebook, YouTube, and Pinterest, through various modalities (e.g., text, image, video, and gif) [11]. Moreover, recent analytic advancements have strengthened the capacity of researchers and practitioners to compute and analyze metrics that evaluate the process of implementing social media, as well as any health-related impacts and outcomes associated with its implementation. As such, new collaborative evaluation methods are being deployed to improve the integration of social media within health-related interventions. While progress is being made, there remain significant challenges inhibiting the widespread acceptance, adoption, and use of social media in health promotion [4,12,13]. Further examining the impact of communication and advocacy within social-media-based interventions and campaigns is central to this endeavor.

Health education specialists play a critical role in creating, managing, and monitoring health promotion programs. As health promotion becomes more deeply rooted in Internet-based programming, health education specialists are tasked with becoming more competent in computer-mediated contexts that optimize both online and offline consumer health experiences. Accordingly, this Special Issue aims to explore social media as a translational health promotion tool by bridging principles of health education and health communication that examine: (1) the method with which social media users access, negotiate, and create health information that is both actionable and impactful for diverse audiences; (2) strategies for overcoming challenges to using social media in health promotion; and (3) best practices for designing, implementing, and evaluating social media campaigns and forums in public health. In this commentary, we discuss updated communication and advocacy roles and responsibilities of health education specialists in the context of using social media in research and practice.

2. Updated Social-Media-Related Roles and Responsibilities of Health Education Specialists

The National Commission for Health Education Credentialing, Inc. (NCHEC) and the Society for Public Health Education (SOPHE) recently co-sponsored a new health education specialist practice analysis. A panel of 17 individuals with diverse backgrounds (i.e., work setting, experience level, education background, demographics, and geographic settings) that affect the practice of health education conducted a validation study, known as *Health Education Specialist Practice Analysis II (HESPA II 2020)* to re-verify the entry- and advanced-level responsibilities, competencies, and subcompetencies that provide the foundation for the professional preparation and development of all health education specialists [14]. A broad cross-section of both certified and noncertified health education specialists from all 50 U.S. states volunteered to participate in the study. Study participants were contacted via existing lists of the sponsoring organizations with additional assistance provided by the Coalition of National Health Education Organization (CNHEO) and national and state affiliates of major health education associations. Two online surveys, one focusing on competencies and one focusing on knowledge areas, were available for a three-month window from November 2018 to January 2019, resulting in 3,851 usable surveys [14].

Findings from this research provided significant implications for professional preparation, continuing education, and practice for the health education profession. Moreover, *HESPA II 2020* produced a new hierarchical model with eight areas of responsibility, 35 competencies, and 193 subcompetencies [13]. Within these new areas of responsibility, Advocacy (Area V) and Communication (Area VI) were designated as standalone areas of responsibility that contained a variety of new competencies and subcompetencies that reflected the increasing importance of using social media in the process and practice of health education. Table 1 outlines these two areas of responsibility with five associated health education specialist competencies and six subcompetencies that directly mention social media use.

Table 1. HESPA II 2020 competencies and subcompetencies that address health education specialist use of social media.

Area of Responsibility	Competency	SubCompetency
Advocacy	Engage coalitions and stakeholders in addressing health issues and planning advocacy efforts	Specify strategies, a timeline, and roles and responsibilities to address the proposed policy, system, or environmental change (e.g., develop ongoing relationships with decision makers and stakeholders, use social media, register others to vote, and seek political appointment)
	Engage in advocacy	Use media to conduct advocacy (e.g., social media, press releases, public service announcements, and op-eds)
Communications	Determine factors that affect communication with the identified audience(s)	Identify communication channels (e.g., social media and mass media) available to and used by the audience(s)
	Deliver the message(s) effectively using the identified media and strategies	Use current and emerging communication tools and trends (e.g., social media, community presentations, annual reports, and patient newsletters)
		Use digital media to engage audience(s) (e.g., social media management tools and platforms)
	Evaluate communication	Assess reach and dose of communication using tools (e.g., paper-based surveys, focus groups, semistructured in-depth interviews, data mining software, social media analytics, and website analytics) [1]

[1] Advanced 1 subcompetency not included in the entry-level, Certified Health Education Specialist (CHES®) examination. Subcompetency will be included in the Master Certified Health Education Specialist (MCHES®) examination.

2.1. Engage Coalitions and Stakeholders in Addressing Public Health Issues Using Social Media

Health education specialists are tasked with specifying strategies, timelines, and roles and responsibilities to address proposed policy, system, or environmental changes through social media. Social media allows for synchronous and asynchronous communication in a centralized, readily accessible digital location where a high degree of transparency exists. Social media can assist health education specialists in building a network of supporters, particularly for advocacy efforts [15]. These interactive, digital tools can be used to effectively expand the reach and inclusivity of advocacy campaigns to engage stakeholders to support public health issues, regardless of geographic location and timing [16]. Specifically, when used with traditional, relationship-building strategies, social media can bolster outreach approaches and reinforce relationships among stakeholders, including public health education coalition groups. This is done through promoting dialogue between leaders and supporters, as well as increasing collaborative communication among stakeholder groups. Additionally, social media tools are highly cost-effective for expanding communication among stakeholders and coalition groups interested in supporting public health education and promotion issue(s) [17,18]. Therefore, social media technologies have potential to improve communication among stakeholders in order to further engage supporters for successful social change. However, building relationships with stakeholders and coalitions through traditional communication channels, while supporting these relationships through the use of social media technologies, is ideal for fostering lasting and productive stakeholder relationships for addressing public health issues [18]. This allows for the opportunity to develop and nurture collaborative relationships among decision makers, which can include diverse stakeholders such as community members, organizations, and policymakers.

2.2. Engage in Health Policy Advocacy Through Leveraging Social Media

Social media has become a critical tool in advocating for health policy, including its development, planning, and reform. Engagement with advocates is a key element in advocating for health policy, and social media provides a platform for new supporters and the general public to become aware of the important issues [19]. In addition, social media tools create widespread access to public officials, many of whom have their own social media websites, for the opportunity to share information regarding health policy issues impacting constituents. While these technologies create the digital platform to increase awareness and evoke support for health policy advocacy, health education specialists must strive to promote actions that results in social change through advocacy efforts. Social media can complement traditional advocacy approaches to shift policy priorities for supporting health policy. In a framework developed by Scott and Maryman [18], social media and advocacy are aligned through empowerment and organization theories for shifting policy priorities. Specifically, the model suggests that quality social media presence must involve 1) critical awareness —engaging supporters through awareness of an issue that drives the desire to actively support the cause, 2) relationship building—creating relationships in a digital space and with face-to-face interactions that move passive supporters to active supporters, and 3) mobilizing action—creating action through both social media-supported online and offline forms of political engagement [18]. Successful social media campaigns for health policy advocacy require health education specialists to utilize planning and evaluation skills to effectively assess the use of social media in this capacity.

2.3. Determine Factors that Affect Health Communication on Social Media with the Identified Audience(s)

It is important for health education specialists to identify communication channels, such as social media, that are available to and used by their intended audience. Being digital-media-proficient means being able to meet priority populations where they are to bring about change within the physical, social, and online environments in which they live, work, and play. There are many challenges to effectively using digital media platforms, such as social media, within health education/promotion interventions and campaigns. These challenges are directly tied to the nature of social media itself, where health education specialists cannot fully control what, when, and how health information is shared. In some respects, social media can be considered the "wild west" for health information. Users can freely engage and interact with health information that may or may not be accurate or supported by empirical evidence. While challenges are to be expected, engagement can be maximized on social media through managing misinformation, reducing agency barriers to use, measuring audience reach and impact of posted messages/content, and keeping up with new trends in social media adoption and use. To effectively engage diverse audiences, there are several steps that can be followed to adopt a more strategic approach to social media use in health promotion: 1) understand how the priority population uses social media, 2) identify evidence-based social media strategies, 3) select appropriate communication times and channels, and 4) determine which types of social media apps will engage your audience most often in a meaningful way [20].

2.4. Deliver Health Message(s) Effectively Using Social Media

As reflected in *HESPA II 2020* competencies and subcompetencies, health education specialists are tasked with fine tuning their message delivery to ensure that intended audiences are being reached. This involves using current and emerging communication tools and digital media (e.g., social media management tools and platforms) to engage audiences. There are various social media tools, guidelines, and best practices that health education specialists can use for this purpose [20,21]. For example, health education specialists should stay abreast of new forms of social media that are accessed regularly (i.e., daily or almost daily) by intended users. Next, consider adopting a social media policy. A formal social media policy on relevant topics such as hashtag use, tagging, communicating, and updating content can limit destructive posts that adversely impact online communities [21]. Moreover, policy implementation facilitates productive interactivity that respects the diversity of user demographics, cultural backgrounds, and opinions. Finally, try to keep social media activity both lively and relevant. Skilled social media moderators are essential for maintaining social media pages and maximizing engagement through scheduling messages and responding promptly to user posts about current public health issues that are of concern. Moderators can provide invaluable social support that clinicians are often unable to offer, such as sharing insight about how to effectively communicate with healthcare providers [20].

2.5. Evaluate Health Promotion Activity Occurring on Social Media

Evaluation is a fundamental element of most all social media activities within the field of health promotion [20]. Process evaluation, or the measurement of factors that influence the success or failure of social media use (i.e., tracking social media analytics and performance indicators), is the most relevant type of evaluation to assess use of social media as part of an intervention or as a standalone tool [19]. Data from process evaluation enables key decision makers and other stakeholders to monitor program inputs (e.g., messages, videos, and chat sessions) and outputs (e.g., number of followers, number of likes, and number of comments left) of social media activity [11]. Tools such as social media analytics and data mining software can assist health education specialists in assessing the reach and dose of communication messages [22]. Analytics also help to extract useful patterns of user activity to measure the engagement, experience, and moderator responsiveness within online communities [23]. This type of social media data enables decision makers to learn from mistakes, make health promotion program modifications, monitor progress towards program goals, and justify the success of achieving desired health-related outcomes [20].

3. Conclusions

Social media provides an outlet to increase and promote translational health communication strategies and effective data dissemination, in ways that allow users to not only utilize but also create and share pertinent health information. Moreover, the use of social media for advocacy and communications in health promotion offers exciting new prospects for broader reach, greater efficiency, and lowered costs of communication and advocacy campaigns. As with other technological innovations in healthcare, these efficiencies may be viewed by those providing funding as an opportunity to decrease budgets and increase the scope of health promotion activity delivered by health education specialists and their organizations. This very may well result in a reduction in the use of more established communication channels (e.g., TV, radio, and print-based media) traditionally used for health promotion.

Although the application of social media in public health and health promotion has yielded some success in terms of generating support structures and networks for effective health behavior change, there are challenges and complications associated with social media use that also need to be addressed (e.g., managing misinformation, ensuring compliance with user privacy protections). While it is relatively straightforward to view social media use as a universal communication channel, especially for those who already use social media, the risk of using social media lies in reducing health information access among those who are not technologically "connected". Social media is not likely to be an effective option for population subgroups include the elderly; the physically and cognitively disabled; and those with low text, technical, and eHealth literacy.

As health education specialists, we need to be wary of designing social media interventions or campaigns that are most suited to population segments that are comfortably well off, and text-, tech- and eHealth-literate. In addition, the use of social media by health education specialists faces significant headwinds from individuals or entities using social media to promote alternative views on health-related issues (e.g., anti-vaccinations, pro fad diets, and advocating for exclusionary healthcare policies). Some social media platforms have belatedly taken action to limit some of these discussions (e.g., Facebook with anti-vaccination groups), but the response is unlikely to be timely. We acknowledge that these types of completing voices are usually far better resourced than health education specialists who have limited resources to support robust social-media-based advertising campaigns. Therefore, we must be vigilant in monitoring and evaluating public health advocacy and communication that occurs on various popular social media websites.

Our Special Issue begins to tackle these important issues by bringing together international, multidisciplinary scholars who employed innovative methodologies to better understand how social media is used by multiple audiences for the purposes of health promotion and engagement. Specifically, these articles delve into the sociocognitive and affective factors that mediate the relationship between social media use, community engagement, and positive health outcomes. This was achieved by augmenting our understanding of traditional health education approaches with theories rooted in the complementary yet distinct disciplines of health communication. We sincerely hope that the new empirical knowledge generated within this Special Issue will help academic health education specialists, as well as other public health professionals, use more pragmatic paradigms for planning, implementing, and evaluating social media interventions and campaigns in the field of health promotion.

Author Contributions: Conceptualization, M.S. and S.R.P.; methodology, M.S. and S.R.P.; formal analysis, M.S., S.R.P., B.H.C., and J.D.C.; writing—original draft preparation, M.S. and S.R.P.; writing—review and editing, B.H.C. and J.D.C. All authors have read and agreed to the published version of the manuscript.

Funding: This research received no external funding.

Acknowledgments: We would like to thank the *IJERPH* editorial staff and manuscript review board members for their support and contributions during the preparation of this Special Issue.

Conflicts of Interest: The authors declare no conflict of interest.

References

1. Edington, D.W.; Schultz, A.B.; Pitts, J.S.; Camilleri, A. The future of health promotion in the 21st century: A focus on the working population. *Am. J. Lifestyle Med.* **2016**, *10*, 242–252. [CrossRef] [PubMed]
2. Number of Social Network Users Worldwide from 2010 to 2021. Available online: https://www.statista.com/statistics/278414/number-of-worldwide-social-network-users/ (accessed on 26 December 2019).
3. Merriam-Webster: Social Media. Available online: http://www.merriam-webster.com/dictionary/socialmedia (accessed on 26 December 2019).
4. A Report on the Use of Social Media to Prevent Behavioral Risk Factors Associated with Chronic Disease. Available online: http://ehidc.org/resource-center/reports/BehavioralRisk.pdf (accessed on 26 December 2019).
5. World Health Organization. E-Health and Public Health-A Perfect Marriage. Available online: http://www.euro.who.int/en/health-topics/Health-systems/e-health/news/news/2017/05/ehealth-and-public-health-a-beautiful-marriage (accessed on 29 January 2020).
6. Welch, V.; Petkovic, J.; Pardo, J.P.; Rader, T.; Tugwell, P. Interactive social media interventions to promote health equity: An overview of the reviews. *Health Pro. Chron. Dis. Prev. Can.* **2016**, *36*, 63–75. [CrossRef] [PubMed]

7. Hunter, R.F.; De La Haye, K.; Murray, J.M.; Badham, J.; Valente, T.W.; Clarke, M.; Kee, F. Social network interventions for health behaviours and outcomes: A systematic review and meta-analysis. *PLoS Med.* **2019**, *16*, e1002890. [CrossRef] [PubMed]
8. Johns, D.J.; Langley, T.E.; Lewis, S. Use of social media for the delivery of health promotion on smoking, nutrition, and physical activity: A systematic review. *Lancet* **2017**, *390*, S49. [CrossRef]
9. Bennett, G.G.; Glasgow, R.E. The Delivery of Public Health Interventions via the Internet: Actualizing Their Potential. *Annu. Rev. Public Health* **2009**, *30*, 273–292. [CrossRef] [PubMed]
10. Neiger, B.L.; Thackeray, R.; Van Wagenen, S.A.; Hanson, C.L.; West, J.H.; Barnes, M.D.; Fagen, M.C. Use of social media in health promotion: Purposes, key performance indicators, and evaluation metrics. *Health Pro. Pract.* **2012**, *13*, 159–164. [CrossRef] [PubMed]
11. Zhao, Y.; Zhang, J. Consumer health information seeking in social media: A literature review. *Heal. Inf. Libr. J.* **2017**, *34*, 268–283. [CrossRef] [PubMed]
12. Cummings, E.; Ellis, L.; Turner, P. The past, the present, and the future: Examining the role of the "Social" in transforming personal healthcare management of chronic disease. *Health Lit. Breakthr. Res. Prac.* **2017**, 287–304.
13. Greenhalgh, T.; Wherton, J.; Papoutsi, C.; Lynch, J.; Hughes, G.; A'Court, C.; Hinder, S.; Fahy, N.; Procter, R.; Shaw, S.; et al. Beyond Adoption: A New Framework for Theorizing and Evaluating Nonadoption, Abandonment, and Challenges to the Scale-Up, Spread, and Sustainability of Health and Care Technologies. *J. Med. Internet Res.* **2017**, *19*, e367. [CrossRef] [PubMed]
14. Cottrell, R. Findings of the Health Education Specialist Practice Analysis II (HESPA II)—2020. In Proceedings of the American Public Health Association (APHA)'s 2019 Annual Meeting and Expo 2019, Wilmington, NC, USA, 4–6 November 2019.
15. Lovejoy, K.; Saxton, G.D. Information, Community, and Action: How Nonprofit Organizations Use Social Media*. *J. Comput. Commun.* **2012**, *17*, 337–353. [CrossRef]
16. Satariano, N.B.; Wong, A. Creating an online strategy to enhance effective community building and organizing. In *Community Organizing and Community Building for Health and Welfare*; Rutgers University Press: New Brunswick, NJ, USA, 2012; pp. 269–287.
17. Obar, J.A.; Zube, P.; Lampe, C.; Lampe, P.Z. Advocacy 2.0: An Analysis of How Advocacy Groups in the United States Perceive and Use Social Media as Tools for Facilitating Civic Engagement and Collective Action. *J. Inf. Policy* **2012**, *2*, 1–25. [CrossRef]
18. Scott, J.T.; Maryman, J. Using social media as a tool to complement advocacy efforts. *Glob. J. Comm. Psych. Pract.* **2016**, *7*, 1–22.
19. Guo, C.; Saxton, G.D. Tweeting social change: How social media are changing nonprofit advocacy. *Nonp. Vol. Sec. Q.* **2013**, *43*, 57–79. [CrossRef]
20. Bensley, R.J.; Thackeray, R.; Stellefson, M. Using social media. In *Community and Public Health Education Methods: A Practical Guide*; Bensley, R.J., Brookins-Fisher, J., Eds.; Jones & Bartlett Learning: Burlington, MA, USA, 2019; pp. 149–167.
21. Centers for Disease Control and Prevention (CDC) Social Media Tools, Guidelines, & Best Practices. Available online: https://www.cdc.gov/socialmedia/tools/guidelines/index.html (accessed on 26 December 2019).
22. Hanson, C.; Thackeray, R.; Barnes, M.; Neiger, B.; McIntyre, E. Integrating Web 2.0 in Health Education Preparation and Practice. *Am. J. Health Educ.* **2008**, *39*, 157–166. [CrossRef]
23. Seering, J.; Wang, T.; Yoon, J.; Kaufman, G. Moderator engagement and community development in the age of algorithms. *New Media Soc.* **2019**, *21*, 1417–1443. [CrossRef]

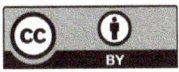

© 2020 by the authors. Licensee MDPI, Basel, Switzerland. This article is an open access article distributed under the terms and conditions of the Creative Commons Attribution (CC BY) license (http://creativecommons.org/licenses/by/4.0/).

MDPI
St. Alban-Anlage 66
4052 Basel
Switzerland
Tel. +41 61 683 77 34
Fax +41 61 302 89 18
www.mdpi.com

International Journal of Environmental Research and Public Health Editorial Office
E-mail: ijerph@mdpi.com
www.mdpi.com/journal/ijerph

www.ingramcontent.com/pod-product-compliance
Lightning Source LLC
LaVergne TN
LVHW070645100526
838202LV00013B/885